# Manual
# Physical Therapy
# of the Spine

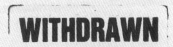

# Manual Physical Therapy of the Spine

**Kenneth A. Olson,** PT, DHSc, OCS, FAAOMPT

Private Practitioner
Northern Rehabilitation and Sports Medicine Associates
DeKalb, Illinois
Adjunct Assistant Professor
Marquette University
Milwaukee, Wisconsin

SAUNDERS

ELSEVIER

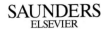

11830 Westline Industrial Drive
St. Louis, Missouri 63146

MANUAL PHYSICAL THERAPY OF THE SPINE                    ISBN: 978-1-4160-4749-0
**Copyright © 2009 by Saunders, an imprint of Elsevier Inc.**

**Library of Congress Cataloging-in-Publication Data**

Olson, Kenneth A.
    Manual physical therapy of the spine / Kenneth A. Olson. – 1st ed.
        p. ; cm.
    Includes bibliographical references and index.
    ISBN 978-1-4160-4749-0 (pbk. : alk. paper)   1. Spine–Diseases–Treatment.   2. Manipulation (Therapeutics)   3. Temporomandibular joint–Diseases.   I. Title.
    [DNLM:   1. Spinal Diseases–therapy.   2. Manipulation, Orthopedic.   3. Physical Therapy Modalities.   4. Spinal Diseases–diagnosis.   5. Temporomandibular Joint Disorders–diagnosis.   6. Temporomandibular Joint Disorders–therapy.   WE 725 O52m 2009]
    RD768.O57 2009
    617.4′7106–dc22

                                                                    2008013022

*Vice President and Publisher:* Linda Duncan
*Executive Editor:* Kathy Falk
*Senior Developmental Editor:* Christie M. Hart
*Publishing Services Manager:* Patricia Tannian
*Senior Project Manager:* Anne Altepeter
*Design Direction:* Renee Duenow

Printed in China

Last digit is the print number:   9   8   7   6   5   4   3   2   1

*To my wife, Janet, and children, Will and Emma,*
*for their love and support, and for bringing joy to my life*

*To my parents, John and Anna Mae, for providing a solid foundation to grow and learn*

*To my grandmother, Miriam, for instilling a passion for helping and teaching*

# Foreword

Dr. Ken Olson's textbook, *Manual Physical Therapy of the Spine*, is a welcome addition to the manual therapy literature. Ken's strong clinical and academic backgrounds provide him with the requisite perspective to write a textbook that is both relevant and practical. Writing a textbook with a broad target audience in mind – physical therapist practitioners, residents and students, physicians, and other manual therapy practitioners – can be very challenging, but I believe Ken has easily met this challenge.

Chapters 1 through 3 are of primary interest to the physical therapy community. Understanding the history of and theories behind manual therapy – thrust joint manipulation in particular – is essential for the appropriate use of such techniques. The history of spinal manipulation clearly provides evidence supporting the claim that no single "modern" health care profession invented or owns this intervention. What makes the various invested professions unique are the underlying rationale and terminology associated with their use of these procedures.

Chapters 4 through 7 provide a fantastic array of examination and treatment techniques that are of interest to all manual therapy practitioners. The illustrations are clear and easy to follow. Learning a technique through drawings and photographs is not easy, but the superb figures in this textbook allow a novice practitioner to begin appreciating the nuances of therapist hand placement, applied direction of force, and patient positioning, thus facilitating student and practitioner skill development and confidence. Video clips on the accompanying DVD further facilitate instruction and learning of the manual examination and manipulation techniques. A great asset to students and clinicians, the video clips highlight patient and therapist position and force application throughout each demonstration.

The textbook provides a thorough theoretical grounding from the perspective of a physical therapist, making it essential background information for physical therapist students, residents, and fellows. The material is also of value to practitioners outside the physical therapy profession, because it promotes better understanding of where we as professions overlap and where we diverge. Dr. Olson's thorough literature review promotes an evidence-based approach to utilization of manual therapy techniques. If this approach is adopted by all interested parties, then similarities between the various professions should increase and the differences over time should disappear.

*Manual Physical Therapy of the Spine* provides readers with the perfect blend between theory and practice. The textbook is a rich teaching resource for physical therapist academic faculty and residency/fellowship instructors. For students, residents, and fellows, the textbook is invaluable not only during their educational experience but also beyond. Dr. Olson is to be commended and applauded for his efforts to provide us with a textbook that is relevant to today's practice and will remain so far into the future.

**William G. Boissonnault, PT, DHSc, FAAOMPT**

# Preface

This textbook has integrated an impairment-based manual physical therapy approach with use of research evidence to support management of spinal and temporomandibular joint (TMJ) conditions. The textbook provides the necessary background information and detailed instructional materials to allow full integration of manipulation and manual physical therapy examination and treatment procedures of the spine into physical therapist professional education and clinical practice. Additionally, the textbook advocates for physical therapists, physicians, and other health professionals to follow the recommendations of high-quality clinical practice guidelines and systematic reviews for management of spinal and TMJ disorders and provides the necessary background and instructional information to assist in skill development to effectively implement the evidence-based treatment recommendations related to manual therapy, manipulation, and therapeutic exercise.

The primary audience for this textbook is physical therapy students and faculty in professional physical therapist education programs. The secondary audience for this textbook is practicing physical therapists, chiropractors, and physicians who wish to keep up with what is being taught in professional physical therapist education programs. Additionally, persons in manual physical therapy residency, fellowship, and post-professional degree programs in orthopaedic and manual physical therapy will find this textbook to be a useful adjunct to other instructional materials.

Although physical therapists have been practicing manipulation since the inception of the profession, all physical therapist professional degree programs in the United States must now demonstrate full integration of both thrust and nonthrust joint manipulation in the curriculum to maintain accreditation. The textbook and accompanying DVD provide physical therapist education faculty and students with detailed instructional materials to effectively instruct and learn manipulation. The textbook also provides the research evidence to successfully integrate the use of manual physical therapy procedures into the management of spinal and TMJ disorders.

Chapter 1 provides an introduction to the components of the textbook, presents the essential elements of an impairment-based manual physical therapy approach, reviews the history of manipulation with the physical therapy profession, and introduces the essential definitions and principles of evidence-based practice and manual physical therapy.

Chapter 2 provides a framework for completing a comprehensive spinal examination, including medical screen, patient interview, disability assessment, and tests and measures. In addition, evaluation of the examination findings and principles involved in arriving at a diagnosis and plan of care are included. The tests and measures presented in this chapter are the basic examination procedures used to screen the spine or are techniques used across anatomical regions to complete a comprehensive spinal examination. Additional special tests and manual examination procedures, such as passive intervertebral motion tests, are presented in detail in subsequent chapters that focus on each anatomical region of the spine.

Chapter 3 includes the principles related to the practice of mobilization/manipulation. Theories are described to explain the effects of manipulation, and the available research to support each theory is presented. A brief overview of evidence to support the use of manipulation is presented; further detail regarding the evidence is provided in the chapters that cover anatomical regions. Potential adverse effects and contraindications to manipulation are discussed, and concepts of learning and teaching manipulation are also presented.

Chapters 4 through 7 provide a review of evidence to support the examination and treatment techniques presented in the chapter as well as the kinematics and functional anatomy of the anatomical areas to be covered in the chapter. Anatomical areas are organized as follows: lumbopelvic, thoracic and rib cage, cervical spine, and temporomandibular joint. Classification of common conditions treated by physical therapists is presented in each chapter to assist with clinical decision making, and patient management principles are addressed for each condition. Detailed descriptions of examination and manual therapy treatment procedures are the primary emphasis of each chapter and the DVD. Common exercises to address each diagnostic classification are also included in each chapter.

In addition to providing the necessary research evidence to support a manual physical therapy approach for management of spinal and TMJ disorders, the book provides detailed descriptions and multiple photographs of each examination and treatment procedure. Many of the manipulation techniques also include alternative methods to match various clinical situations.

Professional photographer Jim Womack took the photographs. Multiple angles are presented of many techniques on live and anatomical models to clearly illustrate hand and body placement. Arrows are also used with many techniques to illustrate direction of force application.

A professional media production team led by Gary Bargholz with Guy Simoneau, PT, PhD, filmed the DVD segments at Marquette University, providing professional-quality clips.

Three cameras were used to film each examination and treatment technique from frontal, lateral, and cranial views, to allow a unique three-dimensional perspective in order to appreciate each procedure. I provide oral step-by-step instruction of each procedure with the demonstrations. In the textbook an icon **DVD** is used to alert readers to procedures that are demonstrated on the DVD. Course instructors can use the DVD to present the techniques, and students can use the DVD to review most of the manual therapy procedures included in the textbook.

The textbook and DVD will be very useful additions to the permanent library of clinicians who practice manual therapy techniques to manage spinal disorders. Although the body of research evidence will continue to evolve over time, the technique descriptions and presentations will remain as valuable resources to reference when practitioners are presented with various spinal and TMJ disorders in the future.

**Kenneth A. Olson**

# Acknowledgments

Professionally, I am indebted to the influence and mentorship of Stanley Paris and the faculty and staff of the University of St. Augustine for Health Sciences who guided my graduate education. Other professional mentors include Bill Boissonnault, Tim Dunlop, Laurie Hartman, Mary Jane Harris, Trish King, David Lamb, Steve McDavitt, Catherine Patla, and Mariano Rocabodo. I am grateful to Guy Simoneau, Elaine Lonnemann, Ron Schenk, and Josh Cleland for reviewing multiple chapters of the textbook and providing useful feedback to improve the quality of the project and to Jacob Slusser, who worked with me when he was a student physical therapist to develop the format used to describe the manipulation techniques. I also acknowledge my colleagues in private practice and my current and past students who have challenged me to find better ways to teach and practice manual physical therapy.

Kathy Falk, Christie Hart, and Anne Altepeter have been helpful and efficient at Elsevier in helping to move this book along in a timely manner. Jim Womack took the photographs used in the textbook. Charlie Cardon provided the mobilization table (Cardon Rehabilitation Products, Niagra Falls, N.Y.) used for the DVD, and the excellent DVD was filmed at Marquette University.

**Kenneth A. Olson**

# Contents

# Introduction

## OVERVIEW

This chapter introduces the purpose of the textbook, describes the history of manipulation, defines common terminology used in the textbook, introduces evidence-based principles, and provides an explanation for use of the textbook and the accompanying DVD.

## OBJECTIVES

- Describe the purpose of the textbook and DVD
- Explain the philosophy of treatment used in orthopaedic manual physical therapy
- Describe the history of manipulation
- Define common terminology used in orthopaedic manual physical therapy
- Explain evidence-based principles for assessment of the reliability and validity of clinical examination procedures and clinical trials
- Explain how to use this textbook and DVD

## PURPOSE

The purpose of this textbook is to provide the necessary background information and detailed instructional materials to allow full integration of manipulation and manual physical therapy examination and treatment procedures of the spine into physical therapist professional education and clinical practice.

The primary audience for this textbook is physical therapy students and faculty in professional physical therapist education programs. The secondary audience is practicing physical therapists, chiropractors, and osteopathic physicians who want to keep current with professional physical therapist education programs. In addition, this textbook is a useful adjunct to other instructional materials for manual physical therapy residency, fellowship, and postprofessional degree programs in orthopaedic and manual physical therapy.

Although physical therapists have been practicing manipulation since the inception of the profession, as of January 2006, all physical therapist professional degree programs must demonstrate full integration of both thrust and nonthrust joint manipulation in the curriculum to maintain accreditation.[1,2]

The intent of this textbook and DVD is to provide physical therapist programs detailed instructional materials for more effective instruction of manipulation.

Prerequisites in the curriculum should include clinical tests and measures for musculoskeletal conditions, including manual muscle testing, muscle length testing, and goniometry. Knowledge of therapeutic exercise, anatomy, physiology, and functional anatomy and biomechanics should also precede instruction in manipulation. Each chapter provides a review of the evidence to support the examination and treatment techniques presented in the chapter and the kinematics and functional anatomy of the anatomic areas covered in the chapter. Classification of common conditions treated by physical therapists is presented in each chapter to assist with clinical decision making, and patient management principles are addressed for each condition. Detailed descriptions of examination and manual therapy treatment procedures are the primary emphasis of each chapter and the DVD. Common exercises to address each diagnostic classification are also included in each chapter.

## HISTORY OF MANIPULATION

Manipulation in recorded history can be traced to the days of Hippocrates, the father of medicine (460-355 BC). Evidence is seen in ancient writings that Hippocrates used spinal traction methods. In the paper "On Setting Joints by Leverage," Hippocrates describes the techniques used to manipulate a dislocated shoulder of a wrestler.[3] Succussion was also practiced in the days of Hippocrates. The patient was strapped in an inverted position to a rack that was attached to ropes and pulleys along the side of a building. The ropes were pulled to elevate the patient and the rack as much as 75 feet, at which time the ropes were released and the patient crashed to the ground to receive a distractive thrust as the rack impacted the ground.[4] Six hundred years later, Galen wrote extensively on manipulation procedures in medicine.[3]

The Middle Ages saw little advance in the practice of medicine and manipulation because of the reliance on the church for most healing.[3] In the Renaissance era, Ambrose Paré emerged. Paré was a famous French physician and surgeon in the 1500s[3] who used armor to stabilize the spine in patients with tuberculosis.[4] His manipulation and traction techniques were similar to those of Hippocrates, but he opposed the use of succussion.[4]

The bone setters flourished in Europe from the 1600s through the late 1800s. Friar Moulton in 1656 published the text *The Complete Bone-Setter*. The book was later revised by Robert Turner.[4] No formal training was required for bone setters; the techniques were often learned from family members and passed down from one generation to the next. The clicking sounds that occurred with manipulation were thought to be the result of bones moving back into place.[4]

In 1871, Wharton Hood published the book *On Bone-Setting*, which was the first such book by an orthodox medical practitioner.[5] Hood's father had treated a bone setter, Richard Hutton. Hutton was grateful for the medical care and offered to teach Hood's father about bone setting. Instead, Wharton Hood accepted the offer. Hood thought that the snapping sound with manipulation was the result of breaking joint adhesions.[5] Paget[6] believed that orthodox medicine should consider the adoption of what was good and useful about bone setting but should avoid what was potentially dangerous and useless.

Osteopathy was founded by Andrew Still in 1874. In 1896, the first school of osteopathy was formed in Kirksville, Mo.[4] Still developed osteopathy based on the "Rule of the Artery," with the premise that the body has an innate ability to heal and that with spinal manipulation to correct the structural alignment of the spine, the blood can flow to various regions of the body to restore the body's homeostasis and natural healing abilities. Still's philosophy placed an emphasis on the relationship of structure to function and used manipulation to improve the spinal structure to promote optimal health.[7] The osteopathic profession continues to include manipulation in the course curriculum but does not adhere to Still's original treatment philosophy. Many osteopathic physicians in the United States do not practice manipulation on a regular basis because they are focused on other specialty areas such as internal medicine or emergency medicine. Osteopathy in many European countries remains primarily a manual therapy profession.

Chiropractic was founded in 1895 by Daniel David Palmer. One of the first graduates of the Palmer School of Chiropractic in Davenport, Iowa, was Palmer's son B.J. Palmer, who later ran the school and promoted the profession. D.D. Palmer was a storekeeper and a "magnetic healer." According to legend, in 1895, he used a manual adjustment directed to the fourth thoracic vertebra that resulted in the restoration of a man's hearing.[8] The original chiropractic philosophy is based on the "The Law of the Nerve" that states that adjustment of a subluxed vertebra removes impingement on the nerve and restores innervation and promotes healing of disease processes.[3] The "straight" chiropractors continue to adhere to Palmer's original subluxation theories and use spinal adjustments as the primary means of treatment. The "Mixers" incorporate other rehabilitative interventions into the treatment options, including physical modalities such as therapeutic ultrasound and exercise.

Physical therapy evolved from medicine to provide physical treatments such as manual physical therapy within the medical model. In 1899, the Chartered Society of Physiotherapy was founded in England.[3] Physical therapists formed their first professional association in the United States in 1921, originally named the American Women's Physical Therapeutic Association.[1] As the Association grew in the 1930s and men became physical therapists, the organization eventually changed its name to the American Physical Therapy Association (APTA).[1]

Between 1921 and 1936, at least 21 articles and book reviews on manipulation were found in the physical therapy literature,[9] including the second edition of the book *Massage and Therapeutic Exercise* by the founder and first President of the APTA, Mary McMillan. In a subsequent editorial,[10] she wrote of the four branches of physiotherapy, which she identified as "manipulation of muscle and joints, therapeutic exercise, electrotherapy, and hydrotherapy."[11] Titles of articles during this period were quite explicit regarding manipulation, such as "The Art of Mobilizing Joints"[12] and "Manipulative Treatment of Lumbosacral Derangement."[13] The articles used phrases such as "adhesion . . . stretched or torn by this simple manipulation"[14] and "manipulation of the spine and sacroiliac joint."[15] This usage helps to illustrate that manipulation has been part of physical therapy practice since the founding of the profession and through the 1930s.[9]

From 1940 to the mid 1970s, the word *manipulation* was not widely used in the American physical therapy literature.[3] This omission may have been due in part to the American Medical Association's Committee on Quackery that was formed in the 1960s and was active for the next 30 years in an attempt to discredit the chiropractic profession. The committee was forced to dissolve in 1990 because of the Wilk's "restraint of trade" case that was upheld in the US Supreme Court.[8] Because physical therapy remained within the mainstream medical model, the terms *mobilization* and *articulation* were used during this timeframe to separate physical therapy from chiropractic.

However, physical therapists continued to practice various forms of manipulation.

Through the mid 1900s, several prominent European physicians influenced the practice of manipulation and the evolution of the physical therapist's role as a manipulative therapist. In 1949, James Mennell published the first edition of his textbook titled the *Science and Art of Joint Manipulation*. Mennell adapted knowledge of joint mechanics in the practice of manipulation and coined the phrase "accessory motion".[16]

James Cyriax published his classic *Textbook of Orthopaedic Medicine* in 1957. He made great contributions to orthopaedic medicine with the development of detailed systematic examination procedures for extremity disorders, including refinement of isometric tissue tension signs, end feel assessment, and capsular patterns.[17] Cyriax attributed most back pain to disorders of the intervertebral disc and used aggressive general manipulation techniques that included strong manual traction forces to "reduce the disc."[17] Cyriax trained many physiotherapists, including Stanley Paris and Freddy Kaltenborn, to carry on the skills and techniques required to effectively use manipulation.

Alan Stoddard[7] was a medical and osteopathic physician in England from the 1950s to the 1970s who used skillful specific manipulation technique and also mentored many physical therapists, including Paris and Kaltenborn. These therapists both believed that the Cyriax approach to extremity conditions was excellent but preferred Stoddard's specific manipulation techniques for the spine.[18,19]

John Mennell, the son of James Mennell, first practiced medicine in England. In the 1960s, he immigrated to the United States, where he held many educational programs for physical therapists through the 1970s and 1980s to promote manipulation within the physical therapy profession. He published several textbooks including *Joint Pain, Foot Pain*, and *Back Pain* and coined the phrase "joint play."[20] Mennell brought attention to sources of back pain other than the intervertebral disc.

In the 1960s, several physical therapists emerged as international leaders in the practice and instruction of manipulation. Physical therapist Freddy Kaltenborn, originally from Norway, developed what is now known as the Nordic approach. He published his first textbook on spinal manipulation in 1964 and was the first to relate manipulation to arthrokinematics.[18] His techniques were specific and perpetuated the importance of biomechanical principles such as the concave/convex and arthrokinematic rules. Kaltenborn also developed extensive long-term training programs for physical therapists to specialize in manual therapy first in Norway and later throughout Europe.

Australian physical therapist Geoffrey Maitland published the first edition of his book *Vertebral Manipulation* in 1964.[21] Maitland was also influenced by the work of Cyriax and Stoddard but further refined the importance of a detailed history and comprehensive physical examination. He also developed the concept of treatment of "reproducible signs" and inhibition of joint pain with use of gentle oscillatory techniques. Maitland

developed the I-IV grading system to further describe oscillatory manipulation techniques.[21]

Physical therapist Stanley Paris was originally from New Zealand. Early in his career, in 1961 and 1962, he was awarded a scholarship to study manipulation in Europe and the United States.[9] He had the opportunity to study with Cyriax, Stoddard, and Kaltenborn during this time and in 1965 published the textbook *Spinal Lesion*.[19] In the late 1960s, Paris immigrated to the United States, where he eventually completed his doctoral work in neuroanatomy of the lumbar spine and developed extensive educational programs for postprofessional physical therapy education in manual physical therapy and manipulation that eventually resulted in the formation the University of St Augustine for Health Sciences in St Augustine, Florida. Paris also played key roles in formation of professional organizations in the United States, including the APTA Orthopaedic Section and the American Academy of Orthopaedic Manual Physical Therapists (AAOMPT), two professional organizations that have played roles in advocating for inclusion of manipulation within the scope of physical therapy practice and that have promoted education, practice, and research in manual physical therapy. Paris worked with physical therapists Maitland, Kaltenborn, and Gregory Grieve of the United Kingdom to form the International Federation of Manipulative Therapists (IFOMT; Figure 1-1).

The IFOMT was founded in 1974 and represents organized groups of manual/manipulative physical therapists around the world that have established stringent postgraduation specialization educational programs in manual/manipulative physical therapy. The Federation sets educational and clinical standards and is a subgroup of the World Confederation of Physical Therapy (WCPT). One organization of each WCPT country can be

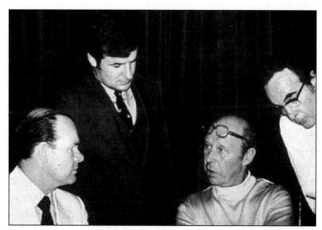

**FIGURE 1-1** Photograph was taken in 1974 in Montreal, Canada, at the successful formation of the International Federation of Orthopaedic Manipulative Therapists (IFOMT). Dr. Paris was Chair of the conference. The other three individuals were consultants to the process and had served in that capacity for 6 years before this event. IFOMT later became a subsection of the World Confederation for Physical Therapy. From *left:* Geoffrey Maitland, Stanley Paris, Freddy Kaltenborn, and Gregory Grieve. (From Paris SV: *Phys Ther* 86(11):1541-1553, 2006.)

recognized by IFOMT to represent that country if the organization meets IFOMT criteria.

The Orthopaedic section of the APTA represents all aspects of musculoskeletal physical therapy and is open to all members of the APTA, including physical therapist assistants. Before formation of the AAOMPT, no organization in the United States could meet the IFOMT criteria because no recognized educational system in manual therapy upheld standards of training and examination in manual therapy for physical therapists in the United States. However, by 1990, at least eight active manual therapy residency programs were operating independently within the United States.

In 1991, Freddy Kaltenborn invited representatives from these eight manual therapy residency programs to meet at Oakland University in Michigan to consider how the United States could develop educational standards in manual therapy and become a member organization of IFOMT.[22] These eight physical therapists, Stanley Paris, Mike Rogers, Michael Moore, Kornelia Kulig, Bjorn Swensen, Dick Erhard, Joe Farrell, and Ola Grimsby, became the founding members of the AAOMPT. The AAOMPT developed a standards document, bylaws, and a recognition process for residency programs. In 1992, the AAOMPT was accepted as the member organization to represent the United States in IFOMT.

Although prominent individuals such as Paris, Kaltenborn, and Maitland played a large role in development and advancement of manipulation and manual therapy within the physical therapy profession over the last half of the twentieth century, the current practice and the future of the specialty area of orthopaedic manual physical therapy are driven by evidence-based practice.[22] A large growing body of research evidence supports and guides the practice of manipulation within the scope of physical therapy practice and for other manual practitioners.

## ORTHOPAEDIC MANUAL PHYSICAL THERAPY TREATMENT PHILOSOPHY

Paris[23] described a nine-point "Philosophy of Dysfunction" that summarizes the components of a traditional orthopaedic manual physical therapy (OMPT) treatment philosophy (Box 1-1). Paris defines "dysfunction" as increases or decreases of motion from the expected normal or as the presence of aberrant movements.[4] Therefore, the primary focus of the orthopaedic manual physical therapist's examination is the analysis of active and passive movement. If hypomobility is noted, joint mobilization and stretching techniques are used; if hypermobility is noted, stabilization exercises, motor control, and postural correction are emphasized. If aberrant movements are noted, a motor retraining exercise approach is appropriate. If localization of tissue reactivity and pain are noted, gentle oscillatory techniques as described by Maitland can be used to attempt to inhibit pain.[21] To use *Guide to Physical Therapist Practice* terminology, this is an impairment-based approach, which is a foundation of physical therapy.

| BOX 1-1 | Philosophy of Dysfunction as Described by Paris |

I. That joint injury, including such conditions referred to as osteoarthritis, instability, and the aftereffects of sprains and strains, are dysfunctions rather than diseases.

II. That dysfunctions are manifest as either increases or decreases of motion from the expected normal or by the presence of aberrant movements. Thus, dysfunctions are represented by abnormal movements.

III. That where the dysfunction is detected as limited motion (hypomobility), the treatment of choice is manipulation to joint structures, stretching to muscles and fascia and the promotion of activities that encourage a full range of movement.

IV. That when the dysfunction is manifest as increased movement (hypermobility), laxity or instability, the treatment of the joint in question is not manipulation but stabilization by instruction of correct posture, stabilization exercises and correction of any limitations of movement in neighboring joints that may be contributing to the hypermobility.

V. That the primary cause of degenerative joint disease is joint dysfunction. Therefore, it may be concluded that its presence is due to the failure or lack of accessibility to physical therapy.

VI. That the physical therapist's primary role is in the evaluation and treatment of dysfunction, whereas that of the physician is the diagnosis and treatment of disease. These are two separate but complementary roles in health care.

VII. That since dysfunction is the cause of pain, the primary goal of physical therapy should be to correct the dysfunction rather than the pain. When, however, the nature of the pain interferes with correcting the dysfunction, the pain will need to be addressed as part of the treatment program.

VIII. That the key to understanding dysfunction, and thus being able to evaluate and treat it, is understanding anatomy and biomechanics. It therefore behooves us in physical therapy to develop our knowledge and skills in these areas, so that we may safely assume leadership in the non-operative management of neuromusculoskeletal disorders.

IX. That it is the patients' responsibility to restore, maintain, and enhance their health. In this context, the role of the physical therapist is to serve as an educator, to be an example to the patient, and to reinforce a healthy and productive lifestyle.

Adapted from Paris SV: *Introduction to spinal evaluation and manipulation*, Atlanta, 1986, Institute Press.

Manual physical therapy approaches place an emphasis on application of biomechanical principles in the examination and treatment of spinal disorders. Motion is analyzed with active and passive motion testing with visualization of the spinal mechanics; the motion is best described with standardized biomechanical terminology. Passive forces are applied, with passive accessory intervertebral motion testing and mobilization/manipulation techniques, along planes of movement parallel or perpendicular to the anatomic planes of the joint surfaces. Therefore, knowledge of spinal anatomy and biomechanics is a prerequisite to learning a manual physical therapy approach for examination and treatment of the spine.

Orthopaedic manual physical therapists use a process of clinical reasoning that includes continual assessment of the patient, followed by application of a trail of manual therapy treatment or exercise, followed by further assessment of the patient's response to the treatment. This intimate relationship between examination, treatment, and reexamination provides useful clinical data for sound judgments regarding the patient's response to treatment and the need to modify, progress, or maintain the applied interventions. Use of examination procedures with proven reliability and validity further enhances the clinical decision-making process.

During the past several years, physical therapists have embraced the principles of evidence-based practice. When research evidence is available to guide clinical decisions, the physical therapist should follow the evidence-based practice guidelines. However, when research evidence is not clear, an impairment-based approach that includes a thorough evaluation and sound clinical decision making should be used, with a focus on restoring function, reducing pain, and returning the patient to functional activities. This textbook attempts to incorporate the best of evidence-based practice with an orthopaedic manual physical therapy approach.

The evidence supports use of a classification system to guide the treatment of patients with spinal disorders.[24,25] The classification system has been well developed for the lumbar spine, and similar principles can be used for other regions of the spine. The classification system recognizes that patients with spinal disorders are a heterogeneous group. However, subgroups of patients can be identified with common signs and symptoms that respond to interventions that can be provided by physical therapists, including manipulation, specific directional exercises, stabilization exercises, and traction. A classification of common disorders is described in great detail for each anatomic region covered in this textbook.

So, for effective treatment of patients with spinal disorders, physical therapists complete a comprehensive physical examination that includes screening for red flags to ensure that physical therapy is appropriate to the patient's condition. The examination includes procedures with proven reliability and validity, and the results of the examination are correlated with patient questionnaire information and the patient's history to determine a diagnosis. The diagnosis places the patient in a classification and includes a problem list of noted impairments that impact the patient's condition. As treatment is implemented, the patient's condition is continually reassessed to determine the results of treatment and to determine whether modifications in diagnosis and treatment are necessary. The primary emphasis of the treatment is integration of manual therapy techniques and therapeutic exercise with principles of patient education to ultimately allow the patient to self-manage the condition.

## Evidence-Based Practice

Evidence-based practice is defined as the integration of best research evidence with clinical expertise and patient values.[26] The research evidence considered in evidence-based practice is meant to be clinically relevant patient-centered research of the accuracy and precision of diagnostic tests, the power of prognostic markers, and the efficacy and safety of therapeutic, rehabilitative, and preventive regimens.[26] Clinical experience, the ability to use clinical skills and past experience, should also be incorporated into evidence-based practice to identify each patient's health state and diagnosis, risks and benefits of potential interventions, and the patient's values and expectations.[26] Patient values include the unique preferences, concerns, and expectations each patient brings to a clinical situation; these values must be integrated into clinical decisions if the therapist is to properly serve the patient.[26]

Evidence-based principles are incorporated throughout this textbook. When studies are identified to illustrate the accuracy and precision of diagnostic tests, this information is reported in the "notes" section of the examination technique description; when clinical outcome studies that use a specific intervention are identified, this information is included as well. The examination and treatment procedures included in this textbook have been chosen based on the research evidence to support their use, on my clinical experience, and on safety considerations. The decision to use the examination and treatment techniques presented in this textbook should be made based on the clinician's knowledge of the evidence, competence in application of the intervention, and clinical experience combined with the patient's values and expectations. Although this textbook can establish a foundation for evidence-based practice for physical therapy management of spinal and temporomandibular disorders, new evidence continues to emerge regarding the best diagnostic and treatment procedures. Therefore, the practitioner's responsibility is to stay abreast of new developments in research findings and to make appropriate changes in practice to reflect these new findings.

Many of the examination tests presented in this textbook have been tested for reliability and validity; this information is reported when available. Reliability is defined as the extent to which a measurement is consistent and free of error.[27] If an examination test is reliable, it is reproducible and dependable to provide consistent responses in a given condition.[27] Validity is the ability of a test to measure what it is intended to measure.[27] Both reliability and validity are essential considerations in determination of what tests and measures to use in the clinical examination of a patient.

Reliability is often reported as both interrater and intrarater reliability. Intrarater or intraexaminer reliability defines the stability or repeatability of data recorded by one individual across two or more trials.[27] Interrater reliability defines the amount of variability between two or more examiners who measure the same group of subjects.[27] For the statistical analysis of interval or ratio data, the intraclass correlation coefficient (ICC) is the preferred statistical index because it reflects both correlation and agreement and determines the amount of variance between two or more repeated measures.[27,28] For ordinal, nominal, or categorical data, percent agreement can be determined and the Kappa coefficient ($\kappa$) statistic applied, which takes into account the effects of chance on the percent

**TABLE 1-1** Kappa Coefficient Interpretation

| KAPPA STATISTIC | STRENGTH OF AGREEMENT |
| --- | --- |
| <0.00 | Poor |
| 0.00-0.20 | Slight |
| 0.21-0.40 | Fair |
| 0.41-0.60 | Moderate |
| 0.61-0.80 | Substantial |
| 0.81-1.00 | Almost perfect |

Data from Landis JR, Koch GG: *Biometrics* 33:159-174, 1977.

**TABLE 1-2** 2 × 2 Contingency Table

| DIAGNOSTIC TEST | DISEASE | NO DISEASE |
| --- | --- | --- |
| Test positive | True | False |
| | Positive A | Positive B |
| Test negative | False | True |
| | Negative C | Negative D |
| | Sensitivity | Specificity |
| | A/(A+C) | D/(B+D) |

Adapted from Sackett DL, Straus SE, Richardson WS, et al: *Evidence-based medicine: how to practice and teach EBM,* ed 2, Edinburgh, 2000, Churchill Livingstone.
Table is used to compare results of reference standard with results of test under investigation; used to calculate sensitivity and specificity.

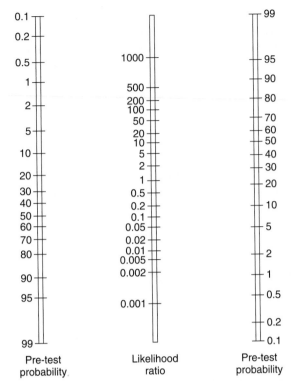

**FIGURE 1-2** Likelihood ratio monogram. (From Sackett DL, Straus SE, Richardson WS, et al: *Evidence-based medicine: how to practice and teach EBM,* ed 2, Edinburgh, 2000, Churchill Livingstone.)

agreement.[27,29] Landis and Koch[30] have established a general guideline for interpretation of Kappa scores (Table 1-1). Because the effect of chance is not affected by prevalence, the Kappa coefficient can be deflated if the prevalence of a particular outcome of the test or measure is either very high or very low.[28] "Acceptable reliability" must be determined by the clinician who uses the specific test or measure and should be based on which variable is tested, why a particular test is important, and on whom the test is to be used.[31]

Results of validity testing examination procedures are reported as sensitivity (Sens), specificity (Spec), positive likelihood ratio (+LR), and negative likelihood ratio (−LR). Sensitivity is the test's ability to obtain positive test results when the target condition is really present, or a true positive.[27] The 2 × 2 contingency table (Table 1-2) is used to calculate the sensitivity and specificity. "SnNout" is a useful acronym to remember that tests with high <u>s</u>e<u>n</u>sitivity have few false negative results; therefore, a <u>n</u>egative result rules <u>out</u> the condition.[26] Specificity is the test's ability to obtain negative test results when the condition is really absent, or a true negative.[27] "SpPin" is a useful acronym to remember that tests with high <u>sp</u>ecificity have few false <u>p</u>ositive results; therefore, a <u>p</u>ositive result rules <u>in</u> the condition.[26]

Likelihood ratios dictate the degree of the shift from the pretest probability that a patient has or does not have a condition to the posttest probability. A positive likelihood ratio is equal to Sensitivity/(1 − Specificity) and represents the amount of increase in odds favoring the condition if the test results are positive.[28] Positive likelihood ratios of greater than 10 generate a large and often conclusive shift in probability; ratios of 5 to 10 generate moderate shifts in probability; and ratios of 2 to 5 generate small but sometimes important shifts in probability.[32] A likelihood ratio nomogram can be used to draw a line from the pretest probability through the likelihood ratio score and continue in a straight line to end at the posttest probability (Figure 1-2).

A negative likelihood ratio is equal to (1 − Sensitivity)/Specificity and represents the decrease in odds favoring the condition if the test results are negative.[28] Negative likelihood ratios of less than 0.1 generate large and often conclusive shifts in probability; ratios of 0.1 to 0.2 generate moderate shifts in probability; and ratios of 0.2 to 0.5 generate small but sometimes important shifts in probability.[32]

Clinical prediction rules (CPR) may be used to enhance the clinician's accuracy in predicting a diagnosis or in determining appropriate treatment strategies.[28] The rule is developed with applying an intervention to a group of patients and then identifying common characteristics in the group of patients who responded favorably to the intervention through calculation of positive and negative likelihood ratios. After the CPR is developed, it must be validated with an investigation of the accuracy of the CPR in a new group of patients with clinical tests or interventions performed by a different group of clinicians other than those who developed the rule.[28,33] Validation should also occur in multiple settings to enhance the rule's generalizability, and an impact study should be completed to determine what impact the rule has had on changing clinical behaviors and to assess whether economic benefits have resulted.[28,33] Clinical prediction rules have been developed to assist in guiding clinical decision making for the use of spinal manipulation and stabilization exercise programs for management of spinal disorders and are presented in subsequent chapters of this textbook.[34-38]

The highest level of evidence to support interventions is based on the recommendations of systematic reviews and clinical practice guidelines, and clinicians should start their search to answer clinical management questions with identification of applicable systematic reviews.[26] A systematic review is a summary of the medical literature that uses explicit methods to systematically search, critically appraise, and synthesize the world literature on a specific issue.[26] The quality of systematic reviews is dependent on the quality of the randomized controlled studies (RCT) that have been done to investigate the effectiveness of the interventions being studied. Sackett et al[26] describe the essential questions to ask when reviewing the validity of randomized controlled trials: (1) Was the assignment of patients to treatment randomized? And was the randomization list concealed? (2) Was follow-up of patients sufficiently long and complete? (3) Were all patients analyzed in the groups to which they were randomized (even those who did not follow through on the prescribed treatment)? (4) Were patients and clinicians kept blind to treatment? (5) Were groups treated equally, apart from the experimental therapy? And (6) Were the groups similar at the start of the trial? If these questions are answered favorably, the results of the RCT can be used to assist with clinical decision making as long as the patient under consideration fits within the parameters of the patient population studied in the RCT.

Lower levels of evidence such as case reports or case series are useful for developing a hypothesis of the effect of a treatment approach, but a true cause and effect from the treatment used in the case reports and case series cannot be assumed without a control group. Often case series studies are used to support the need for an RCT and assist with development of the RCT methodology.

The literature is reviewed in each chapter related to the classification categories for subgrouping disorders commonly treated by physical therapists. One goal of this textbook is to promote an increase in the number of physical therapists, physicians, and other health professionals who follow the recommendations of high-quality clinical practice guidelines and systematic reviews for management of spinal disorders and to provide the necessary background and instructional information to assist in skill development to effectively implement the treatment recommendations related to manual therapy and exercise.

## HOW TO USE THIS BOOK AND DVD

This book and DVD can be used in a variety of ways. The textbook has been organized by anatomic region as a useful and easy to use reference resource for students and clinicians. However, when this textbook is used as a resource to teach a course, students should be taught and tested on the principles and procedures of a detailed spinal examination and in the clinical decision making required to appropriately classify and diagnose spinal disorders before learning and being tested on the motor skills of spinal manipulation. Testing students on the examination procedures before teaching manipulation facilitates safe application of the treatment procedures. In addition, many of the passive intervertebral motion (PIVM) tests used in the spinal examination are converted to manipulation techniques. Therefore, the process of learning and being tested on these PIVM tests facilitates the motor skills required for proper performance of the manipulation techniques. The more proficient students become in the examination procedures, the easier the manipulation techniques are to learn. Instructors may choose to teach and examine students on the examination of multiple regions of the spine before beginning instruction in manipulation techniques.

The DVD can be used to assist the instructor in demonstration of the examination and manipulation techniques. Three cameras were used to film each technique, which provides unique angles of perspective and viewing that an individual viewing a demonstration in a large group of students cannot have. A live demonstration is still valuable, and the DVD may best be used for a second viewing or review of the technique during practice sessions. In addition, because all students will have their own DVD with the textbook, they can check on the proper performance of the technique during practice sessions.

---

### Definitions of Terms from the *Guide to Physical Therapist Practice*

**Arthrokinematic:** The accessory or joint play movements of a joint that cannot be performed voluntarily and that are defined by the structure and shape of the joint surfaces, without regard to the forces producing motion or resulting from motion.

**Assessment:** The measurement or quantification of a variable or the placement of a value on something. Assessment should not be confused with examination or evaluation.

**Diagnosis:** Diagnosis is both a process and a label. The diagnostic process includes integrating and evaluating the data that are obtained during the examination to describe the patient/client condition in terms that will guide the prognosis, the plan of care, and intervention strategies. Physical therapists use diagnostic labels that identify the impact of a condition on function at the level of the system (especially the movement system) and at the level of the whole person.

**Evaluation:** A dynamic process in which the physical therapist makes clinical judgments based on data gathered during the examination.

*Continued*

## Definitions of Terms from the *Guide to Physical Therapist Practice*—cont'd

**Examination:** A comprehensive screening and specific testing process leading to diagnostic classification or, as appropriate, to a referral to another practitioner. The examination has three components: the patient/client history, the systems review, and tests and measures.

**Functional limitation:** The restriction of the ability to perform, at the level of the whole person, a physical action, task, or activity in an efficient, typically expected, or competent manner.

**Impairment:** A loss or abnormality of anatomical, physiological, mental, or psychological structure or function. *Secondary impairment:* Impairment that originates from other, preexisting impairments.

**Intervention:** The purposeful interaction of the physical therapist with the patient/client and, when appropriate, with other individuals involved in patient/client care, using various physical therapy procedures and techniques to produce changes in the condition.

**Joint integrity:** The intactness of the structure and shape of the joint, including its osteokinematic and arthrokinematic characteristics.

**Joint mobility:** The capacity of the joint to be moved passively, taking into account the structure and shape of the joint surface in addition to characteristics of the tissue surrounding the joint.

**Manual therapy techniques:** Skilled hand movements intended to improve tissue extensibility; increase range of motion; induce relaxation; mobilize or manipulate soft tissue and joints; modulate pain; and reduce soft tissue swelling, inflammation, or restriction.

**Mobilization/manipulation:** A manual therapy technique comprising a continuum of skilled passive movements to the joints and/or related soft tissues that are applied at varying speeds and amplitudes, including a small-amplitude/high-velocity therapeutic movement.

**Osteokinematics:** Gross angular motions of the shafts of bones in sagittal, frontal, and transverse planes.

**Passive accessory intervertebral motion (PAIVM) tests:** A type of passive joint mobility assessment that uses passive joint play motions of the spine to induce spinal segment passive motion. The therapist judges the degree of passive mobility at the targeted spinal motion segment by sensing the amount of resistance to the passive joint play movement. Joint mobility, irritability, and end feel can be assessed with these procedures.

**Passive intervertebral motion (PIVM) tests:** A type of passive segmental joint mobility assessment of the spine that might include either passive accessory intervertebral motion tests or passive physiological intervertebral motion tests. The therapist will make judgments of segmental passive motion, end feel, and pain provocation (i.e., irritability) assessment based on these procedures.

**Passive physiological intervertebral motion (PPIVM) tests:** A type of passive joint mobility assessment that uses passive osteokinematic motions of the spine to induce spinal segment passive motion, which is palpated by the therapist to judge the degree of passive mobility at the targeted spinal motion segment.

Adapted from American Physical Therapy Association: Guide to physical therapist practice, *Phys Ther* 81:9-746, 2001, The Association.

## Additional Definitions of Manual Therapy Terminology

**Accessory motion:** Those motions that are available in a joint that may accompany the classical movements or be passively produced isolated from the classical movement. Accessory movements are essential to normal full range-of-motion and painless function.

**Component motion:** Motions that take place in a joint complex or related joint to facilitate a particular active motion.

**Close-packed position:** Position of maximum congruency of a joint that is locked, statically efficient for load bearing but dynamically dangerous.

**Joint dysfunction:** A state of altered mechanics, either an increase or decrease from the expected normal, or the presence of an aberrant motion.

**Joint play:** Movements not under voluntary control that occur only in response to an outside force.

**Kinematics:** The study of the geometry of motion independent of the kinetic influences that may be responsible for the motion. In biomechanics, the two divisions of kinematics are osteokinematics and arthrokinematics.

**Loose-packed position:** Position of a joint where the capsule and ligaments are their most slack, which is unlocked, statically inefficient for load bearing, and dynamically safe.

Data from Paris SV, Loubert PV: *Foundations of clinical orthopaedics,* St Augustine, Fla, 1990, Institute Press.

## REFERENCES

1. APTA: *American Physical Therapy Association,* www.apta.org/About/apta_history/history. Accessed March 22, 2005.

2. APTA, CAPTE, editor: *Evaluative criteria for the accreditation of education programs for the preparation of physical therapists,* Alexandria, Va, 2005, APTA.

3. Paris SV, Loubert PV: *Foundations of clinical orthopaedics,* St Augustine, Fla, 1990, Institute Press.

4. Paris SV: A history of manipulative therapy, *JMMT* 8(2):66-77, 2000.

5. Hood W: On the so-called "bone-setting": its nature and results, *Lancet* 1:336-338, 372-374, 441-443, 1871.

6. Paget J: Cases that bone setters cure, *Br Med J* 1:1-4, 1867.

7. Stoddard A: *Manual of osteopathic practice,* London, 1969, Hutchinson.

8. Peterson DH, Bergmann TF: *Chiropractic technique: principles and procedures,* ed 2, St Louis, 2002, Mosby.

9. Paris SV: 37th Mary McMillan lecture: in the best interest of the patient, *Phys Ther* 86(11):1541-1553, 2006.

10. McMillan M: Change of name [editorial], *PT Rev* 5(4):3-4, 1925b.

11. McMillan M: *Massage and therapeutic practice,* ed 2, Philadelphia, 1925, Saunders.

12. Herman RF: The art of mobilizing joints, *Phys Ther Rev* 16:94-95, 1936.

13. Thornhill MC: Manipulative treatment of lumbosacral derangement: report of a series of cases treated with technic described by Dr. B. S. Troedsson, *Phys Ther Rev* 18:65-67, 1938.

14. Tait R: The place of manipulation and gymnastics in treatment, *Am J Phys Ther* Dec:240-242, 1929.

15. Swenson LL. Study of the intervertebral disc: with special reference to rupture of the nucleus pulposus and its relation to low back pain and to sciatica, *Phys Ther Rev* 21:179-184, 1941.

16. Mennell J: *The science and art of joint manipulation,* London, 1949, Churchill.

17. Cyriax J: *Textbook of orthopaedic medicine,* vol 1, ed 2, London, 1957, Cassell.

18. Kaltenborn FM: *The spine basic evaluation and mobilization techniques,* Oslo, Norway, 1964, Olaf Norlis Bokhandel.

19. Paris SV: *Spinal lesion,* Churchchrist, New Zealand, 1965, Pegasus.

20. Mennell J McM: *Joint pain,* Boston, 1964, Little Brown.

21. Maitland GD: *Vertebral manipulation,* London, 1964, Butterworth.

22. Olson KA: President's message: history is on our side, *Articulations* 11(2):1-3, 8, 2005.

23. Paris SV: *Introduction to spinal evaluation and manipulation,* Atlanta, 1986, Institute Press.

24. Brennan GP, Fritz JM, Hunter SJ, et al: Identifying subgroups of patients with acute/subacute "nonspecific" low back pain: results of a randomized clinical trial, *Spine* 31(6):623-631, 2006.

25. Fritz JM, Delitto A, Erhard RE: Comparison of a classification-based approach to physical therapy and therapy based on clinical practice guidelines for patients with acute low back pain: a randomized clinical trial, *Spine* 28:1363-1372, 2003.

26. Sackett DL, Straus SE, Richardson WS, et al: *Evidence-based medicine: how to practice and teach EBM,* ed 2, Edinburgh, 2000, Churchill Livingstone.

27. Portney LG, Watkins MP: *Foundations of clinical research applications to practice,* ed 2, Upper Saddle River, NJ, 2000, Prentice Hall.

28. Cleland JA: *Orthopaedic clinical examination: an evidence-based approach for physical therapists,* Carlstadt, NJ, 2005, Icon Learning Systems.

29. Cohen J: A coefficient of agreement for nominal scales, *Educ Psychol Meas* 20(1):37-46, 1960.

30. Landis JR, Koch GG: The measurement of observer agreement for categorical data, *Biometrics* 33:159-174, 1977.

31. Rothstein JM, Echternach JL: *Primer on measurement: an introductory guide to measurement issues,* Alexandria, Va, 1999, American Physical Therapy Association.

32. Jaeschke R, Guyatt GH, Sackett DL: How to use an article about a diagnostic test. B: what are the results and will they help me in caring for my patients? *JAMA* 271:703-707, 1994.

33. McGinn T, Guyatt GH, Wyer P, et al: Users' guides to the medical literature XXIIa: how to use articles about clinical decision rules, *JAMA* 284:79-84, 2000.

34. Childs J, Fritz J, Flynn T, et al: A clinical prediction rule to identify patients with low back pain most likely to respond to spinal manipulation: a validation study, *Ann Intern Med* 141(12):922-928, 2004.

35. Cleland JA, Childs JD, Fritz JM, et al: Development of a clinical prediction rule for guiding treatment of a subgroup of patients with neck pain: use of thoracic spine manipulation, exercise, and patient education, *Phys Ther* 87(1):9-23, 2007.

36. Flynn T, Fritz J, Whitman J, et al: A clinical prediction rule for classifying patients with low back pain who demonstrate short-term improvement with spinal manipulation, *Spine* 27:2835-2843, 2002.

37. Hicks GE, Fritz JM, Delitto A, et al: Preliminary development of a clinical prediction rule for determining which patients with low back pain will respond to a stabilization exercise program, *Arch Phys Med Rehabil* 86:1753-1762, 2005.

38. Tseng YL, Wang WTF, Chen WY, et al: Predictors for the immediate responders to cervical manipulation in patients with neck pain, *Man Ther* 11:306-315, 2006.

## CHAPTER 2

# Spinal Examination and Diagnosis in Orthopaedic Manual Physical Therapy

## CHAPTER OVERVIEW

The purpose of this chapter is to provide a framework for completion of a comprehensive spinal examination including systems medical screen, patient interview, disability assessment, and tests and measures. In addition, evaluation of the examination findings and principles involved in a diagnosis and plan of care are included. The tests and measures presented in this chapter are the basic examination procedures used in screening the spine or are techniques used across anatomic regions to complete comprehensive spinal examination. Additional special tests and manual examination procedures such as passive intervertebral motion tests are presented in detail in subsequent chapters that focus on each anatomic region of the spine.

## OBJECTIVES

- Describe the components of a comprehensive spinal examination
- Perform a medical screen as part of a spinal examination
- Describe common red flags and yellow flags that must be evaluated as part of a comprehensive spinal examination
- Explain the components of a patient interview and provide interpretation of common responses to interview questions
- Use and interpret relevant questionnaires for pain, function, and disability
- Perform common tests and measures used in a spinal examination
- Explain the reliability and validity of common tests and measures used in a spinal examination
- Describe the process used in the evaluation of clinical findings, diagnosis, and treatment planning for common spinal disorders utilizing the current best evidence with an impairment-based approach

## DIAGNOSIS IN PHYSICAL THERAPY PRACTICE

Physical therapist diagnostic classifications are based on clusters of patient signs and symptoms to guide treatment decisions. Because physical therapist interventions are designed for correction of physical impairments such as hypomobility or instability, the physical therapy diagnostic classifications are based on impairments that can be treated with physical therapy interventions. Other physical therapy diagnostic classifications may describe symptom location and behavior if these are the primary focus of the physical therapy interventions.

Medical diagnostic classifications focus on identification of disease and are determined by physicians. Although the physi-

cal therapist does not make a medical diagnosis, the physical therapist must determine whether the patient's condition is appropriate for physical therapy or whether the patient should be immediately referred for further medical diagnostic assessment. The physical therapist may also identify signs of conditions that warrant further medical consultation but that may not be severe or progressive in nature so that physical therapy can still proceed while the patient seeks further medical assessment. The patient may also have medical conditions that have been diagnosed and are being appropriately managed. In this situation, physical therapy can proceed, but the condition should be monitored or taken into consideration as physical therapy treatment is implemented.

## MEDICAL SCREEN

Medical screening is the evaluation of patient examination data for the decision of whether a patient referral to a medical practitioner is warranted.[1] Box 2-1 and Table 2-1 list common red flags for which patients must be screened before initiation of physical therapy. With any signs or symptoms characteristic of red flags, patients should be referred to the appropriate medical practitioner for further diagnostic tests. Some comprehensive resources can assist in training clinicians to screen for medical conditions that need to be further assessed by a physician.[1,2] Conditions such as gastrointestinal (GI) disease, psychosocial issues, or cardiovascular disease are cause for caution. If these conditions have not been diagnosed and treated by a physician, a referral is warranted. If these conditions are being medically managed, the physical therapist can proceed with the evaluation and treatment while continuing to monitor these conditions. Life-threatening conditions such as malignant disease are important conditions for identification; if suspected, these conditions warrant an immediate referral to the appropriate physician.

The results of a systematic review for assessment of the accuracy of clinical features and tests used to screen for malignant disease in patients with low back pain found the prevalence rate of malignant disease ranged from 0.1% to 3.5%.[3] A history of cancer (positive likelihood ratio [+LR] = 23.7), an elevated erythrocyte sedimentation rate (ESR; +LR = 18.0), a reduced hematocrit level (+LR = 18.2), and overall clinician judgment (+LR = 12.1) increased the probability of identification of a malignant disease.[3] A combination of age of 50 years or more, history of cancer, unexplained weight loss, and no improvement after 1 month of conservative treatment showed a sensitivity of 100% for identification of malignant disease.[3] Malignant disease is rare as a cause of low back pain, and the most useful features and tests are a history of cancer, an elevated ESR, a reduced hematocrit level, and clinician judgment.[3]

A medical intake form is an essential component of a comprehensive initial patient examination. See Figure 2-1 for an example of a medical intake form. Symptoms of medical conditions such as increased muscle tone and pain may mimic symptoms of musculoskeletal dysfunctions. In addition, identification of risk factors for certain medical conditions impacts the precautions to and progression of physical therapy interventions. For instance, a patient with cardiovascular disease risk factors such as hypertension needs close monitoring as therapeutic exercise programs are initiated and progressed. However, if the patient's hypertension is managed with beta

| BOX 2-1 | Red Flags for the Cervical Spine |
| --- | --- |

**Cervical Myelopathy**
Sensory disturbance of hands
Muscle wasting of hand
Intrinsic muscles
Unsteady gait
Hoffmann's reflex
Hyperreflexia
Bowel and bladder disturbances
Multisegmental weakness or sensory changes

**Neoplastic Conditions**
Age >50 years
History of cancer
Unexplained weight loss
Constant pain; no relief with bed rest
Night pain

**Upper Cervical Ligamentous**
Instability
Occipital headache and numbness
Severe limitation during neck AROM in all directions
Signs of cervical myelopathy

**Inflammatory or Systemic Disease**
Temperature >37°C
Blood pressure >160/95 mm Hg
Resting pulse >100 bpm
Resting respiration >25 bpm
Fatigue

**Vertebral Artery Insufficiency**
Drop attacks
Dizziness
Lightheadedness related to head movements
Dysphasia
Dysarthia
Diplopia
Cranial nerve signs

Adapted from Childs JD, Fritz JM, Piva SR, et al: *JOSPT* 34(11):686-700, 2004.
*AROM*, Active range of motion.

| TABLE 2-1 | Red Flags for Low Back Region | |
| --- | --- | --- |
| **CONDITION** | **RED FLAGS** | |
| Back-related tumor | Age >50 y<br>History of cancer<br>Unexplained weight loss<br>Failure of conservative therapy | |
| Back-related infection (spinal osteomyelitis) | Recent infection (e.g., urinary tract or skin)<br>Intravenous drug user/abuser<br>Concurrent immunosuppressive disorder | |
| Cauda equine syndrome | Urine retention or incontinence<br>Fecal incontinence<br>Saddle anesthesia<br>Global or progressive weakness in lower extremities<br>Sensory deficits in feet (i.e., L4, L5, S1 areas)<br>Ankle dorsiflexion, toe extension, and ankle plantarflexion weakness | |
| Spinal fracture | History of trauma (including minor falls or heavy lifts for individuals who have osteoporosis or are elderly)<br>Prolonged use of steroids<br>Age >70 y | |

From Boissonnault WG: *Primary care for the physical therapist: examination and triage*, Philadelphia, 2005, Saunders.

To ensure you receive a complete and thorough evaluation, please provide us with important background information on the following form. All information is considered confidential and will be released only to your physician unless prior written authorization is given. Thank you.

Name: _____

Occupation: _____

Are you seeing any of the following for your current condition? (Check box.)

☐ Physician (MD, DO)          ☐ Psychiatrist/psychologist          ☐ Attorney

☐ Dentist          ☐ Physical therapist          ☐ Chiropractor

Have you EVER been diagnosed as having any of the following conditions?

☐ Cancer. If YES, describe what kind: _____

| | | | |
|---|---|---|---|
| ☐ Heart problems | ☐ Rheumatoid arthritis | ☐ Prostate problems | ☐ Anemia |
| ☐ Pacemaker | ☐ Other arthritic conditions | ☐ Epilepsy/seizure disorders | ☐ Ulcers |
| ☐ Circulation problems | ☐ Osteoporosis | ☐ Depression | ☐ Liver disease |
| ☐ High blood pressure | ☐ Kidney disease | ☐ Sexually transmitted diseases | ☐ Tuberculosis |
| ☐ Lung disease | ☐ Thyroid problems | ☐ Fibromyalgia | ☐ Allergies |
| ☐ Asthma | ☐ Stroke | ☐ Chemical dependency (i.e., alcoholism) | ☐ Latex allergy |
| ☐ Diabetes | | | ☐ Other: |

Please list any surgeries or other conditions for which you have been hospitalized within the past few years, including the approximate date of the surgery or hospitalization:

Date                    Surgery/hospitalization

_____          _____

_____          _____

Please describe any injuries for which you have been treated (including fractures, dislocations, sprains) within the past few years and the approximate date of injury:

Date                    Injury

_____          _____

_____          _____

Have you recently noted:

Have you fallen within the past 12 months?                                      Yes_____ No_____

During the past month, have you often been bothered by feeling down, depressed, or hopeless?  Yes_____ No_____

During the past month, have you often been bothered by little interest or pleasure in doing things? Yes_____ No_____

How much coffee or caffeine-containing beverages do you drink a day?          _____

How many packs of cigarettes do you smoke a day?                              _____

If one drink equals one beer or glass of wine, how much alcohol do you drink in a week? _____

How are you able to sleep at night?          ☐ Fine          ☐ Moderate difficulty          ☐ Only with medications

**On the scale below, please circle the number that best represents the average level of pain you have experienced over the past 48 hours:**

No pain      0  1  2  3  4  5  6  7  8  9  10      Worst pain imaginable

**FIGURE 2-1** Medical intake form.

**Aggravating factors:** Identify up to three important activities that you are unable to do or are having difficulty with as a result of your problem. List them below:

1. _____
2. _____
3. _____

<table>
<tr><td colspan="2">**Below for the therapist:**</td></tr>
<tr><td>Rating: _____</td></tr>
<tr><td>Rating: _____</td></tr>
<tr><td>Rating: _____</td></tr>
<tr><td>AVG: _____</td></tr>
</table>

| Therapist Use | | |
| --- | --- | --- |
| Unable to perform | 0 1 2 3 4 5 6 7 8 9 10 | Able to perform activity at same level as before |

Body chart: Please mark your present symptoms on the body chart.

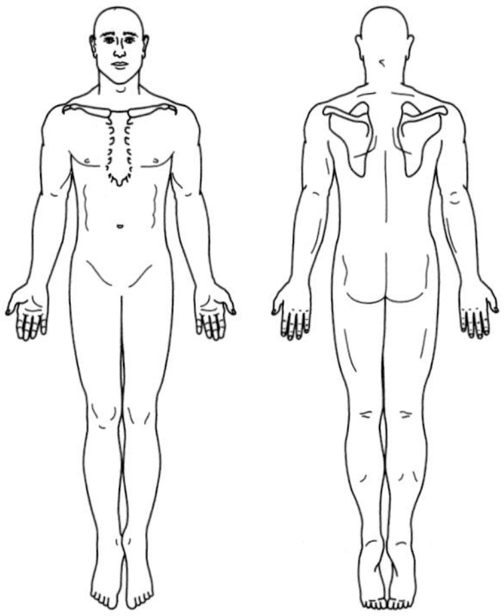

Please list any PRESCRIPTION medication you are currently taking (INCLUDING pills, injections, and/or skin patches):

_____

_____

Which of the following OVER-THE-COUNTER medications have you taken in the past week? (Check box.)

☐ Aspirin   ☐ Laxatives   ☐ Vitamins/supplements

☐ Tylenol   ☐ Antacids   ☐ Advil/Motrin/Ibuprofen

☐ Decongestants   ☐ Antihistamines   ☐ Other

How did you hear about Northern Rehab?

☐ Physician   ☐ Family/friend   ☐ Newspaper

☐ Yellow Pages   ☐ Website   ☐ Drive-by

Therapist Use

Form reviewed with patient?   Yes _____   No _____

Date _____   Therapist signature _____

**FIGURE 2-1, cont'd**

blocker-therapy, which lowers heart rate and dampens or eliminates the pulse response to exercise, the pulse rate is not an effective means for monitoring the patient's response to exercise.[4] Instead, perception of the patient's level of exertion needs to be used to monitor patients who exercise while undergoing beta blocker therapy. Likewise, a diagnosis of osteoporosis is a precaution to excessive strain through the skeletal system with strong stretching or manipulation procedures. However, skilled gentle manual therapy and soft tissue techniques used with precautions to protect the skeletal system and gradual progressive loading of the skeletal system with a monitored exercise program benefit patients with osteoporosis.

A complete list of medications that the patient is taking is also an important component of the medical screen. This information can provide insights into the medical conditions for which the patient is undergoing treatment, and the therapist may find that the combination of prescription and over-the-counter medications is causing an overdosage situation that could result in medical complications. A common example is the use of antiinflammatory drugs. Boissonnault and Meek[5] found that 79% of 2433 patients who were treated in a sample of outpatient physical therapy clinics reported use of antiinflammatory drugs during the week before the survey. Nearly 13% of these patients had two or more risk factors for development of GI disease, and 22% reported combined use of aspirin and another antiinflammatory drug.[5] The risk factors for development of GI complications from nonsteroidal antiinfammatory drugs (NSAIDs) include advanced age (>61 years), history of peptic ulcer disease, use of other drugs known to damage or exacerbate damage to the GI tract, consumption of or high doses of multiple antiinflammatory drugs or aspirin, and serious systemic illness such as rheumatoid arthritis.[6]

The physical therapist should review the medical intake form with the patient for follow-up questions regarding medical conditions and medications to obtain greater detail concerning the nature of each condition. This review can also provide insight into the level of understanding the patient has of the medical conditions and medications. The physical therapist can assist the physician in identification of patient needs regarding further education on the medical management of the patient's conditions; the physical therapist also can make referrals for further consultation regarding identified risk factors for medical complications that may inhibit the rehabilitation process.

Psychosocial issues or yellow flags as listed in Box 2-2 are indications that the rehabilitation approach should be modified.[7] Fear avoidance beliefs associated with chronic low back pain have been shown to be effectively treated with an active exercise program monitored by a physical therapist combined with a behavior modification program that provides positive reinforcement for functional goal attainment.[8] A gradual introduction of activities that the patient fears in a monitored therapeutic environment has yielded favorable results in patients with chronic low back pain.[8]

Patients with chronic whiplash-associated disorder (WAD) with moderate to severe ongoing symptoms have been shown to have higher levels of unresolved posttraumatic stress and high levels of persistent fear of movement and reinjury.[9] Heightened anxiety levels in patients after a whiplash injury have been associated with a greater likelihood of long-term pain and a poorer prognosis.[9] When these factors are identified in a patient with acute WAD, an early psychologic consultation is indicated.[9]

Heightened anxiety and fear avoidance beliefs should not prevent a physical therapist from providing interventions to address the physical impairments identified with these patients but should elevate the clinician's awareness that an active exer-

---

**BOX 2-2    Clinical Yellow Flags That Indicate Heightened Fear Avoidance Beliefs**

**Attitudes and Beliefs**
Belief that pain is harmful or disabling, which results in guarding and fear of movement
Belief that all pain must be abolished before return to activity
Expectation of increased pain with activity or work; lack of ability to predict capabilities
Catastrophizing; expecting the worst
Belief that pain is uncontrollable
Passive attitude toward rehabilitation

**Behaviors**
Use of extended rest
Reduced activity with significant withdrawal from daily activities
Avoidance of normal activity and progressive substitution of lifestyle away from productive activity
Reports of extremely high pain intensity
Excessive reliance on aids (braces, crutches, etc)
Sleep quality reduced after onset of pain
High intake of alcohol or other substances with an increase since onset of back pain
Smoking

Data from Childs JD, Fritz JM, Piva SR, et al: Proposal of a classification system for patients with neck pain, *JOSPT* 34(11):686-700, 2004; and Kendall NAS, Linton SJ, Main CJ: *Guide to assessing psychosocial yellow flags in acute low back pain: risk factors for long-term disability and work loss,* Wellington, New Zealand, 2002, Accident Rehabilitation and Compensation Insurance Corporation of New Zealand and the National Health Committee.

---

cise approach combined with pain management strategies should be incorporated into the treatment plan.

Depression can also impact the health status and the rehabilitation potential of patients. The medical intake form should include the following two questions to screen for depression:

During the past month, have you often been bothered by feeling down, depressed, or hopeless?    Yes    No
During the past month, have you often been bothered by little interest or pleasure in doing things?    Yes    No

If the patient answers "yes" to these two questions, the follow-up "help" question should be asked:

Is this something with which you would like help?    Yes    Yes, but not today    No

Arrol et al[10] reported a sensitivity of 79% and a specificity of 94% for detection of major depression with the two screening questions with the "help" question, for a positive predictive value of 41% and a negative predictive value of 98.8%.[10] If the patient answers "yes" to all three questions, the patient should be referred for further assessment and treatment of the depression as an adjunct to the physical therapy treatment. Major clinical depression has a lifetime prevalence rate of 10% to 25% for women and 5% to 12% for men.[11] Up to 15% of people with major clinical depression commit suicide.[11] In addition, depression is common in patients with chronic back and neck pain, and a multidisciplinary approach that includes counseling, medical management, and exercise is needed to successfully treat these conditions.

## Disability and Psychosocial Impact Questionnaires

Disability, function, and pain indexes have been shown to be more responsive measures of response to treatment for spinal disorders than impairment measures.[12] Disability index forms such as the Fear Avoidance Beliefs Questionnaire (FABQ), the Modified Oswestry Disability Index (ODI), and the Neck Disability Index (NDI) assist in quantification of a patient's perception of disability, the psychosocial impact of the disability, and the prognosis for recovery and, at times, assist in classification of the patient's condition to guide treatment decisions. The Patient-Specific Functional Scale (PSFS) and the Numeric Pain Rating Scale (NPRS) can also assist in quantification of a patient's level of perceived functional limitations and pain perception. These instruments can be used to track outcomes and determine the level of success of a treatment approach for both clinical practice and research situations.

Waddell et al[13] have stated that fear of pain and what we do about it may be more disabling than the pain itself. Individuals react to pain on a continuum from confrontation to avoidance. Confrontation is an adaptive response in which an individual views pain as a nuisance and has a strong motivation to return to normal levels of activity.[14] An avoidance response may lead to a reduction in physical and social activities, excessive fear avoidance behaviors, prolonged disability, and adverse physical and psychologic consequences.[14]

The Fear Avoidance Beliefs Questionnaire (FABQ) was developed and tested by Waddell and colleagues[13] as a way to quantify a patient's fear of physical activity, work, and risk of reinjury and their beliefs about the need to change behavior to avoid pain (Figure 2-2). The questionnaire consists of 16 statements that the patient rates on a scale from 0 (completely disagree) to 6 (completely agree). The FABQ work subscale is calculated with adding items 6, 7, 9, 11, 12, and 15. The FABQ physical activity subscale is calculated with adding items 2, 3, 4, and 5. Test-retest reliability when used with patients with chronic low back pain and sciatica had a Kappa score of 0.74; all results reached a 0.001 level of significance.[14] The Pearson product-moment correlation coefficients for the two scales were 0.95 and 0.88.[14] The FABQ was found to correlate with levels of psychologic distress, and the FABQ work subscale was strongly related to work loss from low back pain over a 1-year period, even with a control for pain intensity and location.[14]

Fear of movement and activity is suspected to be a primary factor in the transition from acute low back pain to chronic long-term disability associated with low back pain. Fritz[14] found that fear avoidance beliefs were present in patients with acute low back pain and were a significant predictor of disability and work status at a 4-week follow-up. In other words, Fritz[14] found that patients with higher levels of fear of work (FABQW > 34; sensitivity = 55%; specificity = 84%; +LR = 3.33; negative likelihood ratio [−LR] = 0.54) at the initial evaluation were less likely to return to full work status after 4 weeks of treatment for the low back pain condition. Higher scores on the FABQ are an indication to use an active exercise–based approach in which the feared activities are gradually introduced to the patient in a controlled environment to assist the patient in overcoming fears.[15] Low scores for the work subscale (FABQW <19) have been associated with an improved likelihood to succeed with lumbopelvic spinal manipulation.[16] Therefore, the FABQ should be completed at the intake of all patients with low back pain–related conditions to assist in guiding treatment decisions. The FABQ can also be used for patients with neck pain.[17]

The Modified Oswestry Disability Index (ODI; Figure 2-3) is a region-specific disability scale for patients with low back pain (LBP). The modified scale substitutes the Employment/Homemaking category for the Sex Life category in the original scale.[18,19] This ODI has been used in numerous LBP studies. The questionnaire consists of 10 items that address different aspects of function and disability, each scored from 0 to 5, with higher values representing greater disability. The total score is obtained with a sum of the responses, which are then expressed as a percentage (range, 0 to 100%). For example, 25/50 = 50%. If all items are answered, the point total can be doubled to obtain the percentage score (i.e., 25 × 2 = 50%).

The purpose of the ODI is assessment of change of perceived disability over time, and the reliability over a 4-week period has been reported as quite good (intraclass correlation coefficient [ICC] = 0.90; 95% confidence interval [CI] = 0.78 to 0.96).[14] Validity and responsiveness are good for construct and content.[14,20] The minimal clinically important difference (MCID) is 6 percentage points (sensitivity = 0.91; specificity = 0.83) and is defined as the amount of change that best distinguishes between patients who have improved conditions and those whose conditions remain stable.[14] The ODI is easy to administer and easy to score. The ODI was developed primarily for patients with acute LBP, and the properties may differ for patients with chronic LBP.

The Neck Disability Index (NDI; Figure 2-4) is a condition-specific questionnaire that has been shown to be reliable and valid with patients with neck pain.[21] This scale has been used in numerous neck pain studies and is structured and scored similarly to the ODI. The questionnaire consists of 10 items that address different aspects of function and disability, each scored from 0 to 5, with higher values representing greater disability. The total score is obtained with a sum of the responses, which are then expressed as a percentage (range, 0 to 100%). For example, 25/50 = 50%. If all items are answered, the point total can be doubled to obtain the percentage score (i.e., 25 × 2 = 50%).

The NDI has also been tested for reliability and responsiveness for patients with cervical radiculopathy.[17] Cleland et al[17] reported test-retest reliability as moderate, with an ICC of 0.68 and a 95% CI of 0.30 to 0.90. The minimal detectable change for the NDI is 10.3 percentage points, and the minimal clinically important change for the NDI was 7.0 percentage points. Cleland et al[22] found that a Patient-Specific Functional Scale (PSFS) exhibited superior reliability, construct validity, and responsiveness in a cohort of patients with cervical radiculopathy as compared with the NDI.

Name: _____    Date: _____

Here are some of the statements that other patients have made to us about their pain. For each statement please circle a number from 0 to 6 to describe how much physical activities such as bending, lifting, walking, or driving affect or would affect your back pain.

| | Completely disagree | | Unsure | | | Completely agree | |
|---|---|---|---|---|---|---|---|
| 1. My pain was caused by physical activity. | 0 | 1 | 2 | 3 | 4 | 5 | 6 |
| 2. Physical activity makes my pain worse. | 0 | 1 | 2 | 3 | 4 | 5 | 6 |
| 3. Physical activity might harm my back. | 0 | 1 | 2 | 3 | 4 | 5 | 6 |
| 4. I should not do physical activities that (might) make my pain worse. | 0 | 1 | 2 | 3 | 4 | 5 | 6 |
| 5. I cannot do physical activities that (might) make my pain worse. | 0 | 1 | 2 | 3 | 4 | 5 | 6 |

The following statements are about how your normal work affects or would affect your back pain.

| | | | | | | | |
|---|---|---|---|---|---|---|---|
| 6. My pain was caused by my work or by an accident at work. | 0 | 1 | 2 | 3 | 4 | 5 | 6 |
| 7. My work aggravated my pain. | 0 | 1 | 2 | 3 | 4 | 5 | 6 |
| 8. I have a claim for compensation for my pain. | 0 | 1 | 2 | 3 | 4 | 5 | 6 |
| 9. My work is too heavy for me. | 0 | 1 | 2 | 3 | 4 | 5 | 6 |
| 10. My work makes or would make my pain worse. | 0 | 1 | 2 | 3 | 4 | 5 | 6 |
| 11. My work might harm my back. | 0 | 1 | 2 | 3 | 4 | 5 | 6 |
| 12. I should not do my normal work with my present pain. | 0 | 1 | 2 | 3 | 4 | 5 | 6 |
| 13. I cannot do my normal work with my present pain. | 0 | 1 | 2 | 3 | 4 | 5 | 6 |
| 14. I cannot do my normal work until my pain is treated. | 0 | 1 | 2 | 3 | 4 | 5 | 6 |
| 15. I do not think that I will be back to my normal work within 3 months. | 0 | 1 | 2 | 3 | 4 | 5 | 6 |
| 16. I do not think that I will ever be able to go back to my normal work. | 0 | 1 | 2 | 3 | 4 | 5 | 6 |

**FIGURE 2-2** Fear Avoidance Beliefs Questionnaire.

The PSFS is a patient-specific outcome measure for investigation of functional status with the patient asked to nominate activities (up to three) that are difficult to perform because of their condition and then to rate the level of limitation for each activity on a 0 to 10 point scale. The ratings are averaged for the three activities. The PSFS has been shown to be valid and responsive to change for patients with several different clinical conditions, including neck pain, knee pain, and low back pain.[23-25] For patients with cervical radiculopathy, the test-retest reliability was high for the PSFS with an ICC of 0.82 and a 95% CI of 0.54 to 0.93.[17] The minimal detectable change for the PSFS was 2.1, and the minimal clinically important change was 2.0 on a 0 to 10 scale.[17] The PSFS can be used for all patients, whereas the ODI is intended to be used with patients with lumbar conditions and the NDI is designed for patients with cervical spine and cervical radiculopathy conditions.

A pain drawing on a body chart is a helpful clinical assessment tool. The patient is advised to complete a body chart as part of a medical screening form (see Figure 2-1), and the therapist should also complete one as part of the initial interview. Patients may draw symptoms in anatomic areas on the body diagram that were not included in the initial medical diagnosis; these symptoms need to be further explored by the therapist to determine whether the symptoms are from a visceral or somatic structure and to determine whether the multiple pain complaints are linked to the same underlying condition or are

**Section 1: To be completed by patient**

Name: _____ Age: _____ Date: _____

Occupation: _____ Number of days of back pain: _____ (this episode)

---

**Section 2: To be completed by patient**

This questionnaire has been designed to give your therapist information as to how your back pain has affected your ability to manage in everyday life. Please answer every question by placing a mark on the line that best describes your condition today. We realize you may feel that two of the statements may describe your condition, but **please mark only the line that most closely describes your current condition.**

**Pain intensity**
_____ The pain is mild and comes and goes.
_____ The pain is mild and does not vary much.
_____ The pain is moderate and comes and goes.
_____ The pain is moderate and does not vary much.
_____ The pain is severe and comes and goes.
_____ The pain is severe and does not vary much.

**Personal care (washing, dressing, etc.)**
_____ I do not have to change the way I wash and dress myself to avoid pain.
_____ I do not normally change the way I wash or dress myself even though doing these tasks causes some pain.
_____ Washing and dressing increase my pain, but I can do these tasks without changing how I do them.
_____ Washing and dressing increase my pain, and I find it necessary to change the way I do these tasks.
_____ Because of my pain I am partially unable to wash and dress without help.
_____ Because of my pain I am completely unable to wash or dress without help.

**Lifting**
_____ I can lift heavy weights without increased pain.
_____ I can lift heavy weights, but doing so causes increased pain.
_____ Pain prevents me from lifting heavy weights off of the floor, but I can manage if they are conveniently positioned (e.g., on a table, etc.)
_____ Pain prevents me from lifting heavy weights off of the floor, but I can manage light to medium weights if they are conveniently positioned.
_____ I can lift only very light weights.
_____ I cannot lift or carry anything at all.

**Walking**
_____ I have no pain when walking.
_____ I have pain when walking, but I can still walk my required normal distances.
_____ Pain prevents me from walking long distances.
_____ Pain prevents me from walking intermediate distances.
_____ Pain prevents me from walking even short distances.
_____ Pain prevents me from walking at all.

**Sitting**
_____ Sitting does not cause me any pain.
_____ I can sit as long as I like provided that I have my choice of seating surfaces.
_____ Pain prevents me from sitting for more than 1 hour.
_____ Pain prevents me from sitting for more than a half hour.
_____ Pain prevents me from sitting for more than 10 minutes.
_____ Pain prevents me from sitting at all.

**Standing**
_____ I can stand as long as I want without increased pain.
_____ I can stand as long as I want, but my pain increases with time.
_____ Pain prevents me from standing for more than 1 hour.
_____ Pain prevents me from standing for more than a half hour.
_____ Pain prevents me from standing for more than 10 minutes.
_____ I avoid standing because it increases my pain right away.

**Social life**
_____ My social life is normal and does not increase my pain.
_____ My social life is normal, but it increases my level of pain.
_____ Pain prevents me from participating in more energetic activities (e.g., sports, dancing, etc.)
_____ Pain prevents me from going out very often.
_____ Pain has restricted my social life to my home.
_____ I have hardly any social life because of my pain.

**Traveling**
_____ I get no increased pain when traveling.
_____ I get some pain while traveling, but none of my usual forms of travel make the pain any worse.
_____ I get increased pain while traveling, but the pain does not cause me to seek alternative forms of travel.
_____ I get increased pain while traveling, and the pain causes me to seek alternative forms of travel.
_____ My pain restricts all forms of travel except that which is done while I am lying down.
_____ My pain restricts all forms of travel.

**Employment/homemaking**
_____ My normal job/homemaking activities do not cause pain.
_____ My normal job/homemaking activities increase my pain, but I can still perform all that is required of me.
_____ I can perform most of my job/homemaking duties, but pain prevents me from performing more physically stressful activities (e.g., lifting, vacuuming).
_____ Pain prevents me from doing anything but light duties.
_____ Pain prevents me from doing even light duties.
_____ Pain prevents me from performing any job or homemaking chores.

---

**Section 3: To be completed by physical therapist/provider**

Score: _____ or _____ % (SEM 11, MDC 16) Initial  FU ____ weeks discharge

Number of treatment sessions: _____ Gender:     Male     Female

Diagnosis/ICD-9 code: _____

Adapted from Hudson-Cook N, Tomes-Nicholson K, Breen A: A revised Oswestry disability questionnaire. In Roland M, Jenner J, editors: *Back pain: new approaches to rehabilitation and education,* New York, 1989, Manchester University Press. [Prepared May 1999]

**FIGURE 2-3** Modified Oswestry Low Back Pain Disability Questionnaire.

Name: _____

Date: _____

This questionnaire has been designed to give your therapist information as to how your neck pain has affected you in your everyday life activities. Please answer each section, marking only ONE box that best describes your status today.

**Section 1 — Pain Intensity**
☐ I have no pain at the moment.
☐ The pain is very mild at the moment.
☐ The pain is moderate at the moment.
☐ The pain is fairly severe at the moment.
☐ The pain is very severe at the moment.
☐ The pain is the worst imaginable at the moment.

**Section 2 — Personal Care (washing, dressing, etc.)**
☐ I can look after myself normally without causing extra pain.
☐ I can look after myself normally, but doing so causes me extra pain.
☐ It is painful to look after myself, and I am slow and careful.
☐ I need help every day in most aspects of self-care.
☐ I do not get dressed, wash with difficulty, and stay in bed.

**Section 3 — Lifting**
☐ I can lift heavy weights without extra pain.
☐ I can lift heavy weights, but doing so gives extra pain.
☐ Pain prevents me from lifting heavy weights off the floor, but I can manage light to medium weights if they are conveniently positioned.
☐ I can lift only very light weights.
☐ I cannot lift or carry anything at all.

**Section 4 — Reading**
☐ I can read as much as I want, with no pain in my neck.
☐ I can read as much as I want, with slight pain in my neck.
☐ I can read as much as I want, with moderate pain in my neck.
☐ I cannot read as much as I want because of moderate pain in my neck.
☐ I can hardly read at all because of severe pain in my neck.
☐ I cannot read at all.

**Section 5 — Headache**
☐ I have no headache at all.
☐ I have slight headaches, which come infrequently.
☐ I have moderate headaches, which come infrequently.
☐ I have moderate headaches, which come frequently.
☐ I have severe headaches, which come frequently.
☐ I have headaches almost all the time.

**Section 6 — Concentration**
☐ I can concentrate fully when I want, with no difficulty.
☐ I can concentrate fully when I want, with slight difficulty.
☐ I have a fair degree of difficulty in concentrating when I want to.
☐ I have a lot of difficulty in concentrating when I want to.
☐ I have a great deal of difficulty in concentrating when I want to.
☐ I cannot concentrate at all.

**Section 7 — Work**
☐ I can do as much as I want.
☐ I can only do my usual work but no more.
☐ I can do most of my usual work, but no more.
☐ I cannot do my usual work.
☐ I can hardly do any work at all.
☐ I cannot do any work at all.

**Section 8 — Driving**
☐ I can drive my car without any neck pain.
☐ I can drive my car as long as I want, with slight pain in my neck.
☐ I can drive my car as long as I want, with moderate pain in my neck.
☐ I cannot drive my car as long as I want because of moderate pain in my neck.
☐ I can hardly drive at all because of severe pain in my neck.
☐ I cannot drive my car at all.

**Section 9 — Sleeping**
☐ I have no trouble sleeping.
☐ My sleep is slightly disturbed (less than 1 hour sleep loss).
☐ My sleep is mildly disturbed (1-2 hours sleep loss).
☐ My sleep is moderately disturbed (2-3 hours sleep loss).
☐ My sleep is greatly disturbed (3-5 hours sleep loss).
☐ My sleep is completely disturbed (5-7 hours sleep loss).

**Section 10 — Recreation**
☐ I am able to engage in all my recreational activities, with no neck pain at all.
☐ I am able to engage in all my recreational activities, with some pain in my neck.
☐ I am able to engage in most but not all of my usual recreational activities because of pain in my neck.
☐ I am able to engage in a few of my usual recreational activities because of pain in my neck.
☐ I can hardly do any recreational activities because of pain in my neck.
☐ I cannot do any recreational activities at all.

**FIGURE 2-4** Neck Disability Index.

separate. In addition, patients may express extreme emotional reactions with their pain symptoms by drawing in pain markings across the entire body or by circling the entire body. In these cases, other questionnaires such as the FABQ should be completed by the patient to further quantify the psychosocial components of the patient's symptoms, and a multidisciplinary approach that includes both active exercise physical therapy and psychologic counseling may be necessary for patient rehabilitation.

The 11-point Numeric Pain Rating Scale (NPRS) is a measure of pain in which patients rate pain ranging from 0 (no pain) to 10 (worst imaginable pain); this scale has been shown to have concurrent and predictive validity as a measure of pain intensity.[26-28] Responsiveness refers to the ability of a measure to detect change accurately when it has occurred.[29] The NPRS shows adequate responsiveness for use in both a clinical and a research setting. A two-point change on the NPRS represents a clinically meaningful change in a patient's perceived level of pain that exceeds the bounds of measurement error.[29]

## Patient Interview and History

The purpose of the initial patient interview is to develop a rapport with the patient, establish a chronology of events, screen for red flags, establish whether physical therapy is appropriate for the patient, develop a hypothesis regarding the cause of the patient's symptoms, and begin to narrow down the appropriate impairment classification or diagnosis for the patient. In the beginning of the interview, open-ended questions should be asked, such as, "When did you first notice this problem?"; "Where did the pain start?"; and "Explain how this problem started."

Next, the location and character of the symptoms should be determined. The therapist should use a body chart to mark interpretation of the pain location, to indicate the focal point of the pain, and to mark where the pain tends to spread. Notes can be made on the body chart regarding the nature of the symptoms, such as sharp pain, burning, numbness, or tingling.

Next, the symptom behavior is determined. The therapist should ask questions such as: "What makes your pain worse?" and "What makes you pain better?" The symptoms associated with common musculoskeletal conditions typically are intensified with certain positions or activities and are relieved with other positions and activities. If the patient is unable to identify positions or activities that affect the intensity and nature of the symptoms, either a strong psychosocial component exists with the pain symptoms or an underlying visceral condition may be causing the symptoms. On occasion, however, the patient is simply a poor historian. These questions also assist with medical screening. For instance, if the patient has throbbing mid-thoracic pain that intensifies in frequency and intensity with exertion such as shoveling snow or climbing stairs, a cardiovascular condition such as an aortic aneurysm may be suspected and should be further evaluated by a physician.

In response to these open-ended questions, more specific follow-up questions should be asked to further outline the symptom behavior as possible diagnostic hypothesis are con-

sidered. For instance, with lumbar spinal stenosis, lower extremity symptoms are commonly provoked with standing and walking and relieved with sitting. In contrast, lumbar radicular symptoms caused by a lumbar herniated disc are commonly provoked with standing and sitting. Specific follow-up questioning to make this distinction can assist in development of the diagnosis.

Another important question is: "How does your pain vary through the course of the day and night?" Most musculoskeletal conditions can be relieved with rest and the use of recumbent positions. If the pain wakes the patient at night, the therapist should inquire whether the patient can quickly return to sleep by changing positions or whether the pain is unremitting regardless of position. The latter answer is a red flag and warrants further medical investigation in most circumstances because malignant diseases can cause intense unremitting night pain. Generally speaking, most musculoskeletal-related pain should improve with rest. However, the patient may feel stiff in the morning, and with activity, a reduction in stiffness is commonly reported. Severe multiple joint morning stiffness is common with rheumatoid arthritis. If the back pain intensifies before meal time and is relieved after eating, a gastric ulcer may be suspected; or if shoulder girdle or thoracic pain is intensified after a heavy meal, a gallbladder problem may be evident.

Determination of functional limitations and establishment of functional goals can assist with documentation and with measurement of progress. Development of a gauge of the level of normal functional activity and how these activities are limited by the current condition can assist in development of the treatment plan, especially regarding duration of treatment. For instance, if the patient wants to return to heavy work or vigorous exercise and currently is very inactive because of a spinal condition, the duration of treatment might be longer than that of a patient who has lesser physical goals.

Inquiries about past treatments for the current condition may assist in development of a treatment plan as well. For instance, if a patient with LBP has received extensive chiropractic "adjustments" for back pain symptoms with minimal benefit, a stabilization exercise program may be indicated, especially if signs and symptoms of instability are noted.

A neurologic screen can also start with the initial interview with the patient asked about any tingling, numbness, or loss of skin sensation. If peripheral symptoms are present, a full neurologic examination is warranted, including deep tendon reflexes, sensation, and myotomal strength testing. In addition, saddle parasthesia or numbness is an indication of a central spinal lesion that causes neurologic involvement of the S4 nerve. Presence of this symptom is a red flag and warrants further diagnostic testing such as magnetic resonance imaging (MRI) for assessment of the integrity of the cauda equina. Follow-up questions regarding bladder function are also indicated with the presence of saddle parasthesia or numbness.

Inquiry about history of similar conditions can provide insight into the underlying diagnosis. For instance, instability and discogenic conditions tend to recur, with intermittent flare-ups reported over many years. Simple muscle and joint sprains and strains are more likely to be a result of a first-time episode of acute back pain.

Medical history can be explored with the patient asked an open-ended question such as, "Other than this problem, how is your overall health?" In addition, the medical intake form should be reviewed with the patient and follow-up questions should be asked for each condition and medication listed to gain further insight into the patient's health status and to screen each system.

Lastly, the patient should be asked to establish functional therapy goals and asked one last open-ended question such as, "Is there anything else you would like to tell me before I begin the examination?" These questions give the patient with another opportunity to provide pertinent medical history that may have been missed to this point.

## TESTS AND MEASURES

### Postural Inspection

Visual inspection of the patient from anterior, posterior, oblique, and lateral views can assist the therapist in determination of postural deviations that may contribute to spinal impairments (Box 2-3). The anterior and posterior views can provide clues of asymmetries in leg length or pelvic height or scoliosis. The lateral view shows alterations in anterior to posterior curves and head, shoulder, and pelvic positions. Kendall's plumb line assessment of posture can be used as a reference standard against which to describe deviations from ideal posture.[30] The oblique views are also important for further analysis of spinal contour. Areas of excessive muscle tone and guarding may also

**BOX 2-3** Postural Inspection

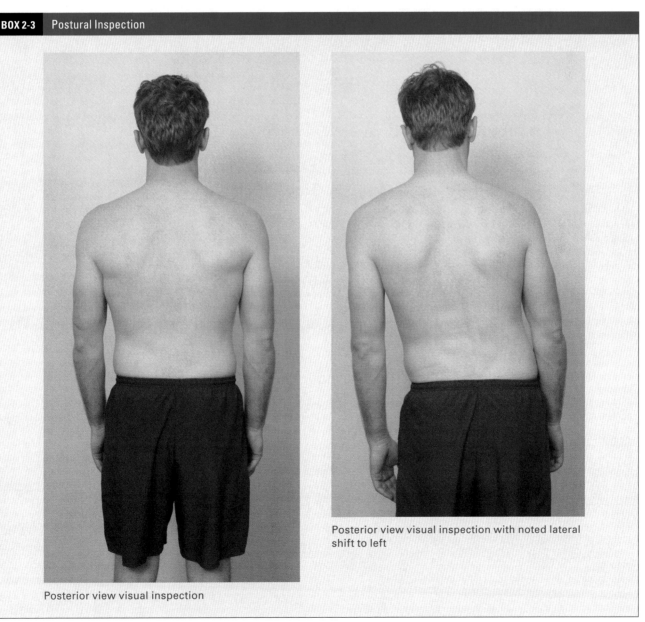

Posterior view visual inspection

Posterior view visual inspection with noted lateral shift to left

*Continued*

**BOX 2-3**    Postural Inspection—cont'd

Anterior view visual inspection

Lateral view visual inspection

**BOX 2-3**   Postural Inspection—cont'd

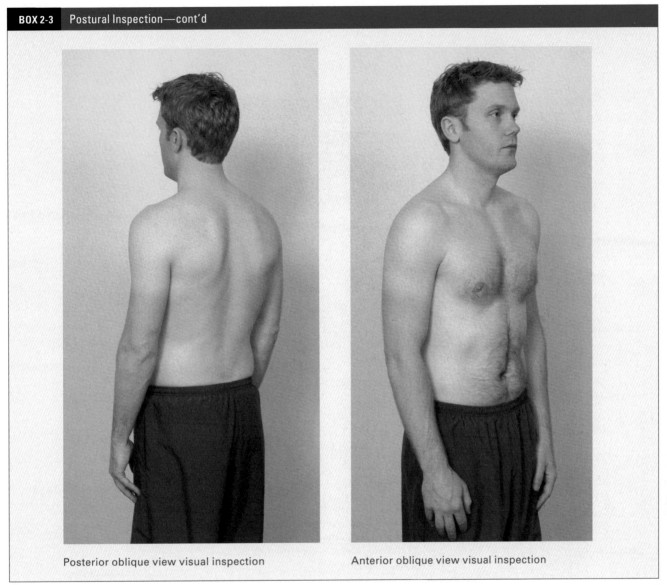

Posterior oblique view visual inspection

Anterior oblique view visual inspection

*Continued*

**BOX 2-3**   Postural Inspection—cont'd

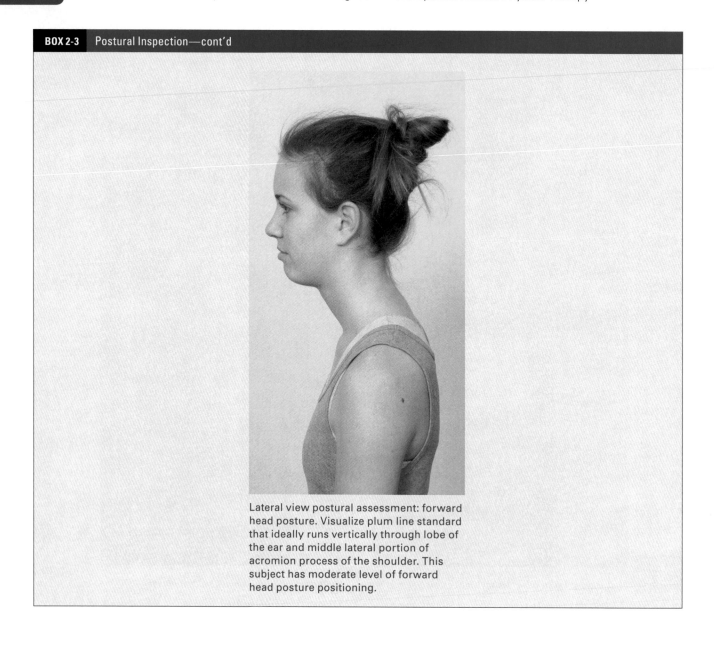

Lateral view postural assessment: forward head posture. Visualize plum line standard that ideally runs vertically through lobe of the ear and middle lateral portion of acromion process of the shoulder. This subject has moderate level of forward head posture positioning.

be noted as signs of underlying instability or tissue irritation. Visual assessment should precede structural examination and palpation.

## Structural Examination

Structural examination is an extension of the visual inspection but involves palpation of bony landmarks for assessment of alteration in symmetry or positioning of the bony structures of the spine and pelvis. Structural examination findings have greater significance in the diagnostic process if the findings can be correlated with other positive examination findings such as limitations in active and passive motion and positive pain provocation testing.

## Level of Mastoid Processes

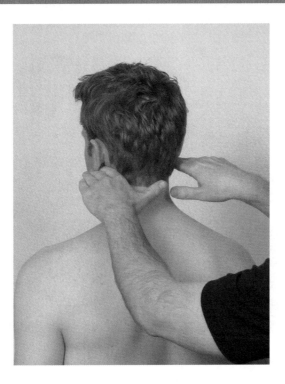

| | |
|---|---|
| **PATIENT POSITION** | The patient stands facing away from the therapist. |
| **THERAPIST POSITION** | The therapist stands directly behind the patient with eyes level with the patient's occiput. |
| **PROCEDURE** | With palms kept parallel to floor and fingers firmly together, the therapist uses the index fingers to palpate the mastoid processes. |
| **NOTES** | The therapist should observe for symmetry in the position of the mastoid processes to assess for a sidebent position of the head that could indicate the presence of a possible craniovertebral dysfunction. |

## Level of Shoulder Girdles and Scapulas

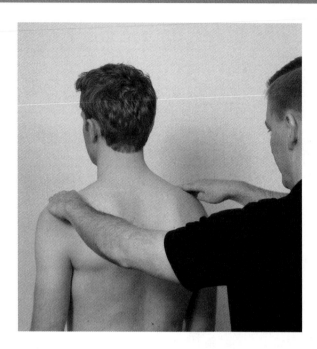
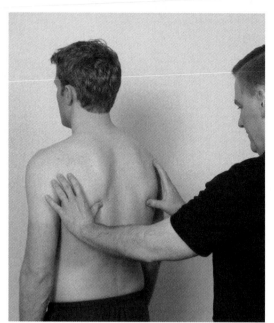

|  |  |
|---|---|
| **PATIENT POSITION** | The patient stands facing away from the therapist. |
| **THERAPIST POSITION** | The therapist stands directly behind the patient with eyes level with the patient's shoulders. |
| **PROCEDURE** | With palms kept parallel to floor and fingers firmly together, the therapist uses the pads of digits 2 to 5 to palpate the superior aspect of the shoulder girdle. Next, the thumbs are used to palpate the inferior angle of each scapula. |
| **NOTES** | The therapist should observe for asymmetry in the position of the shoulder girdles and scapulas that may be a sign of underlying thoracic spine scoliosis or muscle imbalances of the shoulder girdle such as a shortened upper trapezius or levator scapulae muscles and weak lower trapezius or serratus anterior muscles. |

## Palpation of Iliac Crest Height in Standing

(DVD)

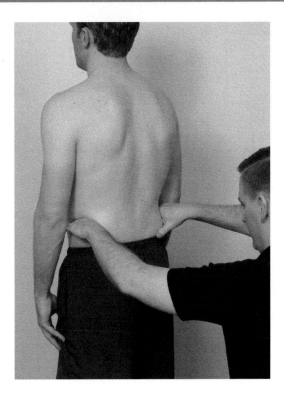

| | |
|---|---|
| **PATIENT POSITION** | The patient stands facing away from the therapist. |
| **THERAPIST POSITION** | The therapist kneels directly behind the patient with eyes level with the patient's iliac crest. |
| **PROCEDURE** | With palms kept parallel to the floor and fingers firmly together, the therapist uses the index fingers to palpate the superior aspect of iliac crests. The therapist should observe for symmetry in heights of iliac crests. |
| **NOTES** | Asymmetry may be an indication of either a leg length difference, a sacroiliac displacement, a structural hip malformation (coxa vara, coxa valga), a hip injury (such a slipped capital epiphysis), or a structural malformation of an innominate bone. Flynn et al[16] reported interexaminer reliability with a Kappa value of 0.23. |

## Palpation of Posterior Superior Iliac Spines in Standing    🔘 DVD

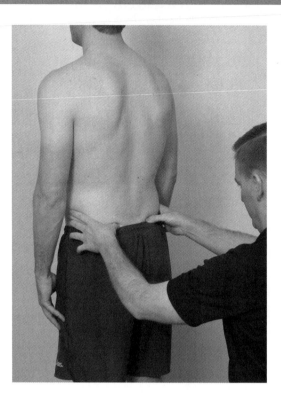

| | |
|---|---|
| **PATIENT POSITION** | The patient stands facing away from the therapist. |
| **THERAPIST POSITION** | The therapist kneels directly behind the patient with eyes level with the patient's posterior superior iliac spines (PSIS). |
| **PROCEDURE** | The therapist first finds the sacral dimples and moves slight lateral and inferior to locate the PSIS on each side with each thumb. The thumbs are used to palpate the inferior aspect of the PSIS (palpate "up and under" PSIS). The therapist should observe for symmetry in heights of the PSIS. |
| **NOTES** | Asymmetry may be an indication of either a leg length difference, a sacroiliac displacement, a structural hip malformation (coxa vara, coxa valga) or hip injury (such a slipped capital epiphysis), or a structural malformation of an innominate bone. Flynn et al[16] reported an interexaminer reliability of 0.13 in standing and of 0.23 in sitting in tests on 71 patients with low back pain referred to physical therapy. |

## Palpation of Greater Trochanter Height   DVD

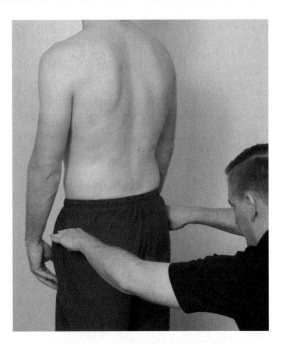

| | |
|---|---|
| **PATIENT POSITION** | The patient stands facing away from the therapist. |
| **THERAPIST POSITION** | The therapist kneels directly behind the patient with eyes level with the patient's greater trochanters. |
| **PROCEDURE** | With palms kept parallel to the floor, the therapist uses the radial aspect of the index fingers to palpate the inferior edge of the greater trochanters (palpate "up and under" the greater trochanters). The therapist may need to ask the patient to sway side to side to help with accurate location of the greater trochanters. The therapist should observe for symmetry in heights of the greater trochanters. |
| **NOTES** | Asymmetry may be an indication of a leg length discrepancy or a structural deviation in the shape of the greater trochanters. A leg length discrepancy of half an inch or greater has been positively correlated with a greater incidence rate of low back pain and should be addressed as part of the treatment program.[31] Palpation of the height of the fibular head and assessment of height of the medial arch of each foot can assist with determination of the portion of the lower extremity where the asymmetry originates. |

## Palpation of Iliac Crest Height in Sitting

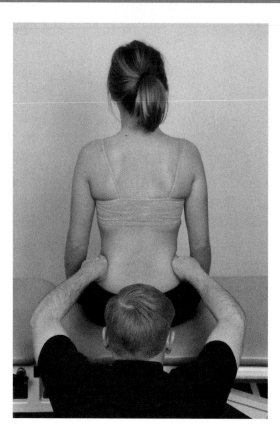

| | |
|---|---|
| **PATIENT POSITION** | The patient sits with legs over the edge of the table and facing away from the therapist. |
| **THERAPIST POSITION** | The therapist kneels directly behind the patient with eyes level with the iliac crests. |
| **PROCEDURE** | With palms kept parallel to the floor and fingers firmly together, the therapist uses the index fingers to palpate the superior aspect of the iliac crests. The therapist should observe for symmetry in height of the iliac crests. |
| **NOTES** | Palpation of the pelvic structures with the patient sitting on a firm level surface can assist with differentiation of the cause of asymmetries noted in the standing structural examination. For example, if the iliac crest height is level in sitting but asymmetry is noted in standing, the cause is likely a lower extremity asymmetry rather than a pelvic dysfunction. However, if the same amount of pelvic height asymmetry is noted both in sitting and in standing, the cause is likely pelvic asymmetry rather than lower extremity structural asymmetry. |

## Palpation of Posterior Sacroiliac Spine in Sitting

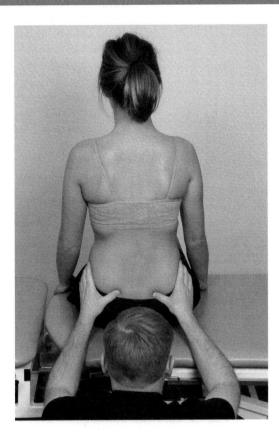

| | |
|---|---|
| **PATIENT POSITION** | The patient sits with legs over the edge of the table and facing away from the therapist. |
| **THERAPIST POSITION** | The therapist kneels directly behind the patient with eyes level with the PSIS. |
| **PROCEDURE** | The therapist first finds the sacral dimples and moves slight lateral and inferior to locate the PSIS on each side with each thumb. The therapist uses the thumbs to palpate the inferior aspect of the PSIS (palpate "up and under" the PSIS). The therapist should observe for symmetry in heights of the PSIS. |
| **NOTES** | Palpation of the pelvic structures with the patient sitting on a firm level surface can assist with differentiation of the cause of symmetries noted in the standing structural examination. For example, if the PSIS height is level in sitting but asymmetry is noted in standing, the cause is likely lower extremity asymmetries rather than a pelvic dysfunction. However, if the same degree of PSIS asymmetry is noted both in sitting and in standing, the cause is likely pelvic asymmetry rather than lower extremity structural asymmetry or leg length difference. |
| | Documentation of structural examination findings can be quickly noted with marking the observed findings on a body chart diagram (Figure 2-5). With writing or describing the findings, consistency with description of the asymmetry by the side that is lower is best. For instance, the structural examination reveals a lowered iliac crest, PSIS, and greater trochanter palpated in the standing position. |

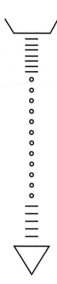

**FIGURE 2-5** Structural examination documentation. Spine diagram can be used to mark structural examination findings. Slash marks can be used to mark relative positions of bony landmarks, and spinal curvatures can be drawn in.

## Active Range of Motion Examination

The purpose of the active range of motion (AROM) examination is to document the amount of motion impairment present at the time of the examination, to identify pain provocation with motion, and to develop a hypothesis on the cause of the pain and limited motion. Signs of spinal instability such as aberrant motion patterns may also be noted with AROM examination. Identification of regions of spinal stiffness with the AROM examination can assist in locating and isolating hypomobile spinal segments that respond favorably to spinal manipulation. The AROM findings are correlated with other examination findings to determine the appropriate spinal disorder classification to guide management of the patient's condition.

## Cervical Forward-Bending Active Range of Motion

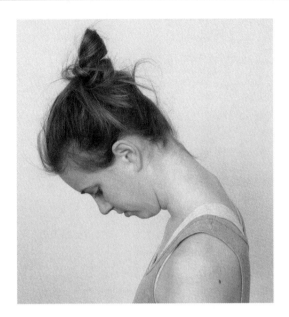 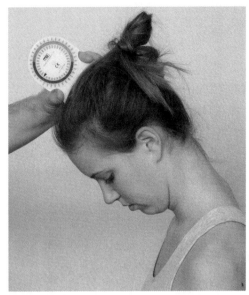

Cervical forward bending measured with inclinometer

| | |
|---|---|
| **PATIENT POSITION** | The patient stands (or sits), with good posture and arms relaxed at the sides. |
| **THERAPIST POSITION** | The therapist stands to the side and slightly behind the patient to clearly observe cervical motion. |
| **PROCEDURE** | The patient is instructed to slowly nod the head and forward bend the cervical spine. The motion should start in the upper cervical spine and continue down to approximately the level of T3. A straightening or reversal of the cervical lordosis should occur on forward bending. The chin should also be near the sternum. Motion can be measured with an inclinometer placed in a midsagittal position on the top of the head. |
| **NOTES** | Whether or not the motion reproduces the patient's symptoms should be noted. If a segmental restriction is due to a unilateral facet restriction, forward bending may deviate to the ipsilateral side of the restriction. Piva et al[32] used a gravity inclinometer to measure cervical forward bending on 30 subjects and found a mean of 60 degrees forward bending, with an ICC of 0.78 (0.59 : 0.89), a standard error of the mean (SEM) of 5.8 degrees, a minimal detectable change (MDC) of 16 degrees, and a Kappa value for symptom reproduction of 0.87 (0.81 : 0.94). |

## Cervical Backward-Bending Active Range of Motion

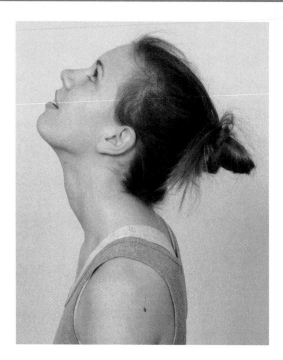 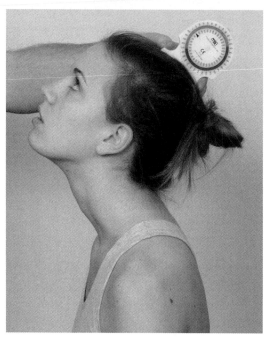

Cervical backward bending measured with inclinometer

| | |
|---|---|
| **PATIENT POSITION** | The patient stands (or sits), with good posture and arms relaxed at the sides. |
| **THERAPIST POSITION** | The therapist stands to the side and slightly behind the patient to clearly observe the cervical motion. |
| **PROCEDURE** | Patient is instructed to slowly look up and backward bend the cervical spine as far as they can move comfortably. Motion can be measured with an inclinometer placed in a midsagittal position on the top of the head. |
| **NOTES** | Whether or not the motion reproduces the patient's symptoms is noted. If a segmental restriction caused by a facet restriction is present, backward bending may deviate to the contralateral side of the restriction. Patients are guarded in case they become dizzy during the backward-bending motion. Reproduction of neck pain may be from facet joint compression/irritation, and a reproduction of referred symptoms into the arm could be from nerve root irritation or from a referral pattern from structures of the cervical spine. Piva et al[32] used a gravity inclinometer to test reliability on 30 subjects and found a mean of 48 degrees of backward bending, an ICC of 0.86 (0.73 : 0.93), an SEM of 5.6 degrees, an MDC of 16 degrees, and a Kappa value for symptom reproduction of 0.65 (0.54 : 0.76). |

## Cervical Side-Bending (Lateral Flexion) Active Range of Motion Right and Left with Shoulder Girdle Supported

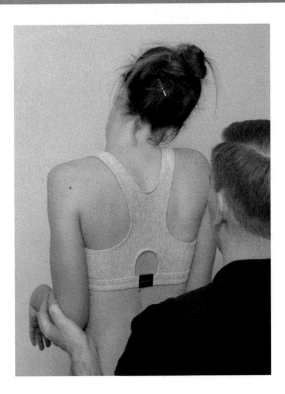

| | |
|---|---|
| **PATIENT POSITION** | The patient stands, with good posture and arms relaxed at the sides. |
| **THERAPIST POSITION** | The therapist stands directly behind the patient. |
| **PROCEDURE** | The patient's arms are supported at the elbows (with elbows flexed to approximately 90 degrees) to passively elevate the patient's shoulders to place the cervical spine soft tissues on slack. The patient is instructed to side bend the cervical spine by slowly dropping the head and neck toward the right shoulder. |
| **NOTES** | The therapist should observe for a smooth curve throughout the cervical spine. Any fulcruming throughout the spinal segments is noted. The therapist observes side bending to the left with the arms supported. The amount of motion available in each direction is compared. The findings of this examination procedure are compared with the findings of the side-bending AROM test with unsupported arms at the side. If the patient is able to achieve significantly greater range of motion with the arms supported, the limitation is most likely the result of soft tissue (i.e., myofascial) tightness. However, if the patient has the same limitation in the amount of range of motion, the limitation is most likely from facet restriction. |

## Cervical Side-Bending (Lateral Flexion) Active Range of Motion Right and Left

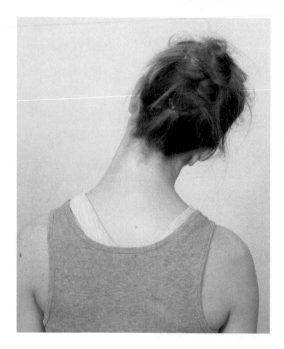

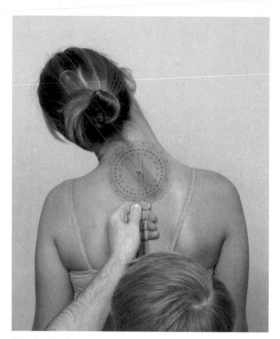

Cervical spine lateral flexion measured with goniometer

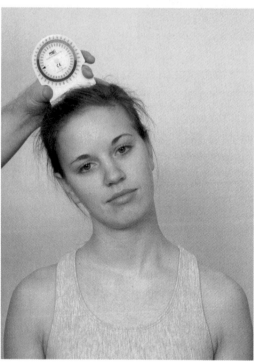

Cervical spine lateral flexion measured with inclinometer

## Cervical Side-Bending (Lateral Flexion) Active Range of Motion Right and Left—cont'd

PATIENT POSITION   The patient stands (or sits), with good posture and arms relaxed at the sides.

THERAPIST POSITION   The therapist stands directly behind the patient.

PROCEDURE   The patient is instructed to side bend (lateral flexion) the cervical spine by slowly dropping the head and neck towards the right shoulder. Motion can be measured with a goniometer (C7 as fulcrum point) or an inclinometer (placed in the frontal plane on top of the head).

NOTES   The therapist should observe for a smooth curve throughout the cervical spine. Any fulcruming throughout the spinal segments should be noted. The amount of motion available in each direction is compared and noted if the motion reproduces the patient's symptoms. Piva et al[32] used a gravity inclinometer to measure cervical side bending on 30 subjects and found a mean AROM of 39 degrees left lateral flexion and of 41 degrees right lateral flexion, with an ICC of 0.85 left and 0.87 right, an SEM of 4.2 left and 3.7 right, an MDC of 12 left and 10 right, and a Kappa value for pain reproduction of 0.28 left and 0.75 right.

## Cervical Rotation Active Range of Motion Right and Left

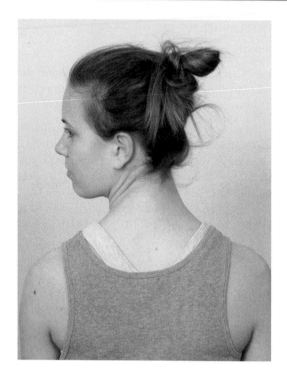

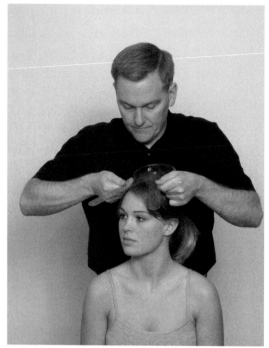

Cervical spine rotation AROM measured with goniometer

| | |
|---|---|
| **PATIENT POSITION** | The patient stands (or sits), with good posture and arms relaxed at the sides. |
| **THERAPIST POSITION** | The therapist stands directly behind the patient. |
| **PROCEDURE** | The patient is instructed to rotate the cervical spine by slowly turning the head and neck to look over the right shoulder. Motion can be measured with a goniometer with the moving arm lined up with the nose, the stationary arm facing straight ahead, and the fulcrum at the center crown of the cranium. |
| **NOTES** | The chin should near the plane of the shoulder with the end range of rotation. The procedure is repeated with rotation to the left. The amount of motion available in both directions is compared and noted if the motion reproduces the patient's symptoms and the location/nature of the symptoms. |
| | Youdas, Carey, and Garrett[33] reported an intraclass correlation coefficient (ICC) for measurements of cervical spine AROM of 60 patients with a universal goniometer that ranged from 0.78 to 0.95 for intratester reliability. When the motion was measured with a cervical range of motion (CROM) inclinometer or universal goniometer, intertester reliability ranged from 0.54 to 0.92. For visual estimates of cervical AROM, ICC values for intertester reliability ranged from 0.42 for flexion/extension to 0.82 for rotation. |

## Upper Thoracic Rotation with One Thumb at C7 and Another at T4

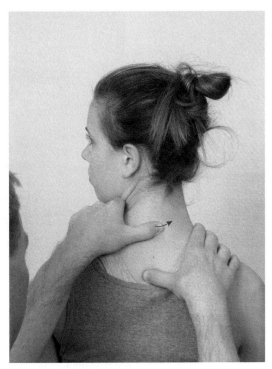

Cervical spine rotation AROM with palpation of upper thoracic rotation

| | |
|---|---|
| **PATIENT POSITION** | The patient stands (or sits), with good posture and arms relaxed at the sides. |
| **THERAPIST POSITION** | The therapist stands directly behind the patient. |
| **PROCEDURE** | With testing of upper thoracic rotation, the therapist uses one thumb to palpate the apex of the patient's C7 spinous process. The other thumb is used to palpate the apex of the patient's T4 spinous process. The patient is instructed to rotate the upper thoracic spine by slowly turning the head and neck to look over the right shoulder. The therapist should observe for the C7 spinous process to move to the opposite side of the rotation with a slight upswing at the end of the movement. The procedure is repeated, with the thumb moved from C7 to T1 and then to T2. |
| **NOTES** | Whether or not the motion reproduces symptoms is noted, as are the location and nature of the symptoms. The thumb position is maintained to assess rotation in the opposite direction. The amount of motion available in each direction at each spinal segment is compared. |

## Active Range of Motion Cervical Spine Rotation in Supine    [DVD]

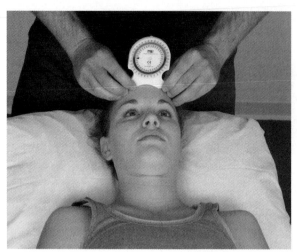

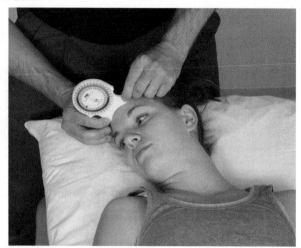

Inclinometer placement for measurement of supine cervical spine rotation

Supine cervical rotation measured with inclinometer

| | |
|---|---|
| **PATIENT POSITION** | The patient is supine with the head resting on a small to medium-sized pillow. |
| **THERAPIST POSITION** | The therapist stands at the head of the table. |
| **PROCEDURE** | The patient is instructed to rotate the cervical spine by slowly turning the head and neck to look over the right shoulder. A gravity inclinometer can be positioned on the forehead and used to measure the motion. |
| **NOTES** | The amount of motion available in both directions is compared. Whether or not the motion reproduces the patient's symptoms is noted, as are the location and nature of the symptoms produced. If neck pain is reported on the ipsilateral side of the most restricted rotation direction, cervical downglide restrictions are suspected on the symptomatic side. If neck pain is reported on the contralateral side of motion restriction, cervical upglide restrictions are suspected on the symptomatic side. Passive intervertebral motion (PIVM) testing must be completed to isolate the passive segmental mobility. Supine rotation testing is a quick way to assess premanipulation and postmanipulation range of motion. Piva et al[32] used a gravity inclinometer to test cervical spine rotation AROM in supine and reported an ICC of 0.86 (0.74 : 0.93) for right rotation and of 0.91 (0.82 : 0.96) for left rotation, a SEM of 4.8 degrees (right) and 4.1 degrees (left), a minimal detectable change of 13 degrees (right) and 11 degrees (left), and a Kappa value of 0.76 (right) and 0.74 (left) for symptom reproduction. |

## Thoracolumbar Forward-Bending Active Range of Motion

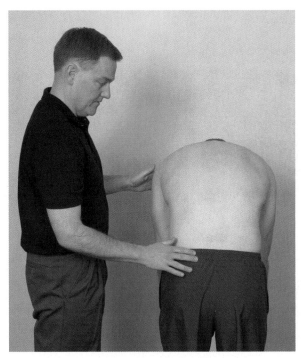

Lumbar and thoracic forward-bending visual inspection

| | |
|---|---|
| **PATIENT POSITION** | The patient stands, with good posture and arms relaxed at the sides. |
| **THERAPIST POSITION** | The therapist stands behind or just lateral to the patient with a clear view of the thoracic and lumbar spine. |
| **PROCEDURE** | The patient is instructed to forward bend the thoracic and lumbar spine by slowly forward bending the head and neck, then the shoulders, followed by the thoracic and lumbar spine. The patient is guarded during the examination to prevent loss of balance and falling forward. The therapist should observe for a smooth forward curve in the thoracic spine and a straightening or reversal of the lordosis in the lumbar spine. |
| **NOTES** | Whether or not the motion reproduces the patient's symptoms is noted. The therapist should observe and palpate for any shaking, juddering, or trick (i.e., aberrant) movements during the motion because these may indicate instability in the lumbar spine. Also, the presence of lateral deviation with forward bending is noted because this may be a sign of a facet joint restriction. The motion may be repeated up to 10 times to determine whether symptoms centralize or peripheralize with the active motion. Once a change in symptoms is noted, the repeated movements are discontinued for that test direction. |

## Lumbar Forward-Bending Measurement

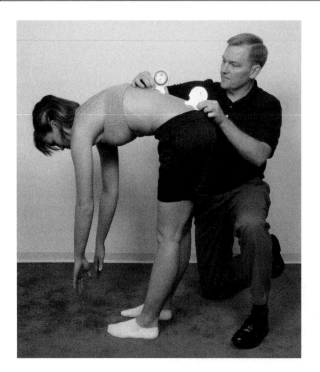
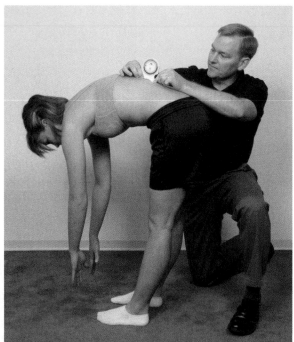

| | |
|---|---|
| **PATIENT POSITION** | The patient stands with feet shoulder width apart, good posture, and arms relaxed at the sides. For the double inclinometer method, inclinometers are placed at midline of the spine in line with the PSIS and 15 cm above the baseline mark. The starting position angles of both inclinometers are zeroed. For the single inclinometer method, place the inclinometer at the T12 spinous process. |
| **THERAPIST POSITION** | The therapist stands just lateral to the patient with a clear view of the thoracic and lumbar spine and inclinometers. |
| **PROCEDURE** | The patient is instructed to forward bend the thoracic and lumbar spine by slowly forward bending the head and neck, then the shoulders, followed by the thoracic and lumbar spine. The angle of both inclinometers at the end position is noted, and the degree of forward bending is calculated with subtracting the angle of the lower inclinometer (represents hip motion) from the upper inclinometer (represents total motion). For the single inclinometer method, simply document the degree of forward bending from the start position. |
| **NOTES** | Nitchke et al[34] found ICC levels for intertester reliability to be 0.35 and for intratester reliability to be 0.52. Maher and Adams[35] found a strong correlation between the inclinometer method of measuring lumbar forward-bending and backward-bending motion and radiographic assessment. A single inclinometer method has also shown good reliability when performed with placing a single inclinometer at the T12 vertebra.[36] |

## Thoracolumbar Backward-Bending Active Range of Motion

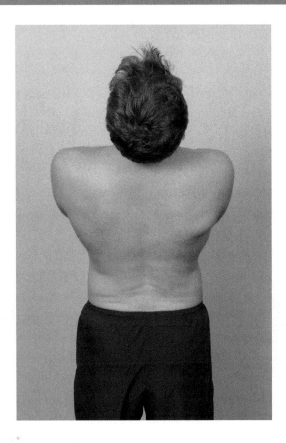

|  |  |
|---|---|
| **PATIENT POSITION** | The patient stands, with good posture and arms folded across the chest. |
| **THERAPIST POSITION** | The therapist stands behind or just lateral to the patient with a clear view of the thoracic and lumbar spine. |
| **PROCEDURE** | The patient is instructed to backward bend the thoracic and lumbar spine by slowly leaning backward as far as comfortable. The therapist should be sure to guard the patient during the examination to prevent loss of balance and falling backward. |
| **NOTES** | The therapist should observe for symmetry in the motion and an increase in lumbar lordosis. Whether the motion reproduces the patient's symptoms is noted. The motion may be repeated up to 10 times to determine whether the symptoms centralize or peripheralize. Once a change in symptoms is noted (i.e., centralization or peripheralization), the repeated movements are discontinued for that test direction. Lumbar backward bending can be measured with either a single or double inclinometer method similar to that described for lumbar forward bending. |

## Thoracolumbar Lateral Flexion Active Range of Motion

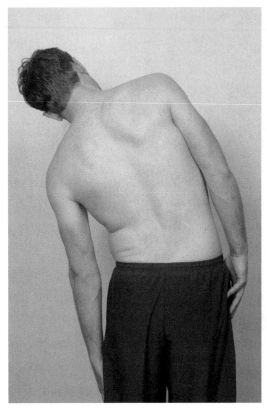

Lumbar and thoracic lateral flexion (side-bending) left

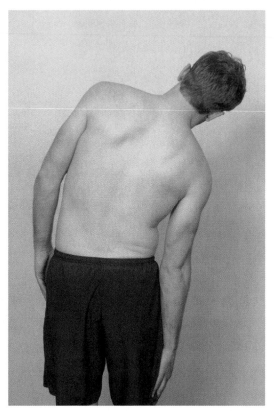

Lumbar and thoracic lateral flexion (side-bending) right

| | |
|---|---|
| **PATIENT POSITION** | The patient stands, with good posture and arms relaxed at the sides. |
| **THERAPIST POSITION** | The therapist stands directly behind the patient. |
| **PROCEDURE** | The patient is instructed to side bend the thoracic and lumbar spine by slowly side bending the head and neck, then the shoulders, followed by the thoracic and lumbar spine to the right. The therapist should observe for a smooth curve throughout the thoracic and lumbar spine. Any fulcruming throughout the spinal segments is noted as is whether the motion reproduces the patient's symptoms. The procedure is repeated with side bending to the left. The amount of motion available in each direction is compared. |
| **NOTES** | A flat area may be an indication of muscle or joint tightness, and a fulcrum point in the range of motion may indicate greater mobility at that spinal level compared with the segments above and below the fulcrum point. |

## Thoracolumbar Rotation

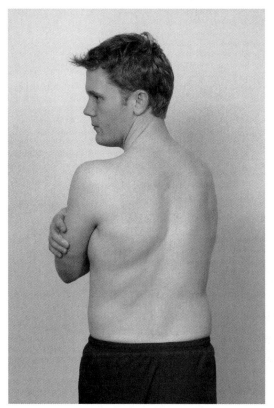

Lumbar and thoracic rotation left

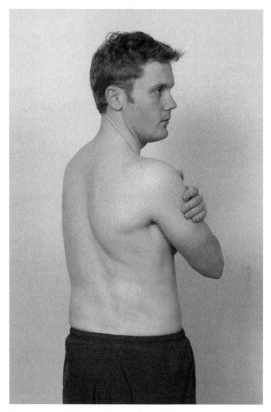

Lumbar and thoracic rotation right

| | |
|---|---|
| **PATIENT POSITION** | The patient stands, with good posture and arms folded across the chest. |
| **THERAPIST POSITION** | The therapist stands directly behind the patient, gently stabilizing the patient's pelvis. |
| **PROCEDURE** | The patient is instructed to rotate the thoracic and lumbar spine by slowly turning the head and neck to look over the right shoulder and by continuing to rotate the shoulders to include the thoracic and lumbar spine. The therapist should observe for side bending of the thoracic and lumbar spine to the left (the opposite direction of the rotation). Whether the motion reproduces the patient's symptoms is noted. The procedure is repeated with rotating to the right. The amount of motion available in each direction is compared. |
| **NOTES** | Overpressure through the pelvis can be provided by the therapist to determine the reactivity of the stretched tissues with this motion. |

## Lumbar Extension–Side-Bending–Rotation Combined Motion

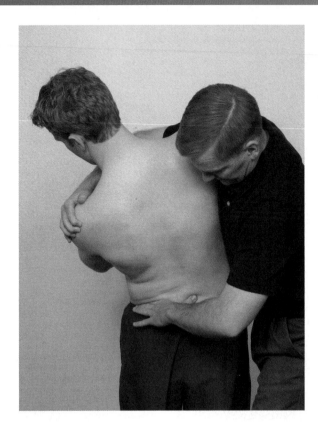

| | |
|---|---|
| **PURPOSE** | The purpose of this motion is to assess the amount of motion and pain provocation with the combined motion of backward bending, side bending, and rotation. |
| **PATIENT POSITION** | The patient is standing. |
| **THERAPIST POSITION** | The therapist stands at the side opposite to the direction of side bending and rotation. |
| **HAND PLACEMENT** | The right hand is positioned with the arm across the patient's chest holding the patient's left shoulder. |
| | The left hand is positioned with the radial aspect of the second digit at the lower lumbar spine to create a fulcrum point for the motion. |
| **PROCEDURE** | The therapist guides the patient into lumbar extension, left side bending, and left rotation with the right arm as the left hand creates a fulcrum point for the motion. |
| **NOTES** | In theory, pain provocation at the low back could result from loading the lumbar facet joints on the side of the combined motions, and leg pain could be provoked with loading and closing the lumbar neuroforamen. Haswell[37] reported a Kappa value of 0.29 (0.06 to 0.52) for intertester reliability in pain provocation with this combined motion test in 35 patients with low back pain. |

## Lumbar Side-Glide (Lateral Shift Correction)

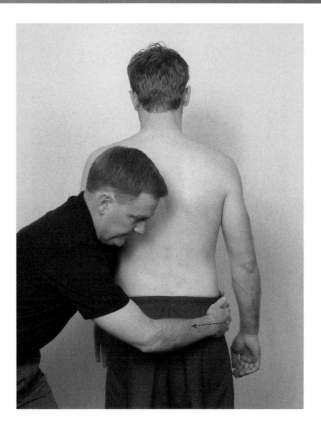

| | |
|---|---|
| **PURPOSE** | The purpose of this motion test is to assess the effects of a manual lateral shift correction on the intensity and location of low back and leg pain. |
| **PATIENT POSITION** | The patient is standing. |
| **THERAPIST POSITION** | The therapist places the left shoulder at the lateral aspect of the thorax on the side of the lateral shift and overlaps the hands at the lateral aspect of the pelvis on the opposite side of the shoulders. |
| **PROCEDURE** | The therapist guides the patient into a lateral shift correction with a force couple of laterally directed forces of the therapist's left shoulder toward the right and hands pulling the pelvis toward the left. The patient is monitored for the effect on symptoms, and the procedure is repeated up to 10 times until determination of whether the correction has no effect, peripherizes symptoms, or centralizes symptoms. |
| **NOTES** | If the lateral shift correction centralizes symptoms, the correction is repeated as part of the treatment program with other repeated movements that have a centralization effect on the patient's symptoms. If symptoms peripheralize into the lower extremity with this maneuver, further assessment is needed to determine whether other repeated movements, manipulation, exercise, or traction are required to affect the symptoms in a more positive way. Although a lateral shift posture is commonly associated with the presence of a herniated disc, other impairments such as spinal facet joint, pelvic, and myofascial system dysfunctions can cause a patient to assume this posture. A thorough analysis of the patient's history and examination of the lumbopelvic structures is needed to develop a treatment plan of care to address the impairments that contribute to a lateral shift posture. |

## Hook-Lying Lower Trunk Rotation    DVD

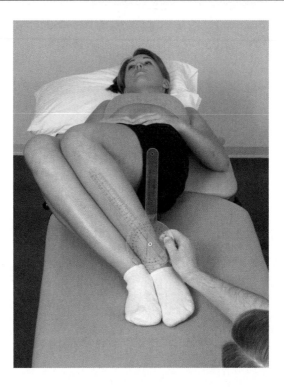

| | |
|---|---|
| **PATIENT POSITION** | The patient is supine hook lying with knees flexed to 90 degrees and feet flat on the table. |
| **THERAPIST POSITION** | The therapist kneels at the foot end of the table. |
| **GONIOMETER ALIGNMENT** | The stationary arm is perpendicular to the table or parallel to a plumb line or straight edge on the wall at the head of the treatment table. |
| | The axis point is 3 inches superior to the talus of the superior lower extremity with the bottom edge of the 14-inch plastic goniometer resting on the talus. |
| | The moving arm is parallel to the shaft of the tibia, pointing to the tibial tuberosity. |
| **PROCEDURE** | The angle of the top leg to the stationary arm represents the degree of lower trunk rotation. The patient can be asked to perform the motion with three repetitions in each direction as a warm-up before the measurement is taken. As the patient moves the legs to the right, a left rotation of the lumbar spine is produced. |
| **NOTES** | Olson and Goerhing[38] tested the reliability of this goniometric measurement and found Pearson correlation coefficients for intrarater reliability that ranged from 0.59 to 0.82 for right rotation ($P < .001$) and 0.76 to 0.82 for left rotation ($P < .001$) and for interrater reliability that ranged from 0.62 to 0.83 with right rotation ($P < 0.001$) and 0.75 to 0.77 for left rotation ($P < 0.001$). Asymmetry in lower trunk rotation is an impairment that can be treated with lumbar rotation manipulation techniques directed in the direction of the limitation. |

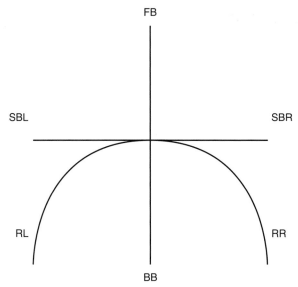

FB

SBL                              SBR

RL                                RR

BB

**FIGURE 2-6** Each line represents 100% of expected range of motion. Slash mark at corresponding length of the line can be made at the observed visual estimate of percent of expected motion in each direction tested. Three slash marks can be used when myofascial limitations are suspected of causing limitation in motion. "X" is used at point of limitation when pain provocation is reported with motion. Additional written notes of pain location with each motion can also be made. Deviations in motion direction or muscle shakiness can also be drawn on motion diagram.

| TABLE 2-2 | PIVM Grading System | |
|---|---|---|
| **GRADE** | **DESCRIPTION** | **TREATMENT** |
| 0 | Ankylosis or no detectable movement | No treatment |
| 1 | Considerable limitation in movement | Mobilization/manipulation |
| 2 | Slight limitation in movement | Mobilization/manipulation |
| 3 | Normal | No treatment |
| 4 | Slight increase in motion | No treatment or stabilization exercises |
| 5 | Considerable increase in motion | Stabilization exercises and treatment of neighboring hypomobility |
| 6 | Unstable | Stabilization exercises and treatment of neighboring hypomobility; external support; fusion |

Adapted from Gonnella C, Paris SV, Kutner M: *Phys Ther* 62(4):436-444, 1982.

## Documentation

When measured with a goniometer or inclinometer, active range of motion can be documented with writing the motion and the corresponding degree measurement. Active range of motion visual estimates are documented with stating the percentage of the expected range of motion that is observed. A chart with lines for each motion can also be used as a shorthand method of documentation, with the end of the stem representing 100% of expected motion (Figure 2-6).

## PALPATION

Palpation is the process of examining the body by means of touch and is a fundamental physical therapist skill that provides information about bony landmark location, tissue temperature, texture, resilience, and motion.[39] Palpation can be divided into palpation for tissue condition, palpation for bony landmark position, and palpation for passive intervertebral motion.

### Palpation for Passive Intervertebral Motion

Physical therapists generally examine passive intervertebral joint motion (PIVM) as part of the examination of patients with spinal disorders. PIVM testing involves the process of passively inducing spinal segmental motion while simultaneously attempting to palpate and judge the amount and quality of

motion. PIVM tests can also be used as pain provocation tests. Some authors separate PIVM tests into two subcategories: passive physiologic intervertebral motion testing (PPIVM) and passive accessory intervertebral motion testing (PAIVM).[40] The PPIVM tests involve induction and palpation of motion in the cardinal planes of movement such as forward bending, side bending, and rotation. PAIVM tests involve induction and judgment of joint play movements that require an outside force to produce the motion such as a posterior to anterior gliding motion of the spinal segment. In addition to being used as a passive motion assessment, PAIVM tests are more likely to be used for assessment of end feel and pain provocation. PPIVM tests are primarily used for assessment of segmental passive movements and at times end feel but less commonly for pain provocation.

The results of PIVM test mobility judgments can be graded and documented simply as hypomobile, normal, or hypermobile for each motion direction and each spinal segment tested. Another common mobility scale first published by Gonnella, Paris, and Kutner[41] incorporates a 7-point (0 to 6) grading scale, with 0 mobility denoting a fused spinal segment and 6 mobility used to describe an unstable joint. A 3/6 on the mobility scale is used to denote a normal degree of mobility judgment for the individual tested. See Table 2-2 for further description of each category on the mobility scale.

The results of pain provocation assessments from PIVM tests are commonly described as the level of tissue or joint reactivity.[42] Table 2-3 outlines three levels of joint reactivity that are based on when the sequence of pain provocation is produced in relation to range of mobility assessment. For instance, a high level of reactivity is described as when pain provocation is reported before resistance to passive motion is detected. A

| **TABLE 2-3** | Reactivity* |
|---|---|
| **LEVEL OF REACTIVITY** | **DESCRIPTIONS** |
| High reactivity | Pain is reported before detection of resistance to passive motion |
| Moderate reactivity | Pain is reported synchronous to detection of resistance to passive motion |
| Low reactivity | Pain is reported after detection of resistance to passive motion (pain only with overpressure to passive motion) |

Adapted from Paris SV: *Introduction to spinal evaluation and manipulation,* Atlanta, 1986, Institute Press.
*Level of reactivity is used to describe relationship of pain provocation as it relates to sense of tissue resistance during passive motion, accessory motion, or PIVM testing.

---

**BOX 2-4    End Feel Classifications**

**Normal End Feel**
Soft tissue approximation: Soft tissue presses against soft tissue at the end of mobility
Tissue stretch: Firm end feel that gives with overpressure at end of expected mobility
Bone to bone: Hard end feel at the end of mobility as a result of normal anatomic structure

**Abnormal End Feel**
Muscle guarding: Muscle holding or tension limiting the passive mobility
Hard capsular: A firm tissue stretch felt before expected passive mobility
Bone to bone: Hard end feel felt before expected passive mobility
Empty: Minimal resistance felt, but motion stopped because of severe pain
Springy block: A springy rebound to passive mobility from internal joint derangement

Data from Paris SV, Loubert PV: *FCO foundations of clinical orthopaedics,* Atlanta, 1990, Institute Press; McGee DJ: *Orthopedic physical assessment,* ed 4, Philadelphia, 2002, Saunders; and Cyriax J: *Textbook of orthopaedic medicine: diagnosis of soft tissue lesions,* vol 1, ed 8, London, 1982, Balliere Tindall.

---

moderate level of reactivity is described as when pain provocation is reported synchronous to detection of resistance to passive motion. A low level of reactivity is described as when pain provocation is reported after resistance to passive motion is detected. In other words, pain is reported only with overpressure to passive motion.

In addition, PIVM tests can be used to make judgments on end feel, which is the quality of resistance that the clinician feels when passively taking a joint to the clinical limits of range. The type of end feel depends on the anatomic structure of the joint tested. The end feel can be judged as normal or abnormal for that joint. The spinal segments typically are restrained by capsular and ligamentous tissues. Therefore, the end feel with performance of PAIVM tests for the spine tends to be a firm capsular or tissue stretch end feel. Box 2-4 outlines and describes normal and abnormal end feels. Olson et al[43] found that the reliability of end feel testing was higher than the reliability for mobility judgments with testing of PIVM for craniovertebral side bending. Patla and Paris[44] showed fair to good interrater reliability for testing end feel of the elbow joint with a Kappa value of 0.40 for testing end feel of elbow flexion and a Kappa value of 0.73 for testing end feel of elbow extension. Most reliability studies on PIVM testing have focused on judgments of mobility or pain provocation or both.

Manual physical therapists use the results of PIVM tests to guide which interventions will be used. Therapists who use the examination of passive intervertebral joint motion as part of the comprehensive examination of spinal conditions are able to formulate intervention plans that achieve positive patient outcomes.[45-53] In addition, clinical prediction rules that predict patient success from lumbar manipulation and lumbar stabilization exercise programs to treat low back pain include the results of posterior to anterior PAIVM tests in the set of criteria that comprise the rules,[15,16] which validates the clinical utility of the PAIVM testing in clinical decision making to enhance treatment outcomes for patients with low back pain. However, when passive intervertebral joint motion testing has been studied in isolation, both interrater and intrarater reliability results have been poor.[41,43,54-56]

In clinical situations, therapists rarely use passive joint mobility examinations in isolation. Rather, they combine the results of passive mobility examinations with other examination procedures, such as patient history, observation, palpation for position and condition, active range of motion, and various other selected special tests. With use of the results of a cluster of examination procedures that have adequate reliability, rather than those of only a single examination procedure, the therapist can determine the patient's specific impairments and generate an intervention plan. Professional standards are not met with an intervention plan based on the results of only one examination procedure. However, most studies that have looked at rater reliability have studied specific examination procedures in isolation.[41,43,54-56]

Gonnella, Paris, and Kutner[41] assessed passive intervertebral forward bending of levels T12 to S1 and found reasonably good intrarater reliability but poor interrater reliability. They suggested that reliability might be increased by better clarifying the patient position and determining whether the therapists were assessing range of motion or end feel during the examination.[41]

In the chiropractic literature, Nansel et al[55] concluded that motion-based palpation showed poor reliability ($z < .05$; Kappa coefficient, 0.013) and found that it may not be an internally valid predictor of vertebral joint dysfunction in otherwise healthy asymptomatic individuals.[56] Strender, Lundin, and Nell[56] looked at seven different examination procedures of the cervical spine, some of which were PIVM tests, and showed poor interrater reliability (Kappa coefficients for mobility testing were C0-C1 = 0.091; C1-C2 = 0.15; C2-C3 = 0.057).

Maher and Adams[35] studied the reliability of pain and stiffness assessments with a posterior-anterior passive accessory intervertebral motion (PAIVM) test of the lumbar spine and found poor reliability in determining stiffness (ICC values of 0.03 to 0.37) but good reliability in pain reproduction. Binkley, Stratford, and Gill[54] studied lumbar posterior-anterior PAIVM testing and showed poor reliability (ICC R = 0.25) and suggested that caution should be used with the results of this assessment in the absence of other data. Hicks et al[57] studied interrater reliability in identification of lumbar segmental instability. Again, the segmental mobility interrater reliability was poor (−0.02 to 0.26), and the interrater reliability for pain provocation was more acceptable (0.25 to 0.55).

Olson et al[43] assessed interrater reliability of craniovertebral side bending in five different positions of 10 healthy subjects and found poor interrater (Kappa values of −0.03 to 0.18) and intrarater (Kappa values of −0.02 to 0.14) reliability in all positions. Interrater reliability of C1-C2 rotation, C2-C3 lateral flexion, C7-T1 flexion/extension, and first rib spring test was assessed by Smedmark, Wallin, and Arvidsson.[58] These results were somewhat better, showing fair to moderate reliability (Kappa scores ranged from 0.28 to 0.43).[58] Patients were used in this study, and efforts were made to standardize the testing protocol.[58]

Jull, Bogduk, and Marsland[59] were able to show excellent symptom reproduction with palpation and isolation of upper cervical facet joints, and validation of the palpation findings was confirmed (100% agreement) with pain relief produced with anesthetic nerve blocks to the targeted symptomatic joints.

In clinical situations, therapists rarely use passive joint mobility examinations in isolation. Rather, they combine the results of the assessment with the results of other examination procedures. Cibulka and Koldehoff[60] showed excellent interrater reliability in assessment of the sacroiliac joint (Kappa value of 0.88) with use of a cluster of four examination procedures, with the requirement that three of the four have positive results to consider the patient to have a sacroiliac dysfunction. However, Potter and Rothstein[61] showed poor reliability when studying each of those same four examination procedures in isolation.

The design of Cibulka and Koldehoff's[60] study more closely emulates how therapists actually assess patients in the clinic. Riddle et al[62] attempted to reproduce Cibulka and Koldehoff's study of the sacroiliac joint examination procedures. They used the same four clinical examination procedures; however, they used multiple pairs of testers and multiple clinical sites. In this study, the testers were given written instructions on the techniques to be performed; whereas the study from Cibulka and Koldehoff did not specify how the testers were trained.[62] Riddle et al[62] had less favorable results than did Cibulka and Koldehoff with Kappa scores ranging from 0.11 to 0.23. This contrast in the results of these two studies points to the need to standardize examination and training programs to enhance the reliability between testers.

Jarett et al[63] assessed the reliability of use of a cluster of four examination procedures to diagnose craniovertebral (CV) dysfunctions if three of four procedures had positive results. The four criteria included resting head position measured with a CROM inclinometer device, a pattern of AROM restriction characteristic of CV dysfunction, asymmetric position of the C1 transverse process with palpation, and limitation of motion or abnormal end feel assessment with passive CV side-bending test. For the composite test results, the Kappa coefficient for the symptomatic group was 0.524, with an 87% agreement between the two therapists. For the individual tests, the Kappa scores ranged from −0.047 (palpation of the transverse process of C1) to 0.516 (resting CROM position), with percent agreements ranging from 77% to 90%. Overall, this study showed higher Kappa values with use of a cluster of examination findings (categorized as fair to moderate) to determine an impairment when compared with the Kappa values of the individual examination findings (categorized as poor to moderate).[63]

In general, the interrater reliability of PIVM testing is poor, and at times, the intrarater reliability has reached a more acceptable moderate level. See Table 2-4 for further review of individual reliability studies for PIVM testing. Use of palpation and PIVM testing for symptom reproduction has shown acceptable and, at times, very good levels of reliability. In addition, inclusion of PIVM testing in a cluster of findings to arrive at a diagnosis has shown more acceptable levels of reliability; and inclusion of posterior to anterior (PA) PAIVM test findings in the clinical prediction rules for lumbar manipulation and stabilization helps to further validate the clinical usefulness of these procedures.[15,16]

The clinical implications of this body of research on reliability of PIVM testing are that PIVM tests that focus on mobility assessment should not be used in isolation to determine an impairment diagnosis or to guide treatment decisions. Instead, these examination procedures must be used as part of a cluster of findings to arrive at a diagnosis; the other examination procedures should include symptom reproduction, AROM testing, results of disability and fear avoidance questionnaires, and symptom location and behavior. In addition, the motor learning processes used by student therapists to master passive intervertebal motion testing can enhance the ease of learning manipulation procedures. Student physical therapists are suggested to develop competence and be tested on the manual examination skills such as PIVM testing before being taught spinal manipulation.[64]

Detailed illustrations and descriptions of passive intervertebral motion tests are included in Chapters 4, 5, and 6 for each region of the spine. When available, the reliability and validity of each test are included with the description of the technique. Box 2-5 outlines general performance recommendations for clinicians to consider when performing passive intervertebral motion testing. Palpation for tissue condition and position procedures are included in this chapter because these procedures are often included as part of the general spinal examination.

## Palpation for Tissue Condition

The layers of connective tissue of the back should be carefully palpated and assessed as part of the comprehensive spinal

**TABLE 2-4**  Segment Mobility Examination

| PROCEDURE | DESCRIPTION AND POSITIVE FINDINGS | POPULATION | KAPPA VALUE AND PEARSON CORRELATION COEFFICIENT (r) (95% CI) | |
|---|---|---|---|---|
| | | | INTRAEXAMINER RELIABILITY | INTEREXAMINER RELIABILITY |
| Motion palpation* | Examiner sits behind subject. Examining hand is placed horizontally on back so that spinous process bisects proximal phalanges. Dorsal aspect of palpating hand is used to determine amount of motion at each respective segment. Examiners record most hypomobile segment. | 32 asymptomatic volunteers | −0.007 to 0.65 | Ranged from $r = 0.021$ in first trial to $r = 0.85$ in second trial. Association not large enough to be considered different by chance. |
| Determination of segmental fixations[†] | As above. However, each segment determined to exhibit hard end feel on examination of passive joint motion is classified as fixated. | 60 asymptomatic volunteers | Kappa, −0.09 to 0.39 | Kappa, −0.06 to 0.17 |
| Passive motion palpation[‡] | Passive motion palpation is performed. Segment is considered fixated if hard end feel is noted during assessment. | 21 symptomatic and 25 asymptomatic subjects | | Kappa, −0.03 to 0.23; mean, 0.07 |
| Segmental mobility testing[§] | Patient lies on one side with hips and knees flexed. Examiner assesses mobility while passively moving patient. Examiner determines whether mobility of segment is decreased, normal, or increased. | 71 patients with low back pain | | Kappa, 0.54 |
| Hypermobility at any level[¶] | Patient is prone. Examiner applies posteroanterior force to spinous process of each lumbar vertebra. Mobility of each segment is judged as normal, hypermobile, or hypomobile. | 49 patients with LBP referred for flexion-extension radiography | 0.48 (0.35, 0.61) | |
| Hypomobility at any level[¶] | | | 0.38 (0.22, 54) | |

From Cleland JA: *Orthopaedic clinical examination: an evidence-based approach for physical therapists*, Carlstadt, NJ, 2005, Icon Learning Systems.
*Love R, Brodeur R: Inter- and intra-examiner reliability of motion palpation for the thoracolumbar spine, *J Manipulative Physiol Ther* 10:261-266, 1987.
[†]Mootz R, Keating J, Kontz H, et al: Intra- and interobserver reliability of passive motion palpation of the lumbar spine, *J Manipulative Physiol Ther* 12:440-445, 1989.
[‡]Keating J, Bergmann T, Jacobs G, et al: Interexaminer reliability of the evaluative dimensions of lumbar segmental abnormality, *J Manipulative Physiol Ther* 13:463-470, 1990.
[§]Strender L, Sjoblom A, Lundwig R, et al: Interexaminer reliability in physical examination of patients with low back pain, *Spine* 22:814-820, 1997.
[¶]Fritz JM, Piva S, Childs JD: Accuracy of the clinical examination to predict radiographic instability of the lumbar spine, *Eur Spine J* 14:743-750, 2005.

| BOX 2-5 | PIVM Technique Considerations |
|---|---|

1. Patient positioning
   a. Relaxed and well supported
   b. Spinal neutral position
2. Position of therapist
   a. Good body mechanics with table at appropriate height
   b. As close to patient as possible
   c. Firm and professional contact
3. Performance of technique
   a. Slow, rhythmic, relaxing movements
   b. Relax palpating hand
   c. Palpate for, do not create or block, movements
   d. Consider starting away from restricted and painful segments

Adapted from Paris SV, Loubert PV: *FCO foundations of clinical orthopaedics,* Atlanta, 1990 Institute Press.

examination. First, the therapist should start with inspection and palpation of the skin. The therapist needs to look for any skin lesions, scars, or areas of discoloration and ask the patient follow-up questions on the history of any significant findings. The skin is palpated for extensibility, temperature, and moisture. Increased temperature is an indication of an inflammatory process. Poor skin extensibility may be an indication of a connective tissue disorder or of a chronically stiff back. Figure 2-7 provides a grid for documentation of PIVM findings and also provides a body diagram and key for shorthand notation of palpation findings.

| KEY | | SEG | FB | SBL | SBR | RL | RR | BB |
|---|---|---|---|---|---|---|---|---|
| | Comments: | | | | | | | |

X tender

Ⓧ centered pain

//// guarding

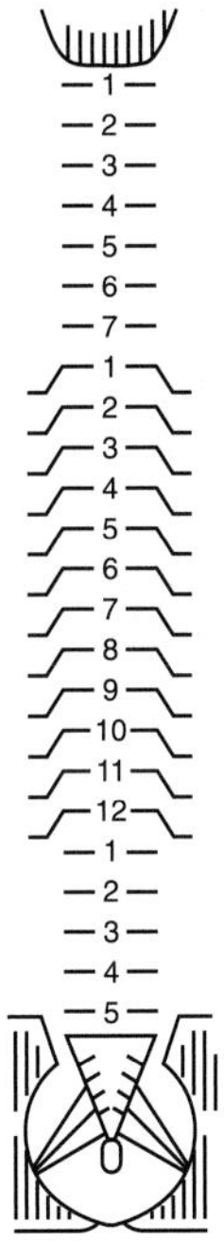

0 Ankylosed
1 Considerable restriction
2 Slight restriction
3 Normal

4 Slight increase
5 Considerable increase
6 Unstable

FIGURE 2-7  Body chart can be used to document palpation findings, and grid can be used to document PIVM test findings.

## Skin Palpation for Temperature and Moisture

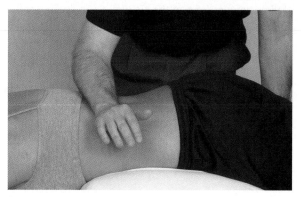

Skin temperature and moisture assessment with forearm

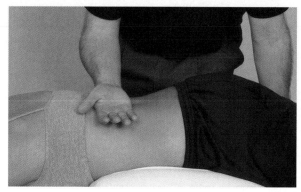

Skin temperature and moisture assessment with dorsum of the hand

| | |
|---|---|
| **PATIENT POSITION** | The patient is prone, with a pillow under the chest/trunk. |
| **THERAPIST POSITION** | The therapist stands next to the patient. |
| **PROCEDURE** | Starting in the cervical region, the therapist uses the dorsum of the hand or the volar aspect of the forearm to palpate the entire length of the spine for temperature and moisture. Both the right and left sides of the back are palpated. |
| **NOTES** | The temperature of the back should be warm in the cervical region, slightly warmer in the thoracic region, and slightly cooler in the lumbar region. The therapist should observe for deviations from this pattern and for differences between right and left sides. Increases in temperature and moisture could be a sign of inflammation, and decreases in temperature and moisture could be a sign of a chronic disorder. |

## Subcutaneous Tissue Assessment

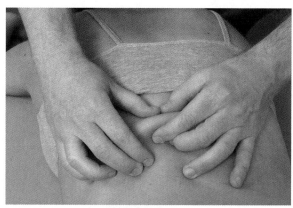

Skin rolling

## Subcutaneous Tissue Assessment—cont'd

| | |
|---|---|
| **PATIENT POSITION** | The patient is prone with a pillow under the chest/trunk. |
| **THERAPIST POSITION** | The therapist stands next to the patient. |
| **PROCEDURE** | The therapist uses the thumb and index finger to gently pinch and lift the skin just lateral to the spine. The skin between the thumb and index finger is gently "rolled" to assess for mobility. The entire length of the spine is assessed, with comparison of right and left sides. |
| **NOTES** | The skin and subcutaneous tissue should be soft and easy to move. The therapist should note any tenderness, abnormal amounts of fat, fluid, edema, or nodules. The skin and subcutaneous tissues are typically more mobile around the lumbosacral junction, the cervical/thoracic junction, and the scapula. Skin extensibility can also be tested with the pads of the index and long fingers to move the skin in small x shapes along the lateral aspect of the spine. |

## Muscle Palpation

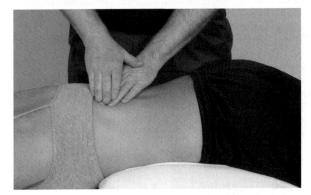

Palpation of specific spinal muscles of various depth

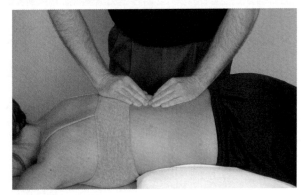

"Muscle splay"

| | |
|---|---|
| **PATIENT POSITION** | The patient is prone, with a pillow under the chest/trunk. |
| **THERAPIST POSITION** | The therapist stands next to the patient. |
| **PROCEDURE** | First, the therapist uses the pads of the index and long fingers to palpate the layers of muscle tissue, with assessment for signs of muscle holding, tenderness, or edema. Next, the index/long fingers and thumbs are used to make a triangle and gently grasp the musculature just lateral to the spine. The therapist assesses how the musculature moves by alternately "pushing" with the thumbs and "pulling" with the fingers. This technique is called "muscle splay." |
| **NOTES** | The muscles should be soft and easy to move. The therapist should note any areas of tenderness or muscle guarding. The right and left sides are compared. See Box 2-6 for an outline of dysfunctional muscle holding states that can be identified with palpation of tissue condition and when found may be an indication to assess the anatomic region for additional impairments. |

---

**BOX 2-6**  Dysfunctional Muscle Holding States

**Muscle Spasm**
  Sudden involuntary muscle contraction
  Observe twitching of the muscle

**Involuntary Muscle Holding**
  Increased muscle tone caused by an underlying dysfunc-
    tion (e.g., instability)
  Disappears when adequately supported
  Hypertonic but otherwise normal to touch

**Chemical Muscle Holding**
  Increased tone remains in multiple positions
  Increased muscle tone to touch that is nonelastic, thick-
    ened, dense tissue
  Limited range of motion and extensibility

  Caused by sustained involuntary muscle holding
  Retention of metabolites and tissue fluids cause fur-
    ther nociception

**Voluntary Muscle Holding**
  Increased muscle tone from pain or fear of pain
  Voluntary movements are restrained

**Adaptive Shortening**
  Normal tone
  Limited range of motion from shortened muscle
  Loss of sarcomeres
  Can be caused by postural adaptation or sustained
    muscle holding states

Adapted from Paris SV, Loubert PV: *FCO foundations of clinical orthopaedics,* Atlanta, 1990, Institute Press.

---

## Palpation of Supraspinous and Interspinous Ligaments

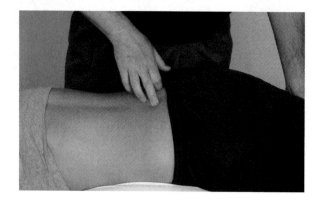

| | |
|---|---|
| **PATIENT POSITION** | The patient is prone with a pillow under the chest/trunk. |
| **THERAPIST POSITION** | The therapist stands next to the patient. |
| **PROCEDURE** | To palpate the supraspinous ligament, the therapist uses the pad of the long finger and palpates the interspinous space. The ligament should be springy and nontender. |
| | To palpate the interspinous ligament, the therapist uses the pad of the long finger and palpates just deep and lateral to the supraspinous ligament. Both right and left sides of the ligament are palpated. The ligament should be springy and nontender. The interspinous ligaments are short and strong and connect the adjoining spinous processes throughout the thoracic and lumbar spine. |
| **NOTES** | Ligaments should normally feel smooth and taut with a springy suppleness. If tenderness is reported, especially if combined with a feeling of swelling, the ligament is likely inflamed. If the ligament feels thickened, hard, and tight, hypomobility is likely at that spinal segment. Strender et al[65] reported a Kappa value of 0.55 for intertester reliability for reproduction of tenderness between spinous processes of the lumbar vertebra in examination of patients with low back pain. |

## Palpation for Position

For diagnosis of a positional fault of a vertebra, stiffness must be noted with PIVM testing with an attempt to move the spinal segment out of the suspected faulty vertebral position. Joint stiffness must be found at the spinal segment to warrant manipulation to correct a positional fault. In theory, a positional fault of a spinal segment may occur when a vertebra is unable to return to its neutral or rest position. Paris[42] describes three suspected theoretic causes:

1. A vertebra may get caught on a rough surface of the joint.

2. An impacted meniscus may lock the facet joints.

3. The facet joints may stiffen in a position after an injury.

Although the three theories are physiologically possible, very little to no evidence is available to prove that positional faults exist, that positional faults can be reliably detected, or that positional faults can be corrected with manipulation techniques. This is likely the result of the lack of a device that can detect and measure positional faults in a reliable and valid manner combined with the fact that a great deal of normal anatomic variability may be misinterpreted as a positional fault.

## Pinch Test: Thoracic and Lumbar Spines

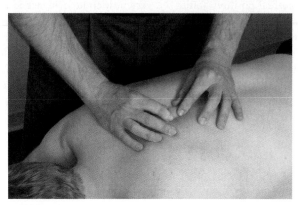

Pinch test for assessment of relative positions of spinous processes

| | |
|---|---|
| **PATIENT POSITION** | The patient is prone with a pillow under the chest/trunk. |
| **THERAPIST POSITION** | The therapist stands next to the patient. |
| **PROCEDURE** | The therapist uses the pad of the long finger to palpate each interspinous space in the lumbar and thoracic spine. Palpation should begin in the lumbar spine and continue cranially. Any forward bent or backward bent positional faults are noted. Also, any swelling or tenderness is noted. The therapist uses the thumb and index finger to pinch adjacent spinous processes in the lumbar and thoracic spine. Any rotational positional faults are noted, as is any swelling or tenderness. |
| **NOTES** | Because anatomic variations in spinous process length and angulation are common, deviations of relative positioning of the spinous processes of the thoracic and lumbar spine must be interpreted with caution. |

# Palpation of Articular Pillars and Facet Joints of the Cervical Spine

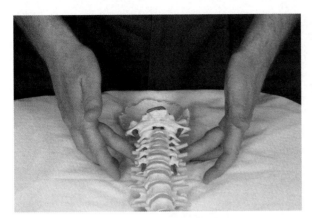 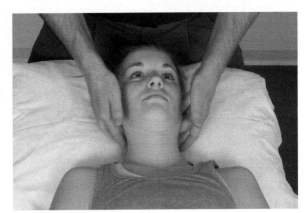

Finger placement for palpation of articular pillars and facet joints of cervical spine

| | |
|---|---|
| **PATIENT POSITION** | The patient is supine with the head on a pillow. |
| **THERAPIST POSITION** | The therapist stands at the head of the patient. |
| **PROCEDURE** | The therapist uses the pads of the long fingers to palpate the spine of the scapula and adjacent soft tissues, noting any tenderness or muscle guarding. For palpation of the articular pillars and facet joints of the cervical spine, the spinous process of C2 is located with the pad of one long finger. With the pads of both long fingers, the therapist slides laterally around the neck until the middle fingers are directly inferior to the mastoid processes. From this position, the pads of the middle fingers are used to palpate the articular pillars and facet joints. The facet joints feel like small peaks and lie deep beneath the muscle tissue. The articular pillars feel like small valleys between each facet joint. Each facet joint and articular pillar are palpated from C2-C3 to C6-C7. |
| **NOTES** | Any swelling or tenderness is noted, and right and left sides are compared. The therapist notes any signs of tenderness, swelling, muscle holding, or tissue thickening. The patient's head should remain on the pillow throughout the procedure. Patient relaxation is the key to palpation of the facet joints and articular pillars. This technique allows for palpation of tissue condition and vertebral position of the cervical spine. Deviations in vertebral position are suspected with comparison of the relative position of the left and right articular pillar of each vertebra as the head and neck rest in the neutral position. |

## Palpate and Spring Test First Rib

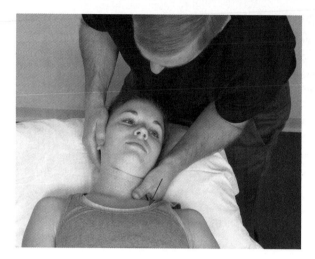

| | |
|---|---|
| **PATIENT POSITION** | The patient is supine with the head on a pillow. |
| **THERAPIST POSITION** | The therapist stands at the head of the patient. |
| **PROCEDURE** | The therapist uses the radial aspect of the index finger and metacarpophalangeal joint to palpate the first rib. The first rib is located in the space lateral to the C7 transverse process, posterior to the clavicle and anterior to the scapula. The position of the rib is noted. To spring test the first rib, the therapist side bends the head and neck towards the side tested to place the scalene muscles on slack and then takes up the tissue slack and gives a slight spring to assess the mobility. |
| **NOTES** | Any stiffness or tenderness is noted, and right and left sides are compared. This evaluation can also be a pain provocation test. The spring test assesses the mobility of the first costo-vertebral, costotransverse, and sternocostal joints. Smedmark, Wallin, and Arvidsson[58] reported a Kappa of 0.35 with testing first rib stiffness in 61 subjects with nonspecific neck problems. |

## Neurologic Examination

The neurologic examination can be divided into tests for sensation, strength, and deep tendon reflex. If positive findings are noted, further diagnostic testing such as a nerve conduction study may be indicated to confirm the findings. See Boxes 2-7 and 2-8 for illustrations of neurologic examination procedures. Sensation testing should include assessment of light touch and sharp/dull perception and should include testing of each dermotomal area. See Figures 2-8 and 2-9 for illustrations of the common dermatomes. Strength tests can be graded on a 0 to 5 scale as described by Kendall, McCreary, and Provance[30] and should include at least one muscle (i.e., myotome) that corresponds to the anatomic nerve roots in the region of the spine assessed. For instance, in the examination of the cervical spine, myotomal strength should be assessed for the cervical nerve roots; and for lumbar spine examination, the lumbar nerve root myotomes should be evaluated. See Tables 2-5 and 2-6 for details on nerve root levels and corresponding muscles for each level.

Deep tendon reflexes are graded 0 to 4, with a grade 2 considered normal, a grade 4 hypertonic, and a grade 0 absent, and should be tested if neurologic involvement is suspected. Boxes 2-7 and 2-8 illustrate proper deep tendon testing (DTR) technique and provide the corresponding nerve root level for each DTR. Vroomen, de Krom, and Knottnerus[66] reported reliability for testing Achilles and patella deep tendon reflexes on patients with lumbar radiculopathy as Kappa values of 0.53 and 0.42.

Lauder et al[67] used the gold standard for diagnosis of nerve root involvement as the cause radiculopathy as needle electrodiagnostic procedures that included a motor nerve conduction study, a sensory nerve conduction study, and a standard 10-muscle electromyogram (EMG) and compared the diagnosis with the results of the history and examination findings. The presence of numbness has a high sensitivity for cervical radiculopathy (79%), and subjects with weakness or a reduced reflex were two to five times more likely to have abnormal results on

---

**BOX 2-7** Upper Quarter Neurologic Examination

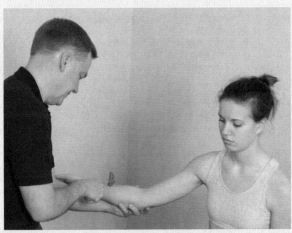

Biceps deep tendon reflex test (C5-C6)

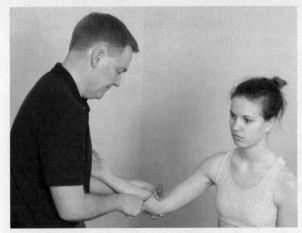

Brachioradialis deep tendon reflex test (C6)

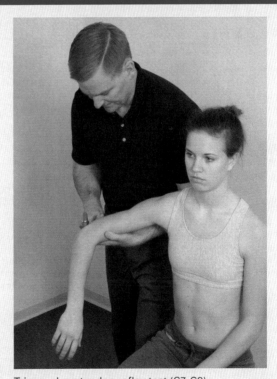

Triceps deep tendon reflex test (C7-C8)

*Continued*

**BOX 2-7** | Upper Quarter Neurologic Examination—cont'd

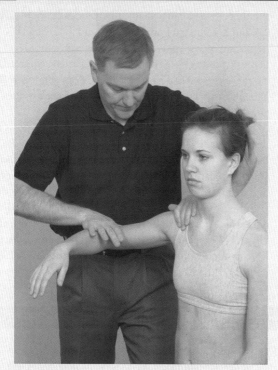

Myotomal testing: manual muscle test

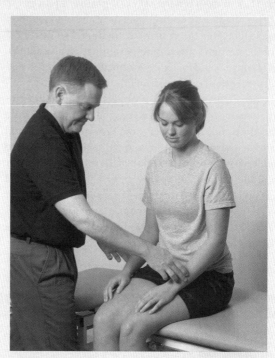

Sensation testing

**TABLE 2-5** | Myotomes of Upper Limb

| NERVE ROOT | TEST ACTION | MUSCLES* |
|---|---|---|
| C1-C2 | Neck flexion | Rectus lateralis, rectus capitis anterior, longus capitis, longus coli, longus cervicis, sternocleidomastoid |
| C3 | Neck side flexion | Longus capitis, longus cervicis, trapezius, scalenus medius |
| C4 | Shoulder elevation | Diaphragm, trapezious, levator scapulae, scalenus anterior, scalenus medius |
| C5 | Shoulder abduction | Rhomboid major and minor, deltoid, supraspinatus, infraspinatus, teres minor, biceps, scalenus anterior and medius |
| C6 | Elbow flexion and wrist extension | Serratus anterior; latissimus dorsi; subscapularis; teres major; pectoralis major (clavicular head); biceps; coracobrachialis; brachialis; brachioradialis; supinator; extensor carpi radialis longus; scalenus antiori, medius, and posterior |
| C7 | Elbow extension and wrist extension | Serratus anterior, latissimus dorsi, pectoralis major (sternal head), pectoralis minor, triceps, pronator teres, flexor carpi radialis, flexor digitorum superficialis, extensor carpi radialis longus, extensor carpi radialis brevis, extensor digitorum, extensor digiti minimi, scalenus medius and posterior |
| C8 | Thumb extension and ulnar deviation | Pectoralis major (sternal head), pectoralis minor, triceps, flexor digitorum superficialis, flexor digitorum profundus, flexor pollicis longus, pronator quadrates, flexor carpi ulnaris, abductor pollicis longus, extensor pollicis brevis, extensor indicis, abductor pollicis brevis, flexor pollicis brevis, opponens pollicis, scalenus medius and posterior |
| T1 | Hand intrinsic | Flexor digitorum profundus, intrinsic muscles of hand (except extensor pollicis brevis), flexor pollicis brevis, opponens pollicis |

From Magee DJ: *Orthopedic physical assessment,* ed 4, Philadelphia, 2002, Saunders.
*Muscles listed may be supplied by additional nerve roots; only primary nerve root sources are listed.

**BOX 2-8** Lower Quarter Neurologic Examination

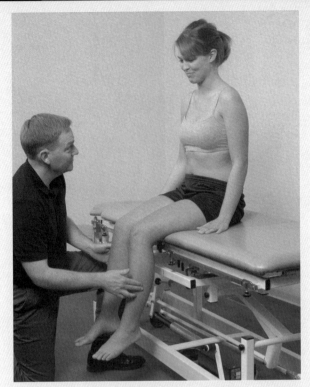

Sensation light touch testing

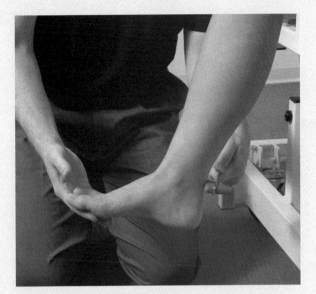

Achilles deep tendon reflex (L4)

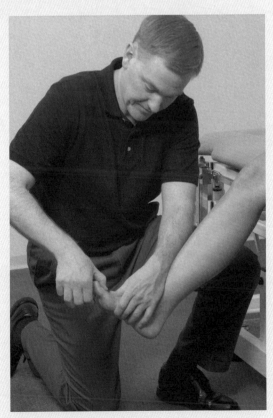

Myotomal strength testing

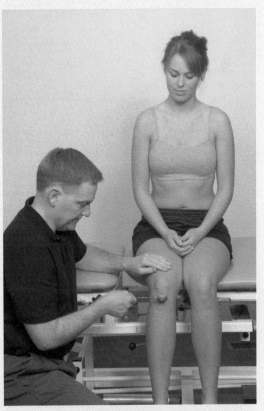

Patella deep tendon reflex (S1)

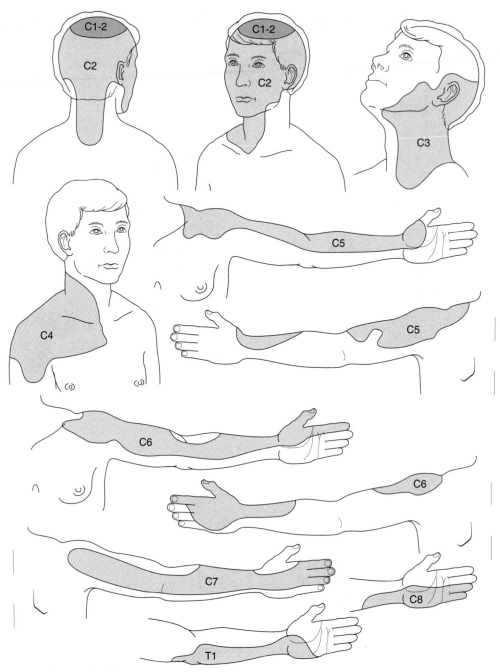

**FIGURE 2-8** Dermatones of cervical spine.

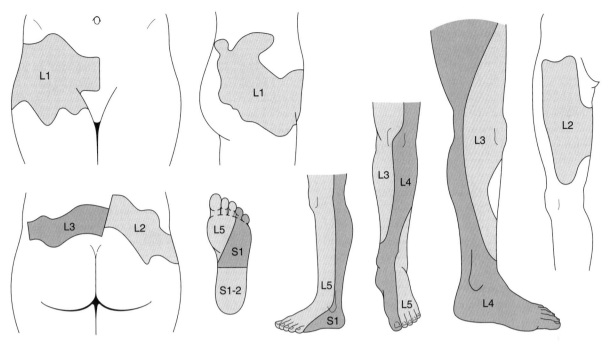

**FIGURE 2-9** Lumbar dermatones.

| TABLE 2-6 | Myotomes of Lower Limb | |
|---|---|---|
| **NERVE ROOT** | **TEST ACTION** | **MUSCLES** |
| L1-L2 | Hip flexion | Psoas, iliacus, sartorius, gracilis, pectineus, adductor longus, adductor brevis |
| L3 | Knee extension | Quadriceps; adductor longus, magnus, and brevis |
| L4 | Ankle dorsiflexion | Tibialis anterior, quadriceps, tensor fasciae latae, adductor magnus, obturator externus, tibialis posterior |
| L5 | Toe extension | Extensor hallucis longus, extensor digitorium longus, gluteous medius and minimus, obturator internus, semimembranosus, semitendinosus, peroneus tertius, popliteus |
| S1 | Ankle plantar flexion<br>Ankle eversion<br>Hip extension<br>Knee flexion | Gastrocnemius, soleus, gluteus maximus, obturator internus, piriformis, biceps femoris, semitendinosus, popliterus, peroneus longus and brevis, extensor digitorum brevis |
| S2 | Knee flexion | Biceps femoris, piriforms, soleus, gastrocnemius, flexor digitorum longus, flexor hallucis, intrinsic foot muscles |
| S3 | Toe plantar flexion | Intrinsic foot muscles (except abductor hallucis), flexor hallucis brevis, flexor digitorum brevis, extensor digitorum brevis |

From Magee DJ: *Orthopedic physical assessment*, ed 4, Philadelphia, 2002, Saunders.

electrodiagnosis.[67] Reduced reflexes combined with weakness are associated with subjects having a nine-fold increase in the likelihood of cervical radiculopathy, and subjects with a reduced biceps reflex were 10 times more likely to have a cervical radiculopathy with needle EMG.[67] For DTR testing, the biceps muscle sensitivity was 0.10, the specificity was 0.99, the +LR was 10.0, and the −LR was 0.91. For DTR testing, the triceps muscle sensitivity was 0.10, the specificity was 0.95, the +LR was 2.0, and the −LR was 0.95. For DTR, the brachioradialis muscle sensitivity was 0.08, the specificity was 0.99, the +LR was 8.0, and the −LR was 0.93.[67] Neurodynamic tension tests are also considered part of the standard neurologic exami-

nation, and detailed descriptions are included in the lumbopelvic and cervical spine chapters.

# EVALUATION OF EXAMINATION FINDINGS AND THE DIAGNOSIS

Clinical decision making in orthopaedic manual physical therapy should be based on an evidence-based approach. Research evidence supports the effectiveness of treating spinal disorders by subgrouping patients based on identification of key physical impairments, patient characteristics, and symptoms.[68] The treatment is based on the subgroup classification that the patient fits into at the time of the examination, and the subgrouping may change through the course of the treatment duration based on reexamination findings. With clinical situations in which the research evidence is not clear, use of an impairment–based approach is the foundation of physical therapy treatment of musculoskeletal disorders.

An impairment-based approach can guide clinical decision making when specific physical impairments such as joint stiffness, joint hypermobility, and muscle weakness or tightness are identified through the clinical examination, and appropriate interventions are administered based on the examination findings. For instance, identification of joint stiffness or hypomobility is an indication for spinal manipulation, and joint hypermobility and weakness are indications for spinal stabilization exercises. The presence of muscle or myofascial tightness is an indication for soft tissue mobilization techniques and stretching. In this way, a problem list can be generated, and a specific intervention for each impairment can be included in the plan of care. The overall management of the patient's condition is based on identification of clusters of signs and symptoms characteristic of a diagnosis or classification. Clinical prediction rules have been developed for several spine disorders and can assist in guidance in the classification and identification of the best possible interventions.[16,17]

Fritz, Whitman, and Childs[69] showed a correlation between patients that were judged as having lumbar hypomobility with passive accessory intervertebral motion (PAIVM) testing to respond favorably to spinal manipulation. In other words, patients with lumbar stiffness are more likely to respond favorably to spinal manipulation. In addition, a strong correlation for a positive response to a spinal stabilization exercise program was correlated with hypermobility noted with posterior to anterior (PA) PAIVM testing of the lumbar spine. This correlation helps to link an impairment-based approach with an evidence-based approach and validates the use of PA PAIVM testing as an important component of a physical therapist examination scheme to determine the most effective intervention for spinal disorders.[69]

Typically, medical practitioners have based a diagnosis either on the patient's symptoms (such as neck pain or low back pain) or on results of imaging studies such as degenerative disc disease or osteoarthritis of the neck. Both of these types of diagnoses are inadequate to guide clinical decision making in physical therapy. The location of symptoms is only one finding that must be correlated with the behavior of the symptoms with activity and other important clinical findings such as movement restrictions, joint restrictions, muscle length impairments, and muscle recruitment patterns. The location of the symptoms alone cannot be the sole guide for determination of the most effective intervention.

In a recent report, patients were given a symptom-based diagnosis at 64% of all visits to family physicians and emergency departments (EDs).[70] A symptom-based diagnosis was given at 91% of all ED visits for neck pain.[70] When a physician cannot identify a serious pathology, the physician makes a diagnosis of sprain, strain, neck pain, or back pain 90% of the time, which is a symptom-based diagnosis that does nothing to guide the proper intervention.[70] These findings suggest that classification systems are needed to guide interventions for neck and back pain.

Likewise, the findings on imaging studies such as MRI and radiographs are commonly provided as the primary diagnosis. Although degenerative changes found on imaging studies of the spine could be contributing factors to the patient's set of signs and symptoms, they are unlikely to be the only factor. The presence or absence of degenerative changes in the spine cannot be the sole finding to guide physical therapy interventions. A wide range of spinal pathology has been shown on MRI results of asymptomatic persons including degenerative changes, disk protrusions, disk herniations, free fragments, and annular tears.[26,71-74]

Most physical therapy interventions do not likely change the degenerative findings seen on imaging studies, but often improvements in mobility, pain, and function can be attained with physical therapy. The imaging findings often are the same at the end of the duration of the physical therapy treatment even when significant clinical improvements are noted. Therefore, the imaging findings cannot be used to guide nonsurgical treatment in most cases.

Most evidence-based guidelines for treatment of spine conditions suggest use of imaging only when a patient has a red flag, has a recent history of significant trauma, or has not responded to at least 4 weeks of conservative management.[75] In these circumstances, imaging is indicated and typically starts with plain radiographs. If the patient has neurologic signs, an MRI may be indicated.

Completion of a comprehensive physical examination to determine whether the symptom behavior and physical impairments follow a typical musculoskeletal pattern can greatly assist in the medical screening and diagnostic process. In the evaluation, the physical therapist must state the clinical impression that best classifies or diagnoses the patient's condition. Next, a problem list should be included that outlines the most significant impairments that contribute to the perpetuation of the patient's primary symptoms. The impairment-based classification system affords a great deal of guidance in clinical decision making in patients with spinal and temporomandibular disorders and is described in detail in Chapters 4 through 7.

## PLAN OF CARE AND PROGNOSIS

Interventions must be identified in the plan of care to address the impairments and to best manage the patient's diagnosed condition. These clinical decisions should be based first on research evidence to support the interventions within the therapist's scope of practice and based on the therapist's clinical knowledge and experience regarding how to best address the impairments and manage the patient's condition. For each anatomic area addressed in Chapters 4 through 7, the clinical research is presented to assist in the clinical decision making for each classification.

The decision regarding frequency and duration of treatment is also based on clinical experience and research evidence. Typically, 4 to 6 weeks is needed to make significant progress in reducing the intensity of pain and severity of disability associated with many spinal conditions. An additional 4 to 6 weeks may be needed to fully restore strength and function. The duration of treatment and the prognosis are influenced by the general health and the psychosocial status of the patient as much as by the diagnosis. For instance, a patient who smokes, is diabetic, or has cardiovascular risk factors tends to recover at a slower rate. Psychosocial factors such as elevated fear avoidance beliefs, anxiety, and depression can impact the rehabilitation process and delay return to work.[76] Job satisfaction before injury can impact the likelihood of recovery from a spine injury and return to work.[77] In addition, patient compliance with the therapist's recommendations and the patient's level of motivation to return to the prior level of function can impact the rate of recovery. All these factors must be considered as a prediction of duration of treatment and prognosis are made at the time of the initial examination.

In explanations of the findings of the examination and treatment plan to the patient with back or neck pain, efforts should be made to offer reassurance of a favorable prognosis and to assure the patient that most back injuries are not serious. The impact of reassurance and patient education provided by a healthcare worker has been shown to effect positive outcomes in treatment of back pain.[78] Spending time with the patient to answer questions, to reassure that conservative treatment can help improve the condition, and to explain the plan of care can assist in development of rapport with the patient and in creating a favorable treatment outcome.

## REFERENCES

1. Boissonnault WG, Goodman C: Physical therapists as diagnosticians: drawing the line on diagnosing pathology, *JOSPT* 36(6):351-353, 2006.

2. Boissonnault WG: *Primary care for the physical therapist: examination and triage,* Saunders, 2005, Philadelphia.

3. Henschke N, Maher CG, Refshauge KM: Screening for malignancy in low back pain patients: a systematic review, *Eur Spine J* 2007. Epub ahead of print.

4. Boissonnault WG, Koopmeiners MB: Medical history profile: orthopaedic physical therapy outpatients, *JOSPT* 20(1):2-10, 1994.

5. Boissonnault WG, Meek PD: Risk factors for anti-inflammatory-drug or aspirin-induced GI complications in individuals receiving outpatient physical therapy services, *JOSPT* 32(10):510-517, 2002.

6. Wolfe MM, Lichtenstein DR, Singh G: Gastrointestinal toxicity of nonsteroidal anti-inflammatory drugs, *N Engl J Med* 340:1888-1899, 1999.

7. Childs JD, Fritz JM, Piva SR, et al: Proposal of a classification system for patients with neck pain, *JOSPT* 34(11):686-700, 2004.

8. George SZ, Fritz JM, Bialosky JE, et al: The effect of a fear-avoidance-based physical therapy intervention for patients with acute low back pain: results of a randomized clinical trial, *Spine* 28:2551-2560, 2003.

9. Sterling M, Jull G, Kenardy J: Physical and psychological factors maintain long-term predictive capacity post-whiplash injury, *Pain* 122:102-108, 2006.

10. Arrol B, Goodyear-Smith F, Kerse N, et al: Effect of the addition of a "help" question to two screening questions on specificity for diagnosis of depression in general practice: diagnostic validity study, *BMJ* dio:10.1136/bmj.38607.464537.7C, 2005.

11. American Psychiatric Association (APA): *Diagnostic and statistical manual of mental disorders,* ed 4, Washington, DC, 2000, American Psychiatric Association.

12. Pengal LHM, Refshauge KM, Maher CG: Responsiveness of pain, disability, and physical impairment outcomes in patients with low back pain, *Spine* 29(8):879-883, 2004.

13. Waddell G, Newton M, Henderson I, et al: A fear-avoidance beliefs questionnaire (FABQ) and the role of fear-avoidance beliefs in chronic low back pain and disability, *Pain* 52:157-168, 1993.

14. Fritz JM: A comparison of a modified Oswestry low back pain disability questionnaire and the Quebec Back Pain Disability Scale, *Phys Ther* 81(2):776-788, 2001.

15. Hicks GE, Fritz JM, Delitto A, et al: Preliminary development of a clinical prediction rule for determining which patients with low back pain will respond to a stabilization exercise program, *Arch Phys Med Rehabil* 86:1753-1762, 2005.

16. Flynn T, Fritz J, Whitman J, et al: A clinical prediction rule for classifying patients with low back pain who demonstrate short-term improvement with spinal manipulation, *Spine* 27:2835-2843, 2002.

17. Cleland JA, Fritz JM, Whitman JM, et al: The reliability and construct validity of the Neck Disability Index and the patient specific functional scale in patients with cervical radiculopathy, *Spine* 31(5):598-602, 2006.

18. Fairbank JC, Couper J, Davies JB, et al: The Oswestry low back pain disability questionnaire, *Physiotherapy* 66:271-273, 1980.

19. Hudson-Cook N, Tomes-Nicholson K, Breen A: A revised Oswestry disability questionnaire. In: Roland MO, Jenner JR, editors: *Back pain: new approaches to rehabilitation and education,* New York, 1989, Manchester University Press.

20. Beurskens AJ, de Vet HC, Koke AJ: Responsiveness of functional status in low back pain: a comparison of different instruments, *Pain* 65(1):71-76, 1996.

21. Vernon H, Mior S: The neck disability index: a study of reliability and validity, *J Manipulative Physiol Ther* 14:409-415, 1991.

22. Cleland JA, Childs JD, Fritz JM, et al: Development of a clinical prediction rule for guiding treatment of a subgroup of patients with neck pain: use of thoracic spine manipulation, exercise, and patient education, *Phys Ther* 87(1):9-23, 2007.

23. Chatman A, Hyams S, Neel J, et al: The patient-specific functional scale: measurement properties in patients with knee dysfunction, *Phys Ther* 77:820-829, 1997.

24. Stratford P, Gill C, Westaway M, et al. Assessing disability and change in individual patients: a report of a patient-specific measure, *Physiother Can* 47:258-263, 1995.

25. Westaway M, Stratford P, Binkley J: The patient-specific functional scale: validation of its use in persons with neck dysfunction, *JOSPT* 27:331-338, 1998.

26. Jensen MC, Brant-Zanwadzki MN, Obuchowski N, et al: Magnetic resonance imaging of the lumbar spine in people without back pain, *N Engl J Med* 331:69-73, 1994.

27. Jensen MP, Turner JA, Romano JM: What is the maximum number of levels needed in pain intensity measurement? *Pain* 58:387-392, 1994.

28. Jensen MPT, Turner JA, Romano JM, et al: Comparative reliability and validity of chronic pain intensity measures, *Pain* 83:157-162, 1999.

29. Childs JD, Piva SR, Fritz JM: Responsiveness of the numeric pain rating scale in patients with low back pain, *Spine* 30(11):1331-1334, 2005.

30. Kendall FP, McCreary EK, Provance PG: *Muscles testing and function fourth edition with posture and pain,* Baltimore, 1993, Williams and Wilkins.

31. Giles L, Taylor J: Low back pain associated with leg length inequality, *Spine* 6(5):510-521, 1981.

32. Piva SR, Erhard RE, Childs JD, et al: Inter-rater reliability of passive intervertebral and active movements of the cervical spine, *Manual Ther* 11(4):321-330, 2006.

33. Youdas JW, Carey JR, Garrett TR: Reliability of measurements of cervical spine range of motion: comparison of three methods, *Phys Ther* 71(2): 98-106, 1991.

34. Nitchke J, Nattrass C, Disler P, et al: Reliability of the American Medical Association Guides' model for measuring spinal range of motion, *Spine* 24:262-268, 1999.

35. Maher C, Adams R: Reliability of pain and stiffness assessments in clinical manual lumbar spine examination, *Phys Ther* 74(9):809-811, 1984.

36. Cleland JA: *Orthopaedic clinical examination: an evidence-based approach for physical therapists,* Carlstadt, NJ, 2005, Icon Learning Systems.

37. Haswell K: Interexaminer reliability of symptom-provoking active sidebend, rotation and combined movement assessments of patients with low back pain, *J Manual Manipulative Ther* 12:11-20, 2004.

38. Olson KA, Goerhing M: Intra and inter-rater reliability of a goniometric lower trunk rotation measurement, *JMMT* 2008 (in review).

39. Downey BJ, Taylor NF, Niere KR: Manipulative physiotherapists can reliably palpate nominated lumbar spinal levels, *Manual Ther* 4(3):151-156, 1999.

40. Maitland G: *Vertebral manipulation,* ed 5, London, 1986, Butterworth.

41. Gonnella C, Paris SV, Kutner M: Reliability in evaluating passive intervertebral motion, *Phys Ther* 62(4):436-444, 1982.

42. Paris SV: *Introduction to spinal evaluation and manipulation,* Atlanta, 1986, Institute Press.

43. Olson K, Paris S, Spohr C, et al: Radiographic assessment and reliability study of the craniovertebral sidebending test, *J Manual Manipulative Ther* 6(2):87-96, 1998.

44. Patla C, Paris SV: Reliability of interpretation of the Paris classification of normal end feel for elbow flexion and extension, *JMMT* 1(2):60-66, 1993.

45. Bigos S, Bowyer O, Braen G, et al: Acute low back problems in adults. In *Clinical practice guideline no. 14 AHCPR,* Publication No 95-0642, Rockville, MD, 1994, Agency for Health Care Policy and Research, Public Health Service, US Department of Health and Human Services.

46. Blomberg S, Hallin G, Grann K, et al: Manual therapy with steroid injections: a new approach to treatment of low back pain, *Spine* 19(5):569-577, 1994.

47. DiFabio R: Manipulation of the cervical spine: risks and benefits, *Phys Ther* 79(1):50-65, 1999.

48. Koes B, Bouter L, VanMameren H, et al: The effectiveness of manual therapy, physiotherapy, and treatment by the general practitioner for nonspecific back and neck complaints, *Spine* 17(1):28-35, 1992.

49. Meade T, Dyer S, Browne W, et al: Low back pain of mechanical origin: randomised comparison of chiropractic and hospital outpatient treatment, *BMJ* 300:1431-1437, 1990.

50. Nilsson N, Christensen H, Hartvigsen J: The effect of spinal manipulation in the treatment of cervicogenic headache, *J Manipulative Physiol Ther* 20(5):326-330, 1997.

51. Nwuga V: Relative therapeutic efficacy of vertebral manipulation and conventional treatment in back pain management, *Am J Phys Med* 61(6):273-278, 1982.

52. Schoensee S, Jensen G, Nicholson G, et al: The effect of mobilization on cervical headaches, *JOSPT* 21(4):184-196, 1995.

53. Twomey L, Taylor L: Spine update: exercise and spinal manipulation in the treatment of low back pain, *Spine* 20(5):615-619, 1995.

54. Binkley J, Stratford PW, Gill C: Interrater reliability of lumbar accessory motion mobility testing, *Phys Ther* 75(9):786-792, 1995.

55. Nansel D, Peneff A, Jansen R, et al: Interexaminer concordance in detecting joint-play asymmetries in the cervical spines of otherwise asymptomatic subjects, *J Manipulative Physiol Ther* 12(6):428-433, 1989.

56. Strender L, Lundin M, Nell K: Interexaminer reliability in physical examination of the neck, *J Manipulative Physiol Ther* 20(8):516-520, 1997.

57. Hicks GE, Fritz JM, Delitto A, et al: Interrater reliability of clinical examination measures for identification of lumbar segmental instability, *Arch Phys Med Rehabil* 84:1858-1864, 2003.

58. Smedmark V, Wallin M, Arvidsson I: Inter-examiner reliability in assessing passive intervertebral motion of the cervical spine, *Manual Ther* 5(2)97-101, 2000.

59. Jull G, Bogduk N, Marsland A: The accuracy of manual diagnosis of for cervical zygopophyseal joint pain syndromes, *Med J Australia* 233-236, 1988.

60. Cibulka M, Koldehoff R: Clinical usefulness of a cluster of sacroiliac joint tests in patients with and without low back pain, *J Orthop Sports Phys Ther* 29(2):83-92, 1999.

61. Potter N, Rothstein J: Intertester reliability for selected clinical tests of the sacroiliac joint, *Phys Ther* 65(11):1671-1675, 1985.

62. Riddle DL, Freburger JK: Evaluation of the presence of sacroiliac joint region dysfunction using a combination of tests: a multicenter intertester reliability study, *Phys Ther* 82(8):772-781, 2002.

63. Jarett LL, Olson KA, Bohannon RW: *Reliability in examining craniovertebral sidebending,* Masters thesis, St Augustine, Fla, 2005, University of St Augustine.

64. Manipulation Education Committee: *Manipulation education manual for physical therapist professional degree programs,* Alexandria, Va, 2004, APTA.

65. Strender L, Sjoblom A, Ludwig R, et al: Interexaminer reliability in physical examination of patients with low back pain, *Spine* 22(7):814-820, 1997.

66. Vroomen PCAJ, de Krom MCTFFM, Knottnerus JA: Consistency of history taking and physical examination in patients with suspected lumbar nerve root involvement, *Spine* 25(1):91-97, 2000.

67. Lauder TD, Dillingham TR, Andary M, et al: Predicting electrodiagnostic outcomes in patients with upper limb symptoms: are the history and physical examination helpful? *Arch Phys Med Rehabil* 81:436-441, 2000.

68. Brennan GP, Fritz JM, Hunter SJ, et al: Identifiying subgroups of patients with acute/subacute "nonspecific" low back pain: results of a randomized clinical trial, *Spine* 31(6):623-631, 2006.

69. Fritz J, Whitman JM, Childs JD: Lumbar spine segmental mobility assessment: an examination of validity for determining intervention strategies in patients with low back pain, *Arch Phys Med Rehabil* 86:1745-1752, 2005.

70. Riddle DL, Schappert SM: Volume and characteristics of inpatient and ambulatory medical care for neck pain in the United States: data from three national surveys, *Spine* 32(1):132-140, 2007.

71. Gore DR: Roentgenographic findings in cervical spine in asymptomatic persons: a ten-year follow-up, *Spine* 26:2463-2466, 2001.

72. Petren-Mallmin M, Linder J: MRI cervical spine findings in asymptomatic fighter pilots, *Aviat Space Environ Med* 70:1183-1188, 1999.

73. Siivola SM, Levoska S, Tervonen O, et al: MIR changes of cervical spine in asymptomatic and symptomatic young adults, *Eur Spine J* 11:358-363, 2002.

74. Stadnik TW, Lee RR, Coen HL, et al: Annular tears and disk herniation: prevalence and contrast enhancement on MR images in the absence of low back pain or sciatica, *Radiology* 206:49-55, 1998.

75. Koes BW, van Tulder MW, Oselo R, et al: Clinical guidelines for the management of low back pain in primary care: an international comparison, *Spine* 26(22):2504-2514, 2001.

76. Fritz JM, Delitto A, Erhard RE: Comparison of classification-based physical therapy with therapy based on clinical practice guidelines for patients with acute low back pain: a randomized clinical trial, *Spine* 28:1363-1371, 2003.

77. Hoogendoorn WE, van Poppel MNM, Bongers PM, et al: Systematic review of psychosocial factors at work and private life as risk factors for back pain, *Spine* 25:2114-2125, 2000.

78. Waddell G: *The back pain revolution,* Edinburgh, 2004, Churchill Livingstone.

## CHAPTER 3

# Manipulation: Theory, Practice, and Education

## CHAPTER OVERVIEW

The purpose of this chapter is to present principles related to the practice of mobilization/manipulation. Theories are described that attempt to explain the effects of manipulation. A brief overview of the evidence that supports the use of manipulation is presented, but further detail on the evidence is provided in the anatomic regional chapters. In addition, potential adverse effects and contraindications to manipulation are discussed. Concepts of learning and teaching manipulation are also presented.

## OBJECTIVES

- Describe the theories that explain the effects of manipulation
- Present an overview of the evidence for the effectiveness of manipulation
- Explain the likelihood of adverse effects and contraindications and precautions to manipulation
- Describe the guiding principles of hand/body placement and handling skills for the performance of manipulation technique
- Describe the components of effective motor learning principles that facilitate learning performance of manipulation

## INTRODUCTION OF MANIPULATION

The *Guide to Physical Therapist Practice*[1] states that *manipulation* is an interchangeable term with *mobilization* and defines mobilization/manipulation as a manual therapy technique comprising "a continuum of skilled passive movements to joints and/or related soft tissues that are applied at varying speeds and amplitudes, including a small amplitude/high velocity therapeutic movement."[1] The American Physical Therapy Association (APTA) Manipulation Education Committee further refined the definition of high-velocity thrust manipulation as "high velocity, low amplitude therapeutic movements within or at end range of motion."[2] These definitions are used throughout this textbook.

An infinite variety of manipulation procedures is possible throughout the spine. Slight variations in hand placement and patient positioning combined with variations in velocity, rhythm, and depth of force application can be made to meet the therapeutic goals of the manual therapy procedure. The techniques included in this text have been chosen based on application of biomechanical principles, their ability to be modified to meet specific patient needs, the evidence to support the use of

the techniques, and the clinical usefulness and safety of the techniques. Maitland[3] has provided a framework for description of various grades of mobilization/manipulation based on the depth within the range of motion that the force is applied and the rate of oscillation application. Table 3-1 provides further description of the grades of mobilization/manipulation. Figure 3-1 has useful diagrams to assist in understanding the application of various depths of force with each grade of manipulation. Grades I and II are within the range that is free of resistance, and grades III and IV are passive movements that move up to the point of resistance. Grades III+ and IV+ are passive movements that stretch into the resistance of a stiff joint.

Paris[4] has described a progressive oscillation manipulation force application that provides a useful way to sequentially gradually increase the force deeper into the range of allowable passive mobility. Once the end of the available range is reached, further end-range oscillations (i.e., grade III+ or IV+), sustained stretch, or short amplitude, high-velocity thrust may be applied. The treatment effect of reducing pain and restoring mobility can be attained with end-range oscillatory techniques, progressive oscillation, or small amplitude, high-velocity

| TABLE 3-1 | Types of Mobilization/Manipulation Techniques |
|---|---|
| **TYPE** | **DESCRIPTION** |
| Grade I oscillation | Small amplitude movement performed near starting position of range |
| Grade II oscillation | Large amplitude movement performed within range but not reaching limit of range; can occupy any part of range that is free of stiffness or muscle guarding |
| Grade III oscillation | Large amplitude movement performed up to limit of range and moves into stiffness or muscle guarding |
| Grade IV oscillation | Small amplitude movement performed at limit of range stretching into stiffness or muscle guarding |
| High velocity thrust | High velocity, low amplitude therapeutic movements within or at end range of motion |
| Isometric | Where patient's muscles are used to mobilize joint by performing isometric contraction against operator's resistance |

thrust. Grade I and II mobilization/manipulation techniques tend to be used for neurophysiological effects of manipulation. The advantage of the thrust manipulation is that the patient is less able to actively guard against a thrust and the mechanical and neurophysiological effects of the manipulation can be maximized.

Isometric manipulation, or muscle energy technique (MET), is a form of manipulative treatment in which the patient actively uses muscles on request from the therapist as the therapist holds the patient's joint in a precisely controlled position, in a specific direction, and against a specific counterforce.[5] The technique is carried out with gradually increasing tension and the technique application is similar to a hold relax stretch technique as described by Knott and Voss,[6] but increased emphasis on positioning focuses the forces at a targeted joint. The joint is positioned at the point of a barrier to further movement. This position is held as the patient is asked to actively move out of the position but is held in the position by the therapist. After the isometric contraction, the joint is moved actively or passively further into the desired range of motion. Isometric manipulations use the local muscles attached at the motion segment to stretch the joint and reflexively inhibit the local muscle tone at the spinal segment to allow easier application of an end-range manipulation.

## EVIDENCE FOR MANIPULATION

The highest level of evidence to support interventions is based on the recommendations of clinical practice guidelines, systematic reviews, and metaanalysis.[7] Numerous clinical practice guidelines have recommended manipulation for the treatment of spinal disorders.[8-10] The strongest support in the literature

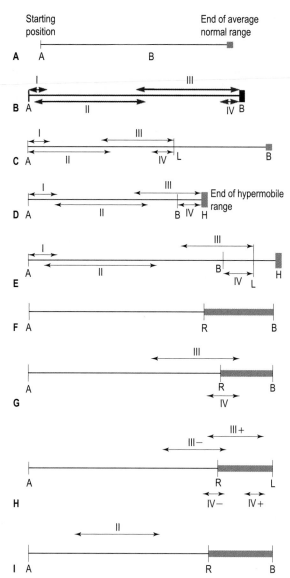

**FIGURE 3-1 A,** Depiction of range of movement. **B,** Grades in normal range with hard end feel. **C,** Grades in hypermobile joint. *L,* Pathologic limit of range (hard end feel). **D,** Grades in relation to hypermobile asymptomatic range. *B,* Range of movement beyond normal average range; *N,* normal hypermobile range. **E,** Grades in hypermoible range with slight limitation and hard end feel. **F,** Depiction of soft end feel. *R,* Beginning of resistance. **G,** Grades III and IV under soft end feel. **H,** Depiction of techniques taken into resistance in grades III and IV under soft end feel. **I,** Grade II movements are always resistance-free movements. From Maitland G, Hengeveld E, Banks K, et al: *Maitland's vertebral manipulation,* ed 7, Edinburgh, 2005, Elsevier.

for thrust manipulation is for the treatment of acute low back pain. Box 3-1 provides a sampling of clinical practice guidelines that recommend manipulation for acute low back pain (LBP). Numerous clinical practice guidelines recommend the inclusion of manipulation within the first 4 to 6 weeks of acute low back pain without radiculopathy.[8-10] The first such guideline to recommend manipulation for acute LBP was the U.S. Agency for Health Care Policy and Research,[8] which provided the highest ranking of evidence for manipulation for any intervention included in the review. Since that time, multiple clinical practice guidelines have arrived at the same conclusion.[8-10]

In regard to treatment of neck pain, the clinical practice guidelines tend to support a multimodular approach that combines nonthrust or thrust manipulation with specific therapeutic exercise programs.[11] Greater evidence is found in the literature to support the use of manipulation and therapeutic exercise than any other intervention provided by physical therapists. The evidence for manipulation is reviewed in greater detail in Chapters 4 to 7, which address each region of the spine and the temporomandibular joint (TMJ).

## EFFECTS OF MANIPULATION

During the past 150 years, many theories have been developed and perpetuated that attempt to explain the effects of manipulation. From the bone setter explanation that the cracking sound associated with a manipulation is a "bone being put back into place" to the modern exploration of the hypoalgesic effects of manipulation, practitioners have attempted to establish theories to explain the mechanism for the beneficial effects of skilled passive movements to joints and surrounding soft tissues.

From a physical therapist's perspective, the two primary indications for spinal manipulation are pain and hypomobility. Therefore the two primary effects of spinal manipulation are

improvement in mobility and reduction of pain. Paris[12] has outlined the effects of manipulation into three main categories: mechanical, neurophysiological, and psychologic. This outline establishes a useful framework for exploration of the evidence to support the theoretic effects of manipulation. The physiology and clinical significance of an audible joint sound that sometimes occurs with a manipulation are also discussed.

## Mechanical Effects

The mechanical effects of manipulation include the restoration of tissue extensibility and range of motion of hypomobile joints. The evidence to support the mechanical effects of manipulation can be divided into studies that show that manipulation can increase range of motion and animal studies that examine how joints and connective tissues respond to immobilization, injury/repair, and mobilization/manipulation.

Many studies have shown improved range of motion after spinal mobilization/manipulation; the following are a sampling of these studies. Nansel,[13] who reported on a study of 24 asymptomatic subjects with asymmetric neck side-bending motion, showed a significant increase in cervical range of motion after thrust joint manipulation to the lower cervical spine compared with subjects who received placebo manipulation. In another study of 16 subjects with chronic neck pain, subjects showed an improvement in cervical range of motion after a thrust joint manipulation to restricted C56 and C67 segments.[14] In a randomized trial of 100 subjects with neck pain, one group received thrust manipulation and the other nonthrust techniques to the cervical spine; both groups had similar improvements in range of motion.[15]

The effect of a single thoracic spine thrust manipulation was studied in 78 asymptomatic subjects who were randomly assigned to receive thrust manipulation to a restricted segment, mobility testing only, or no intervention. Thoracic manipulation was associated with an increase in range of motion, but no improvements were noted in the two other groups.[16] Sims-Williams et al[17] reported on 94 subjects who were randomly assigned to receive a lumbar manipulation or a placebo. Improvements in range of motion were noted after the treatment, but no differences in range of motion were noted compared with the placebo group at a 1-year follow-up examination.

In theory, the mechanical effects of manipulation occur when techniques are used that apply adequate force to apply tensile loads to the connective tissues that comprise and surround the joint capsule and to stretch capsular adhesions that may have formed in response to the injury and repair process.

Connective tissues are made up of a framework of collagen and elastin fibers, and the proportion of collagen and elastin fibers varies from tissue to tissue depending on tissue function.[18] If the tissue's primary function is to transmit loads, such as tendons, or to restrain joint displacement, such as a ligament or joint capsule, the tissue framework is almost exclusively collagen; but if a great degree of elasticity is needed, such as in the ligamentum flavum, a greater percentage of the tissue is made up of elastin.[18] These connective tissue structures respond to a tensile load with various degrees of viscoelastic properties depending on the structural framework.

Woo et al[19] have described the effects of prolonged immobilization (9 weeks) as creation of a loss of extracellular molecules and water in the ground substance that leads to an increase in the number of collagen cross links, which creates inhibition of free-gliding collagen fibers and resultant loss of range of motion. Forced passive motion restores range of motion of the immobilized joint of an animal model with the greatest amount of force necessary with the first cycle of passive range of motion.[19] Woo et al[19] explain that the first cycle of passive motion disrupts the cross linkages between the collagen fibers, which allows the fibers to glide more freely with subsequent passive motion cycles.

Viscoelastic properties are illustrated with a stress/strain or load/elongation (Figure 3-2) curve that illustrates the effect on tissue elongation or strain that is created with a gradually increasing load or stress. The first phase of the stress/strain curve is the toe region; this initial elongation in the tissue occurs with the application of a low load and is created by the straightening of the collagen crimp or waviness of the fibers. Once the fibers are straightened and oriented in the direction of the stress, an increase in load is needed to create a proportional lengthening of the tissue. This second linear phase represents the elastic component of the tissue; if the load is released during this phase, the tissue returns to its original length. Therefore, if a stretch is applied to a tissue with just enough force to elongate the tissue into the elastic phase, the tissue returns to its original length once the stretch is released without producing a long-term increase in tissue length.

If the intensity of the load is gradually increased over time, microfailure of the collagen begins to occur, and when the load

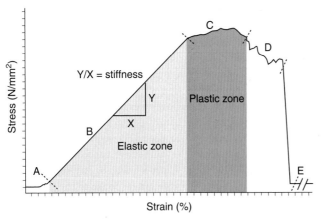

**FIGURE 3-2** Stress-strain curve of an excised ligament that has been stretched to a point of mechanical failure (disruption). The ligament is considered an elastic tissue. *Zone A* shows the nonlinear region. *Zone B* (elastic zone) shows the linear relationship between stress and strain, demonstrating the stiffness of the tissue. *Zone C* indicates the mechanical property of plasticity. *Zones D* and *E* demonstrate the points of progressive mechanical failure of the tissue. From Neumann DA: *Kinesiology of the musculoskeletal system: foundations for physical rehabilitation,* St Louis, 2002, Mosby.

is removed, a proportional increase in tissue resting length remains.[18] This third phase of the stress/strain curve is referred to as the plastic phase. The plastic phase must be reached with stretching/mobilizing to create a long-lasting increase in length of connective tissue. The viscoelastic property of hysteresis occurs when the tissue is stressed into the plastic phase. Hysteresis is characterized by a greater amount of energy being absorbed by the tissue during the loading than is dissipated during the unloading.[20] This energy is likely absorbed by the connective tissues in the form of heat. Warren, Lehmann, and Koblanski[21,22] have shown that heat can be used to decrease the amount of force needed to elongate collagen tissue. The heat production associated with hysteresis can be used to assist in tissue elongation.

With further increase in the strain over time, a progressive failure of collagen bundles occurs. Eventually, the tissue continues to elongate without needing an increased load,[20] which is referred to as the creep phase. If the load is sustained past the creep phase, tensile mechanical failure or rupture of the tissue occurs.[20] Therefore, when a stretch/mobilization is applied to a tissue for the purpose of creating permanent elongation of that tissue, the load must be of sufficient intensity and duration to reach the plastic phase on the stress/strain curve but the failure point must be avoided if excessive tissue damage or rupture is to be prevented.

The stress/strain curve varies between tissues depending on the proportion of collagen and elastin in the tissue. A more elastic tissue tends to elongate to a greater extent before microfailure occurs, but complete failure occurs abruptly with a shorter plastic phase.[23] If a tissue is stretched only within the elastic phase and the plastic phase is never reached, permanent elongation of the tissue does not occur. With repetition of the stretching in the elastic range of the tissue, the connective tissue progressively becomes stronger and more resistant to microfailure. This phenomenon was shown by Tipton et al,[24] who found that dogs that received regular exercise needed a greater degree of force to create failure and rupture of the experimental group's muscle tendon units as compared with a control group. However, Tipton et al[24] also found that dogs that had been immobilized for 6 weeks had a significantly weaker transitional zone in bone-tendon-bone and bone-ligament-bone preparations. The results of this study need to be considered in the stretching of connective tissues. On the basis of this animal research, caution must be taken to avoid rupture of previously immobilized tissues.

Precautions must be taken in attempts to stretch traumatized connective tissues depending on the stage of inflammation and repair. The stages of repair of dense connective tissue include acute inflammation, fibroplastic, and remodeling phases. Acute inflammation lasts 2 to 14 days and is characterized by pain, redness, heat, swelling, and loss of function. A vascular/chemical response occurs with vasodilation, exudate formation, and clotting and a cellular response with phagocytosis to clean the wound. Cummings, Crutchfield, and Barnes[25] recommend resting damaged tissues for the first 24 to 48 hours after trauma to allow the repair process to begin and to avoid excessive inflammation and bleeding. As the repair process continues, the wound is invaded by fibroblasts, which lay down collagen fibers in a random arrangement.[25] The new collagen fibers are held together by weak hydrogen bonds during the first 8 to 10 days, and the collagen can be easily stretched and molded during the first 8 to 10 days.[25]

The fibroplastic phase begins at day 4 and lasts up to 21 days. As the wound matures, the hydrogen bonds are replaced by covalent bonding that strengthens the scar.[25] Reepithelialization and fibroplasia with neovascularization occur during this phase with random strands of fibrin being laid down.[26] Myofibroblasts also enter the wound site as early as 3 to 5 days after trauma and bond to collagen fibers to create shrinkage of the wound.[25,27]

The final phase of healing is the remodeling phase and includes consolidation (day 21 to day 60), with a change from cellular to more fibrous tissue, and finally, maturation (day 60 to day 360), in which collagen fibers are slowly aligned and strengthened, and the weak hydrogen bonds transition to stronger covalent bonds. Loading and stressing the connective tissue during the maturation phase affects the shape, strength, and pliability of the tissue. The collagen bundles organize along lines of stress, and the fibroblasts also orient to stress. Stress to the connective tissue stimulates glycoaminoglycan and proteoglycan production.[26] However, too much stress pulls apart newly formed collagen bundles and causes acute inflammation.

On the basis of this knowledge of the healing process of injured dense connective tissues, Box 3-2 outlines general clinical guidelines to facilitate healing of the connective tissues. Excessive scar tissue formation and myofibroblastic activity are created by excessive inflammation at the area surrounding the wound site; therefore, overstressing a healing wound site with an excessive amount of stretching or exercise could potentially create excessive inflammation and adhesion formation of the adjacent connective tissues.[25] Adhesions could cause a progressive loss of motion for as long as 6 months to 1 year as the scar tissue matures.[25] Mechanical principles such as an understanding of the stress–strain curve can be applied clinically to stretch joint capsular adhesions.

Other theories to explain the mechanical effects of manipulation that have less evidence for support include correc-tion of a facet joint meniscoid entrapment and positional faults.

Acute facet joint locking is a condition with a sudden loss of joint mobility that is often caused by a nontraumatic event. The joints that tend to lock have meniscoids. The mechanism of the locking seems to involve either entrapment of a meniscoid in a groove formed in the articular cartilage or a piece of meniscus that may break loose and form a loose body, with the loose body creating the entrapment.[28,29] Intracapsular meniscoid structures are present in spinal facet joints. Facet menisci are believed to be capable of becoming entrapped, or impinged, between the two facet surfaces, causing the joint surfaces to lock, which is associated with pain with movements that downglide and load the facet joint. Manipulation techniques that gap the joint or isometric manipulation techniques that theoretically pull the facet joint capsule laterally are believed to dislodge the impingement, and patients show immediate improvement in joint motion and reduction of pain with movement.[28,29] No studies have specifically addressed the effect of spinal mobilization/manipulation on meniscoid impingement.[30] However, anatomic plausibility of the meniscoid impingement or entrapment theory has been refuted by anatomists after a review of the literature on the topic.[31,32]

Although traditional chiropractic philosophy is based on detection and correction of spinal subluxations and realignment of these spinal subluxations, no valid research has shown that subluxations/positional faults correlate with pain or are a cause of hypomobility in the spine.[30] Spinal facet subluxations of less than 4.5 mm are not detectable with radiography. In comparison of premanipulation and postmanipulation radiographic results, clinicians were not capable of detecting a change in vertebral position after a chiropractic spinal thrust joint manipulation. In another study by Tullberg et al,[33] joint manipulation did not cause a detectable change in the relative position of the ilium on the sacrum, when measured with roentgen stereophotogrammetric analysis.

Therefore, although the positional fault and meniscoid theories are somewhat plausible, no reliable valid measurement tool is sensitive enough to detect and measure the presence of these impairments in clinical practice. Thus, these conditions are considered theoretic.

## Neurophysiological Effects of Manipulation

In live human subjects, active range of motion is influenced by many variables, including the effects of pain, fear of pain,[34] and neuromotor control, in addition to joint capsule, connective tissue, and myofascial mobility. The ability to restore active range of motion of the spine after a manipulation could potentially be affected by all of these factors. Therefore the neurophysiological effects of manipulation likely provide the most feasible explanation for the beneficial effects of manipulation. The neurophysiological effects of manipulation result in reduction of pain and influence muscle tone and motor control. Some of these effects occur both in the anatomic region where the manipulation has been performed and in other regions systemically. Before a sampling is provided of the research on the

---

| BOX 3-2 | General Clinical Guidelines to Facilitate Healing of Dense Connective Tissues After Severe Injury or Surgery |
| --- | --- |

- Relative rest for the first 24 to 48 hours
- Low load, high repetition exercise can stimulate healing
- Only very gentle range of motion first 10 to 14 days (grade I and II mobilizations)
- Four to 8 weeks is often needed before loading injured tissue to end range (grade III or IV)
- Use pain as a guide because with increased pain is often increased inflammation
- Continue to exercise and stretch for 1 year

neurophysiological effects of manipulation on the sympathetic nervous system and motor system, an explanation of the involved neuroanatomy and physiology is necessary.

The tissues of the spine, including the skin, fascia, muscle, tendon, joints, ligaments, and intervertebral disc (outer annulus), are well innervated and provide afferent input to the central nervous system.[35] Extensive numbers of type I and II mechanoreceptors and free nerve endings (type IV receptors) have been noted in the cervical facet joints[36] and in the muscle spindles of the cervical spine.[37,38] Similar receptors are found in the thoracic and lumbar spine, but in fewer numbers and with a more inconsistent distribution than in the cervical spine.[39] The type I mechanoreceptors provide afferent input to the central nervous system regarding static joint position and increase their rate of firing in response to movement. The type II mechanoreceptors remain inactive as long as joints are immobile; when joints are moved actively or passively, they emit brief bursts of impulses.[40] Therefore, with joint movement caused by spinal manipulation, these receptors fire and provide afferent input to the central nervous system.

The afferent nerves from the receptors terminate in the spinal cord, synapsing in the laminae and ventral horn to signal both proprioceptive and nociceptive information.[41] As spinal manipulation produces movement of the vertebral column and its associated structures, multiple receptors are influenced to generate afferent input to the spinal cord. In the cervical spine, additional complex interactions occur with other systems, such as vestibular and optic systems, that may also activate in response to manipulation techniques.[42] As a result, a neuroanatomic basis is seen through which a multifaceted neurophysiological response may occur with manipulation.

Both animal and human studies have shown that a key locus of control for mediation of endogenous analgesia is the periaqueductal grey area of the midbrain (PAG).[43-45] The PAG plays an important integrative role for behavioral responses to pain, stress, and other stimuli by coordinating responses of a number of systems, including the nociceptive system, autonomic nervous system, and motor system.[46-48] Animal studies have shown that when key regions of the PAG are stimulated, a sympathetic nervous system (fight or flight) response is evoked combined with a nonopioid form of analgesia.[42] Type I and II mechanoreceptors from joints and muscles project to the PAG.[49] A series of studies is presented to show a postmanipulation sympathetic response (skin conductance) combined with analgesia (pressure pain threshold) in symptomatic and asymptomatic subjects, which provides strong evidence that the analgesic response to spinal manipulation is likely the result of the stimulation of mechanoreceptors that provide afferent impulses to the central nervous system (CNS) to trigger descending pain inhibitory pathways originating from the periaqueductal grey area of the midbrain.[50] Many of these studies use double-blind controls and placebo groups to compare the therapeutic effects of manipulation; the systemic and local hypoalgesic effects of manipulation are measured with the use of a mechanical pain threshold devise. A valid measure of hypoalgesia is an increase in mechanical pain pressure threshold. Skin conductance is

monitored as a measure of sympathetic nervous system response to manipulation; when this response is increased, it is a measure of the sympathetic nervous system excitatory response of manipulation.

Sterling, Jull, and Wright[51] studied 30 subjects with cervical pain of insidious onset. These subjects received an anterior glide grade III mobilization to the C5 facet on the painful side, a placebo condition that consisted of manual contacts, or a control condition that consisted of no physical contact between subject and clinician. After the mobilization technique, subjects had a significant increase in pressure pain thresholds and a decrease in visual analog scores compared with the other two conditions.

Terrett and Vernon[52] studied 50 asymptomatic subjects who were randomly assigned to receive either nonthrust or thrust manipulation. A significant elevation in pain tolerance to an experimentally induced electrical pain stimulus was found after the thrust manipulation compared with the nonthrust manipulation. Dhouldt et al[53] randomly assigned 30 subjects with rheumatoid arthritis to receive 12 minutes of mobilization or rest. Mobilization consisted of grade I and II oscillations to T12 and L4. The subjects who received the mobilizations had an increase in pain threshold in the spine, knees, and ankles as compared with the group that received rest.[53]

Peterson, Vicenzino, and Wright[54] evaluated the effect of grade III posteroanterior (PA) mobilization to the C5-C6 spinal segment and showed an increase of skin conductance of 60% from baseline during the treatment intervention versus a 20% increase for the placebo group, with a significant difference between groups. This study showed that PA mobilization produces an initial immediate sympathoexcitatory effect that starts within 15 seconds after initiation of treatment.[54]

Additional studies have considered the influence of a cervical lateral glide manipulation technique[55] and a cervical PA mobilization[56] on mechanical pain thresholds in healthy painfree subjects. Mechanical pain thresholds were measured with a digital pressure algometer. In both studies, the manipulation was shown to produce a significant increase in mechanical pain threshold, which indicates a relative hypoalgesic effect. The lateral glide procedure produced a mean increase in mechanical pain threshold measured at the head of the radius of 25% and measured over the lateral articular pillar of the C5 level after the PA mobilization of 15%. In both cases, the treatment effect was greater than in the control and the placebo groups, both locally and regionally.

Vicenzino et al[55] tested the interaction between changes in mechanical pain threshold and skin conductance during the cervical lateral gliding procedure and found a significant correlation between the time taken to achieve the maximum increase in peripheral skin conductance and the increase in mechanical pain thresholds. Those subjects who had the most rapid sympathoexcitatory response also showed the greatest increase in pain threshold (relative hypoalgesia),[55] which may explain why some individuals respond more dramatically to manipulation than others. The authors hypothesize that those individuals with more direct neural connections from the peripheral to the

PAG have the more rapid symphathoexcitatory response and the greater hypoalgesia effect with manipulation.[55]

Another proposed explanation of the analgesic effect of joint manipulation is stimulation of release of endogenous opioid peptides that bind to receptor sites in the nervous system and produce analgesia. One such opiate is beta-endorphin. Vernon et al[57] measured the plasma levels of beta-endorphin at 5-minute intervals after thrust manipulation of the cervical spine of asymptomatic subjects. The findings showed an increase in the plasma levels of beta-endorphin in the experimental group 5 minutes after the thrust as compared with a control group that received a similar but less aggressive mobilization technique.[57] At 15 minutes after thrust manipulation, the beta-endorphin level was back to a baseline level.[57] However, other investigators have performed similar studies and have been unable to measure differences in beta-endorphin levels after a spinal manipulation as compared with control and sham treatment groups in both symptomatic and asymptomatic groups.[58,59]

For further investigation of the premise that endogenous opioids are involved in analgesia after spinal manipulation, Zusman, Edwards, and Donaghy[60] compared the effects of a spinal manipulation on visual analog scale (VAS) pain scores for subjects who were given Naloxone or a saline solution control. Naloxone is an opioid antagonist and reverses the effect of endogenous opioids. Equal improvements in VAS pain scores were seen for both groups, which suggests that endogenous opioids are not the physiologic mechanism of postmanipulation analgesia.[60] Similar results were noted by Vicenzino et al[61] in a similar study design that used Naloxone with the experimental group and found that after lateral glide cervical mobilization techniques, the hypoalgesia response was the same between the experimental, sham, and control groups.

Animal studies with rats and injections of various medications to either block or enhance the effects of neurotransmitters found that the hypoalgesic affects of manipulation likely involve the descending pain inhibitory mechanisms that use serotonin and noradrenaline rather than opioid or gamma-aminobutyric acid (GABA) receptors.[62] These studies taken together suggest very little evidence to support the involvement of the opioid system in manipulation-induced analgesia.

McGuiness, Vicenzino, and Wright[63] showed a highly significant increase in both respiratory rate and blood pressure after a grade III PA mobilization applied to the C5-C6 motion segment; the placebo group showed a slight decrease in these measures. Vicenzino et al[64] measured factors related to the sympathetic nervous system (SNS) function, including heart rate and blood pressure, during application of a C5-C6 lateral glide nonthrust manipulation on 24 asymptomatic subjects and found a significant increase in heart rate and blood pressure of 14% compared with 1% to 2% in the placebo and control conditions. The respiratory rate increased 36%. These studies further confirm a sympathoexcitory response to manipulation procedures.

The effect of cervical lateral glide manipulation has also been evaluated in patients with lateral epicondylitis.[65] Measures of mechanical pain threshold, pain-free grip pressure, range of shoulder abduction in upper limb neurodynamic (ULND) test 2b, and visual analog scale measures of pain and function were obtained before and after treatment and placebo and control interventions. Treatment resulted in significant improvements in most measures obtained, which indicates that lateral glide cervical manipulation procedures produced a relative hypoalgesic effect of the lateral elbow region a few minutes after the treatment. The mean increase in mechanical pain threshold was approximately 26%, the mean increase in pain-free grip pressure was 29%, and the mean increase in shoulder abduction with ULND 2b was 44%.[65]

In a retrospective analysis of 112 patients who underwent treatment for lateral epicondylalgia, Cleland, Whitman, and Fritz[66] found that patients who received manual therapy to the cervical spine combined with local treatment for the lateral epicondylalgia were seen for significantly fewer visits with positive outcomes as compared with the patients who only received local therapy for the lateral epicondylalgia.

These studies support the concept that manual therapy procedures can produce a hypoalgesic effect both in healthy subjects and in patients. Because this response is coupled with a sympathoexcitatory response and the hypoalgesic effect is both local and systemic, convincing support exists that the mechanism for the neurophysiological effects of manipulation lies in the stimulation of descending pain inhibitory systems of the central nervous system projecting from the midbrain to the spinal cord.

Several studies have investigated the effect of manipulation (usually thrust) on the motor system to determine whether spinal manipulation can inhibit muscle tone, increase muscle tone, or enhance muscle performance. The findings have been variable. Theoretically, muscle tone inhibition occurs with a strong end range stretch of a joint from firing type III joint mechanoreceptors, which create a reflexive inhibition of the local muscle tone of the muscles overlying the joint.

The effect of thrust manipulation of the thoracic and lumbar spine was studied on 34 subjects with joint hypomobility with and without musculoskeletal pain. Subjects were randomly assigned to either receive the thrust manipulation or no intervention. Subjects who received the manipulation had on average a 20% reduction in paraspinal muscle activity as measured with electromyographic activity compared with control subjects.[67] Similar results have been reported in reduction of hamstring muscle activity in subjects with unilateral low back pain, with comparison before and after a lumbar thrust manipulation.[68]

Dishman, Cunningham, and Burke[69] used electrodiagnostic testing to compare the effects of spinal manipulation at the cervical and lumbar spines on the tibial nerve H-reflex to investigate the relationship between potential cortical and segmentally controlled responses to spinal manipulation. A clinician performed a unilateral manipulation at either L5-S1, C5-C6, or both levels. They showed a small but significant decrease in the size of the H-reflex after the lumbar manipulation, but this effect only lasted 60 seconds after the manipulation and no effect was noted from the cervical manipulation.[69] The authors suggest a segmental rather than a global effect produced by spinal manipulation on the motoneuron pool.[69]

Speculation also exists that spinal manipulation can increase muscle strength. In one study performed on 16 subjects with chronic neck pain, biceps muscle strength improved after a thrust joint manipulation to restricted C5-C6 and C6-C7 spinal segments.[14] An increase in lower trapezius strength occurred after a thoracic spine mobilization in a study of 40 asymptomatic subjects.[70] These subjects were randomly assigned to receive either grade IV or grade I anterior glide mobilizations to T6-T12. Subjects who received grade IV mobilization had a significant increase in lower trapezius muscle strength compared with subjects who received grade I mobilizations.[70] Cleland et al[71] were able to show a significant increase in strength output (14%) of the lower trapezius muscle immediately after a thoracic spine thrust manipulation as compared with a control group, and the authors suggest that manipulation techniques may be beneficial in reducing lower trapezius muscle inhibition commonly associated with many postural syndromes. Suter et al[72] studied 18 subjects with knee pain and sacroiliac joint dysfunctions. After correction of the sacroiliac joint dysfunction with a manipulation, a significant increase in knee extension torque occurred on the symptomatic side.

Sterling, Jull, and Wright[51] used nonthrust manipulation of the cervical spine in patients with neck pain to assess the effects on motor responses, sympathetic nervous system function, and analgesia. The effect of PA cervical technique on the craniocervical flexion test (see Chapter 6) was assessed. A decrease activation of superficial muscles of the cervical spine was reported with the craniocervical flexion test and was interpreted as facilitation of the deep neck flexor muscles.[51] This result provides preliminary evidence that spinal manipulation can alter motor responses and facilitate muscle function that was previously inhibited because of pain or impairment.

The effect of spinal manipulation on the motor system is inconclusive. Some studies support both facilitation and inhibition of the motor system after manipulation. The response may vary depending on the technique, the location and nature of the pain, and the muscles that are tested.[42] A growing body of knowledge exists regarding the effects on the sympathetic nervous system in response to spinal manipulation and the hypoalgesic effects that accompany the sympathetic responses. However, absolutely no scientific validation supports the long-held tenet of the chiropractic profession that spinal manipulation alters autonomic nervous system outflow to the organs and viscera and that this rectifies dysfunction of the end organs.[42,73]

Use of isometric manipulation, also known as muscle energy technique (MET), has been advocated for treatment of joint hypomobility conditions. Schenk, MacDiarmid, and Rousselle[74] showed improvements in lumbar backward-bending range of motion in a group of 13 asymptomatic subjects after lumbar isometric manipulation techniques performed two times per week for 4 weeks as compared with a control group. The same researchers[75] showed improvement in cervical range of motion in a group of asymptomatic subjects who received isometric manipulation to the cervical spine two times per week for 4 weeks compared with a control group.

Speculation exists that the isometric manipulation, similar to a hold relax stretch technique, causes the golgi tendon organ to fire, which inhibits the antagonistic movement pattern to allow a greater degree of movement into the agonist movement pattern.[20,76] The effect of isometric manipulation techniques is also explained by Sherrington's principle of reciprocal innervation, which states that with an isometric contraction of the agonistic muscles the antagonistic muscles are inhibited to allow greater freedom of movement into the agonist movement pattern.[77] In addition to these possible explanations of the effects of an isometric manipulation, speculation exists that an isometric contraction of the local muscles attached to the targeted spinal facet joint (e.g., multifidus muscle) applies a stretch to the joint capsule[4] or corrects slight positional faults by either pulling directly on the joint capsule or moving the adjacent bone.[78] Further research is needed to fully understand the mechanical and neurophysiological effects of isometric manipulation techniques.

## Psychological Effects

Very few studies have specifically addressed and measured the psychological effects of manipulation. However, many controlled studies on the effects of manipulation have used a sham or placebo treatment that might include manual touch or positioning for a manipulation without actually imparting a manipulative force. In these studies, slight improvements can often be measured in pain and disability levels for the subjects in the sham treatment groups. The placebo effect is estimated to be 10% to 25% of the benefit of the manipulation as a result of the psychological effects. The effect of touch and reassurance from a medical professional can have powerful effects on easing the patient's fear and anxiety, which can translate into reduced pain and disability. Clinicians and researchers need to be aware of these effects as they assess the benefit of manipulation, which is why high quality clinical research studies use sham treatment and control groups.

## THE AUDIBLE JOINT "POP"

The physiology of an audible joint pop or crack phenomenon associated with a joint manipulation has been investigated in two principal studies: Roston and Haines[79] and Unsworth, Dowson, and Wright.[80] With application of increasing tension at the metacarpal-phalangeal joint of the third finger and monitoring of the amount of joint separation with intermittent radiographs, Roston and Haines[79] were able to show that the amount of joint separation increases very gradually in a linear fashion as the tension on the joint is increased. However, when a critical amount of tension is reached to produce a joint "pop," a sudden increase in the amount of joint separation is noted. Roston and Haines[79] interpreted the space noted after the cracking as a "partial vacuum occupied by water vapor and blood gases under reduced pressure." A joint that has been "cracked" is not capable of being recracked for approximately

20 minutes,[79,80] which is referred to as the refractory period; the belief is that gas must be reabsorbed before the joint can be cracked again.[79]

Unsworth, Dowson, and Wright[80] performed a similar study and described the formation of vapor-filled bubbles in the joint as a result of cavitation, which is the process of fluid converted to gas from a critical reduction in pressure. In the case of the joint, the synovial fluid is vaporized once negative 2.5 atmospheric pressure is reached as a result of tension placed on the joint.[80] Unsworth, Dowson, and Wright[80] further explain the cracking phenomenon as the result of not just the formation of a gas bubbles in the joint cavity from negative pressure but the explosion of these gas bubbles to cause the noise. The gas bubbles seem to collapse instantly once formed as the bubbles come into contact with the remaining synovial fluid, which is of a higher pressure. Unsworth, Dowson, and Wright[80] also identified a sudden jump in joint separation just after the crack and noted that the reloading and noncracking joints have a more gradual separation but separate to the same distance.

The joint surfaces must be close to give the correct preloading conditions for cavitation to occur, and Unsworth, Dowson, and Wright[80] found that the joint separation takes 15 minutes to return to its precracking value. They calculated that reabsorption of the gas, which is believed to be primarily carbon dioxide, may take 30 minutes.[80] These factors may help to explain the refractory period. Unsworth, Dowson, and Wright[80] noted that the joints that did not crack in the study had a resting joint separation 25% greater than the cracking joints. The joints that did not crack separated when under tension in a similar fashion as the cracking joints in their refractory period, and the common denominator seems to be the amount of joint separation before application of the load.

Flynn et al[81] compared the immediate effects of a lumbopelvic manipulation for patients who were noted as having an audible joint sound with the manipulation and for those who did not. In comparison of the response between the two groups, Flynn et al[81] reported no difference in outcomes (disability, pain, lumbar flexion active range of motion [AROM]) between the group of patients who had an audible pop with the manipulation and the group of those who did not. On the basis of Flynn et al's[81] study, the beneficial effects of manipulation do not appear to be dependent on the production of a joint sound. Therefore, creation of a joint sound should not be the primary goal of a manipulation technique. Other outcome measures are more important, including reduction in pain, reduction in perceived disability, and improvement in mobility and function.

## CLINICAL DECISION MAKING IN USE OF SPINAL MANIPULATION

### An Impairment-Based Biomechanical Approach to Clinical Decision Making

*Biomechanical approach* is a term for an impairment-based approach of management of spinal disorders in which clinical decisions are based on the results of clinical tests and measures that analyze active and passive motion. The clinical decisions on the depth, location, and direction of manipulation procedures are based on knowledge of spinal mechanics for interpretation of these clinical findings. Pain provocation and tissue reactivity are assessed in a similar manner, and this clinical information is factored into the decision of manipulation technique selection. For instance, if a joint is both stiff (i.e., hypomobile) and highly reactive, techniques are selected with adequate depth and force to stretch the joint, but less vigorous techniques (grades I and II) may precede the stretch manipulation procedure to first attempt to inhibit pain, especially if the patient reflexively holds against the manipulation forces. A thrust technique can often be successful in this situation because the speed of the technique can proceed the muscle guarding reaction, and if successful, pain reduction and muscle inhibition result at the targeted spinal segment. If a spinal segment is found to be hypermobile, it is treated with stabilization exercises, and perhaps grade III or IV manipulation techniques may be used at hypomobile regions above or below the hypermobile spinal segment.

Cleland and Childs[82] have recently challenged the validity of use of a biomechanical model as a basis for clinical decision making in manual physical therapy. Historically, a biomechanical model has been the basis for most manual physical therapy clinical approaches, and the foundations of these approaches are what clinicians have used to show positive outcomes from manual therapy interventions applied in clinical trials.[83-85] Therefore, one could argue that the biomechanical model works well clinically, but the rationale for the effectiveness is now being challenged.

One argument against the use of a biomechanical model relates to recent evidence with use of dynamic magnetic resonance imaging (MRI) that accessory PA manipulation forces directed to the spine are less localized than originally thought. Kulig, Landel, and Powers[86] assessed spinal dynamics with PA mobilization (grade IV force) techniques of the lumbar spine and showed that sagittal plane motion occurs at all the lumbar spinal levels with this technique.

The results of the study from Kulig, Landel, and Powers[86] revealed a consistent pattern of lumbar spine motion during PA mobilization procedures. The amount of motion was greatest at the targeted spinal segment where the PA force was applied, and the PA force produced motion directed toward extension. In addition, two patterns of motion were observed at the nontargeted segments. With force applied at L5, L4, or L3, all lumbar segments generally moved toward extension. With force applied at L2 or L1, the three most cranial lumbar segments (L1-L2, L2-L3, and L3-L4) moved toward extension, and the two most caudal segments (L4-L5 and L5-S1) moved toward flexion. The magnitude of extension motion was greatest at the targeted segment.[86]

Although the dynamic MRI study illustrates that more than one spinal segment moves with PA force application, the pattern of induced passive motion to the lumbar spine was unique with each targeted segmental application. As an assessment tool, unique information is obtained with assessment of PA mobility at each spinal level and clinical decisions can still be based on this information. Further, if a particular spinal level is painful with PA force application, oscillatory techniques can be applied to adjacent spinal levels to induce some motion at the painful segment. Likewise, if mechanical effects are desired, the greatest extension movement can be applied by mobilizing at the targeted stiff segment. If passive motion is contraindicated at a spinal level, such as after a recent lumbar fusion, PA mobilization techniques should not be used at the adjacent spinal segments. Therefore, the manual physical therapist can use this knowledge to enhance the biomechanical approach but, at the same time, must understand that the ability to be segment specific with manual therapy assessment and treatment procedures has limitations.

The forces applied to specific vertebrae create a motion at more spinal levels than just the targeted segment. At the same time, the pattern and magnitude of motion is unique to localization of force application. Clinically useful information can be attained by applying forces at each vertebrae to assess mobility and reactivity. These results must be interpreted as spinal *region* specific versus spinal *segment* specific. However, for documentation purposes and for the purpose of finding the location to reapply the technique in the future, documentation of the segment where the force was applied is still acceptable. In the end, correlation of findings is needed to determine the best intervention. Clinicians should never rely on the results of one assessment to make a clinical decision. In the case of PA passive accessory intervertebral motion (PAIVM) tests, this examination finding should be correlated with symptom behavior, AROM, tissue palpation, muscle strength/length testing, and other passive intervertebral motion (PIVM) tests.

A second argument against the use of a biomechanical model is the recent evidence that random selection of manipulation techniques may be just as effective as techniques selected based on a clinical assessment that incorporates a biomechanical model.[82] Chiradejnant et al[87] completed a randomized controlled trial to determine the immediate effects on pain level and active range of motion of patients with low back pain treated with a PA lumbar mobilization technique either at the therapist selected level or at a randomly selected level. The study found no difference in short-term outcomes between these two groups, and both groups reported improvements in pain level and lumbar range of motion. Further data analysis revealed better outcomes in patients who received the mobilization technique to the lower lumbar levels compared with the upper lumbar levels. The results of this study confirm that lumbar mobilization treatment has an immediate effect on relief of pain but also suggest that the specific technique used may not be important.[87]

The results of the study of Chiradejnant et al[87] are not surprising after a review of the Kulig, Landel, and Powers[86] MRI study, but the results should not be extrapolated to hold true for all manipulation techniques of the spine. The results should only be interpreted for the PA mobilization technique, which has shown with MRI studies to move multiple

levels, and the PA lumbar mobilization technique should be considered a general lumbar mobilization/manipulation technique.

Haas et al[88] found a similar result in comparison with the short-term effects of cervical spine manipulations that were randomly selected versus those techniques that were selected due to results of cervical passive intervertebral motion (PIVM) testing. Both groups of patients showed same-day reduction in pain and stiffness, but no difference in results could be attributed to the results of PIVM testing.[88] Long-term effects of a random approach to manipulation technique selection have not been studied. The data suggest that pain modulation may not be limited to mechanisms associated with manipulation of joints with restricted motion. In addition, there is evidence of systemic and regional hypoalgesia resulting from a variety of spinal manipulation techniques, which is presented in greater detail in the neurophysiological effects of manipulation section of this chapter.

A third argument against the use of a biomechanical model is that evidence suggests that manipulation techniques are not segment specific.[82] Studies have investigated the accuracy and precision of spinal thrust manipulation techniques as determined by location of cavitations. Ross, Bereznick, and McGill[89] investigated the accuracy of manipulation directed at the lumbar and thoracic spine with skin sensors for detection of the cavitation, and engineering principles were used to determine the distance of the cavitation from the targeted spinal segment. The results showed that thoracic spine manipulation was accurate (i.e., cavitation occurred at the targeted segment) 53% of the time and that lumbar spine manipulation was accurate 46% of the time.[89] Most of the manipulation resulted in multiple cavitations, which usually included the targeted segment, but the authors included the multiple cavitation techniques in their calculations as being not segment specific.[89] This study assumes that joint cavitation is vital to localization of force and success of manipulation. Neither premise has been proven. In fact, Flynn et al[81] showed that the successful outcome with a lumbopelvic region manipulation had little to do with production of an audible joint sound during the manipulation. In addition, multiple techniques are typically used during any one treatment session, which further increases the odds of manipulating the targeted segment.

In summary, preliminary evidence shows that manual therapists are unable to be as specific with segmental manual therapy assessment and manipulation techniques as they have purported to be in the past. As manual therapy procedures are taught and practiced clinically, consideration of these limitations must be taken into account. However, the refinement of manual therapy skill and the application of successful techniques to produce favorable outcomes are dependent on efforts to strive to be as specific as possible. Undue claims of supernatural palpation skills are unwarranted, but as the evidence emerges to guide clinical practice with clinical prediction rules, the identification of patients who will benefit from manipulation continues to be dependent on skillful manual examination and manipulation procedures.[90-92]

Fritz, Whitman, and Childs[92] showed a correlation between patients who had passive lumbar hypomobility with central posterior to anterior PAIVM testing and the patients who responded favorably to spinal manipulation. In other words, patients with lumbar stiffness are more likely to respond favorably to spinal manipulation. In addition, a strong correlation for a positive response to a spinal stabilization exercise program was correlated with hypermobility noted with central PA PAIVM testing of the lumbar spine. This correlation helps to link an impairment approach with an evidence-based approach and validates the use of PA PAIVM testing as an important component of a physical therapist examination scheme to determine the most effective intervention for spinal disorders.[92]

Clinical decision making in orthopaedic manual physical therapy is based on an evidence-based approach. Research evidence supports the effectiveness of treatment of spinal disorders by subgrouping patients based on identification of key physical impairments, patient characteristics, and symptoms. With clinical situations in which the research evidence is not clear, use of a biomechanical impairment-based approach is the foundation of physical therapy treatment of musculoskeletal disorders. An impairment approach can guide clinical decision making where specific physical impairments such as joint stiffness, joint hypermobility, muscle weakness, or tightness are identified through clinical examination, and appropriate interventions are administered based on the examination findings. This textbook presents the evidence for clinical decision making, such as clinical prediction rules, but also includes a biomechanical impairment-based approach in the assessment and treatment of spinal disorders. Patient classifications also are presented to assist in management of common signs and symptoms.

## Adverse Effects, Safety, and Contraindications with Spinal Manipulation

Cervical spine manipulation techniques pose a risk of adverse effects that range from mild soreness to severe neurovascular injury. Adverse reactions to cervical spine manipulation may include temporary increase in neck pain, radiating arm pain, headache, dizziness, impaired vision, or ringing in the ears.[93] Hurwitz et al[93] surveyed 280 participants in a chiropractic cervical spine manipulation clinical trial 2 weeks after the trial was started, and 25% of the participants reported increased neck pain or stiffness/soreness that most commonly lasted less than 24 hours after the manipulation. Patients who received nonthrust techniques reported significantly fewer adverse reactions.[93] Participants with histories of neck trauma, pain less than 1 year, worsening of pain since onset, pain ratings of 8+ on a 0 to 10 scale, neck disability index (NDI) scores of 16 or more, moderate or severe headache, nausea during the past month, and lack of confidence in the treatment were more likely than others to report unpleasant symptoms or discomfort with the chiropractic manipulation.[93] Based on these results, Hurwitz et al[93] suggest that nonthrust manipulation techniques may be preferable in most patients with neck pain over thrust tech-

| BOX 3-3 | Factors That Affect Increased Likelihood of Adverse Reactions to Cervical Spine Thrust Manipulation |
|---|---|

History of neck trauma
Pain less than 1 year
Worsening of pain since onset
Pain ratings of 8+ on a 0 to 10 scale
NDI scores of 16 or more
Moderate or severe headache
Nausea during the past month
Lack of confidence in the treatment

Data from Hurwitz EL, Morgenstern H, Vassilaki M, et al: *Spine* 30(13):1477-1484, 2005.

niques, especially when the patient has high levels of pain and disability associated with an acute neck pain episode. Cagnie et al[94] surveyed 465 patients treated by 59 manipulative physical therapists after the first visit, and 60% reported at least one postmanipulation reaction. The most common reactions were headache (19%), stiffness (19.5%), local discomfort (15.2%), radiating discomfort (12.1%), and fatigue (12.1%). Most of these reactions began within 4 hours and generally disappeared within 24 hours. Women were more likely to report adverse effects than were men. Use of upper cervical manipulations, use of medication, gender, and age were independent predictors of headache after manipulation (Box 3-3). Upper cervical spine manipulation was 3.17 times more likely to cause headache than manipulation of the lower cervical spine, and for every 1 year increase in age, a 2.4% decrease was seen in risk of headache after manipulation.[94]

Although minor temporary adverse reactions to cervical spine manipulation are fairly common, catastrophic complications from cervical manipulation are extremely rare. The most catastrophic complication is vertebral artery dissection or vertebral basilar insufficiency (VBI), which is a condition characterized by occlusion or injury to the vertebral artery that causes loss of blood flow to the hindbrain. The vertebrobasilar system provides 10% to 20% of the blood supply to the brain and branches to many vital neural structures, including the brain stem, cerebellum, spinal cord, cranial nerves III to XII and their nuclei, and portions of the cerebral cortex.[95]

Vertebral basilar insufficiency may cause dizziness, lightheadedness, nausea, or numbness to the face. It could also result in slurred speech, nystagmus, or blurred vision. More severe cases of VBI can present as a cerebrovascular accident and even on occasion can cause death. The signs of VBI complications commonly reported include dizziness, diplopia, dysphagia, drop attaches, difficulty in swallowing, and nausea.[96] The vertebral artery is particularly susceptible to injury at the atlas because of its orientation and position at this mobile spinal level. Vigorous rotation of the neck is thought to potentially "kink" the vertebral artery along its course, which could cause dissection of the artery or trauma that may cause formation of a blood clot.[97] End range and forceful cervical spine rotation forces, especially when combined with cervical extension, have been implicated as the most likely source of injury to this portion of the vertebral artery.[98] Also important to note is that a patient with a vertebral artery dissection may initially have only a symptom of neck pain.[99,100]

DiFabio[101] completed an extensive review of the literature and found reports in the literature of 177 patients (from 1925 to 1997) with adverse events to manipulation. The primary diagnosis was arterial dissection/spasm and brain stem lesions, and 32 cases (18%) resulted in death.[101] Physical therapists were involved in less than 2% of the cases, and no deaths were attributed to cervical spine manipulation provided by physical therapists.[101] The type of manipulation was not described in 46% of the cases, but the largest percentage of cases in which the technique was reported included rotation (23%).[101] Only 10% of the cases reported that the injury occurred during the first manipulation.[101] DiFabio[101] concluded that because the potential risks of VBI from manipulation are catastrophic and because a lack of evidence showed that cervical spine thrust manipulation techniques are more effective than nonthrust manipulation techniques, the more gentle nonthrust mobilization/manipulation techniques are recommended to treat the cervical spine.

The exact risk of serious complications from cervical spine manipulation is not known. Rivett and Milburn[102] reported that the incidence rate of severe neurovascular compromise was estimated to be within a wide range of 1:50,000 manipulations to 1:5 million manipulations. Other estimates of risk of VBI from cervical spine manipulation have been stated as being 6 in 10 million manipulations or 0.00006%,[98,103] and the risk of death has been stated as 3 in 10 million manipulations.[103] Haldeman, Kohlbeck, and McGregor[98] found 367 cases of vertebral artery dissection or occlusion reported in the literature between 1966 and 1993 regardless of the mechanism of injury and reported that 43% of these cases were the result of spontaneous events such as standing up from a nap, 31% were from cervical spine manipulation, 16% were from trivial trauma such as a sudden head movement, and 10% were from major trauma such as a motor vehicle accident. Prediction of which patients may have VBI after cervical spine manipulation is difficult. Haldeman and Rubinstein[104] reviewed 64 cases of VBI (two deaths) after cervical spine manipulation and were unable to identify risk factors in the patient's history or physical examination that could predict the likelihood of a VBI event. Haldeman, Kohlbeck, and McGregor[98] concluded that vertebral artery dissection should be considered a rare, random, and unpredictable complication associated with activities such as neck movement, trauma, and manipulation.

The level of risk of serious injury from cervical spine manipulation compared with serious complications from other interventions commonly used to treat neck pain is very low. For instance, the likelihood of a serious gastrointestinal (GI) bleed from nonsteroidal antiinflammatory medications (NSAIDs) is 1 per 1000 versus 6 per 10 million cervical manipulations.[97] The death rate for NSAID-associated GI problems is estimated at 0.04% per year among patients with osteoarthritis who receive

NSAIDs, with 3200 deaths per year. Likewise, the risk of complication after cervical surgery is 16 per 1000.[103] Therefore, if the level of risk is put in this context, the risk associated with cervical manipulation is extremely low and the potential for successful outcomes is fairly high.

Currently no clinical prediction rule can accurately identify patients at risk for VBI, and little evidence supports the accuracy of historic information, physical examination screening procedures, or diagnostic imaging procedures to accurately identify patients at risk for VBI.[105] With screening examination procedures designed to occlude the vertebral artery test for potential risk of VBI, clinicians must recognize the strong possibility of a false-negative finding from the test. Cote et al[106] showed that the extension-rotation test has a sensitivity of approximately zero, which indicates a high likelihood of false-negative results from this commonly performed screening examination procedure (see Chapter 6). Reports are found in the literature of clinicians who performed these screening examination procedures and obtained a negative finding and still the patient had a VBI caused by the manipulation.[107,108] The suggestion is that no compelling evidence shows that either clinical examination or diagnostic imaging such as ultrasound scan can identify patients at risk for VBI.[105]

Mitchell et al[109] used transcranial Doppler sonography to show occlusion of the contralateral vertebral artery in 30 young healthy female subjects with a VBI test that used sustained end range cervical rotation with no symptoms reported by the subjects. Therefore, this study supported the use of cervical rotation to assess the collateral blood flow in the vertebral basilar system to screen for underlying vascular pathology. However, blood flow studies such as this do not support the validity, sensitivity, or specificity of the VBI test to predict patients who may be at risk of vertebral artery injury caused by a cervical spine manipulation. This type of blood flow study suggests that VBI manifests only with concomitant vascular anomaly or predisposing vascular pathology of the ipsilateral vertebral artery.[95]

If the primary patient symptom with cervical rotation is dizziness, the cause of the dizziness could be a vestibular disturbance, sensorimotor disturbance related to cervical joint mechanoreceptor dysfunction, or a VBI problem. The validity, sensitivity, or specificity of clinical tests to differentiate these conditions has not been tested. One such test is to hold the head still as the patient rotates the body to induce cervical rotation without moving the head (see Chapter 6). In theory, this test prevents stimulation of the vestibular system but still stresses the vascular and cervical joints.

Some argue that premanipulative testing should be abandoned because of its doubtful predictive validity and because the risk caused by the test is potentially greater than the level of force that is used in many cervical spine manipulation techniques.[95,100,110] Other authors contend that if testing occasionally prevents a stroke, then its use is warranted.[95,111,112]

Whether or not a clinician uses a VBI test for premanipulation screening, ongoing patient assessment is needed throughout cervical spine manipulation technique application. This assessment should include holding the manipulation position (10 seconds) before application of the thrust while monitoring for nystagmus, slurred speech, nausea, or dizziness. If the patient tolerates the neck position well, the technique can be used. If the patient does not tolerate it well, other procedures should be used. In addition, safety should be built into technique selection and application for all patients. Haldeman, Kohlbeck, and McGregor[98] reported that 84% of the 115 cases of vertebral artery injury from manipulation involved end range cervical rotation as a component of the technique. Use of multiple planes of movement can assist in finding a manipulative barrier for an effective technique while avoiding end range rotation with the manipulation procedure. Also, maintenance of slight cervical spine forward bending with application of cervical manipulation may facilitate safety. Thoracic spine manipulation techniques can also be used to relieve cervical spine pain,[113] and thoracic manipulation is generally safe. A trial of more gentle nonthrust cervical manipulation techniques is wise, especially in patients with risk factors for adverse reactions to thrust manipulation, including higher pain scores (8+), higher NDI scores (16+), female gender, and treatment of the upper cervical spine. Use of the gentlest forces to the cervical spine to accomplish the therapy goals can assist in patient comfort and safety.

No replacement exists for ongoing assessment of the patient as manual physical therapy techniques are used to assure a safe patient response. If minor signs of VBI are noted during manual therapy examination or treatment procedures, the manual physical therapy must be immediately discontinued; the patient's head should be supported on a pillow, with the patient resting supine and the legs elevated to enhance blood flow to the brain. The patient must be closely monitored until full recovery.

In summary, severe adverse responses to thrust manipulation of the cervical spine are extremely rare. Thorough ongoing patient assessment is necessary to identify signs of VBI throughout the examination and treatment sessions, and thrust manipulation techniques to the cervical spine must not be used when positive signs of VBI are noted during the screening examination or treatment session. Manual physical therapy techniques that use nonthrust forces are less likely to cause adverse reactions compared with thrust manipulation techniques for the cervical spine. When in doubt, therapy should start with the gentler cervical spine techniques and use of thoracic thrust manipulation techniques to assist in the treatment of neck pain should be considered.

Serious or severe complications of lumbar spinal manipulation are extremely rare.[114] The most serious potential complication from lumbar manipulation is development of cauda equina syndrome. Cauda equina syndrome is a medical emergency that should be treated surgically as soon as possible for decompression of the cauda equina. The signs and symptoms of cauda equina syndrome may include urinary retention, fecal incontinence, widespread neurologic signs and symptoms in the lower extremities that may include gait abnormality, saddle area numbness, and a lax anal sphincter.[115]

Haldeman and Rubenstein[104] reviewed the literature in a 77-year period and could only find 10 reports of cauda equina syndrome after lumbar manipulation. The risk of cauda equina syndrome from lumbar manipulation has been estimated to be less than 1 in 100 million manipulations.[116,117] This level of risk of serious harm can be put into perspective relative to other common interventions for low back pain. With use of NSAIDs, the chance of development of serious gastrointestinal bleeding as a consequence is 1% to 3%; 7600 deaths and 76,000 hospitalizations annually in the United States are attributable to NSAIDs. If NSAIDs are used for more than 4 weeks, the chance of development of a GI bleed is 1/1000.[118-120] Compared with exercise, spinal manipulation is safer as well, with a risk of sudden death from exercise estimated to be 1 : 1.5 million episodes of vigorous physical exertion.[121] The risk of a serious complication of lumbar spinal manipulation compares favorably with other common interventions used to treat low back pain.

Minor short-lived side effects of lumbar manipulation are more common. Senstad, Leboeuf-Yde, and Borchgrevink[117] surveyed 1058 patients seen for 4712 treatment sessions by chiropractors in Norway, and 75% of all treatments included manipulation to the lumbar spine. No severe complications were noted, but 55% reported at least one minor side effect. The most common side effects included local discomfort (53%), headache (12%), fatigue (11%), and radiating discomfort (10%). Reactions were mild or moderate in 85% of the cases. Sixty-four percent of the reactions appeared within 4 hours of treatment, and 74% had disappeared within 24 hours. Uncommon reactions were dizziness, nausea, hot skin, or "other" symptoms, each accounting for 5% or less of the reactions.[122] Symptoms that began later than the day of or the day after treatment or symptoms that caused reduced activities of daily living were unusual.[117]

Leboeuf-Yde et al[123] surveyed 625 patients treated with 1856 spinal manipulations by chiropractors in Sweden. No severe complications or injuries were noted, but 44% reported at least one side effect, such as local discomfort, fatigue, or headache. The symptoms resolved in less than 48 hours in 81% of the cases.[123] The two studies on minor adverse effects of manipulation both surveyed patients who were treated with chiropractic manipulation. Similar data have not been collected on other practitioners, such as physical therapists who regularly practice spinal manipulation.

Contraindications to spinal manipulation can be separated into two categories: relative and absolute. The first contraindication to consider is a lack of indications. If other interventions have evidence of greater effectiveness for a particular disorder, manipulation should not be used. In addition, the patient must be screened for red flags, and appropriate referrals must be made if the patient has any of the red flags listed in Box 3-4. The absolute contraindications involve a situation in which the forces to be used for the manipulation are likely to cause harm regardless of modification in technique (Box 3-5). Relative contraindications are situations in which the potential exists for harm with manipulation but with adequate technique

---

**BOX 3-4    Red Flags**

The following are considered red flags to proceeding with treatment and are indications for further medical investigations such as imaging studies and referral to a specialists:

- Significant trauma
- Weight loss
- History of cancer
- Fever
- Intravenous drug use
- Steroid use
- Patient age >50 years
- Severe unremitting nighttime pain
- Pain that worsens on lying down

Adapted from Kendall NAS, Linton SJ, Main CJ: *Guide to assessing psychosocial yellow flags in acute low back pain: risk factors for long-term disability and work loss,* Wellington, New Zealand, 2002, Accident Rehabilitation and Compensation Insurance Corporation of New Zealand and the National Health Committee.

---

**BOX 3-5    Absolute Contraindications to Manipulation**

Lack of indications
Poor integrity of ligamentous or bony structures from recent
    injury or disease process
        Unstable fracture
        Bone tumors
        Infectious disease
        Osteomyelitis
Vertebral basilar insufficiency (cervical spine)
Rheumatoid arthritis (upper cervical spine)
Use of anticoagulant medication

---

**BOX 3-6    Relative Contraindications to Manipulation**

Osteoporosis
Herniated disc with radiculopathy
Signs of spinal instability
Rheumatoid arthritis
Pregnancy

---

modification, skill, and special care, the technique may still be effective and cause no harm (Box 3-6).

## GUIDING PRINCIPLES OF MANIPULATION PERFORMANCE

The patient must be positioned in a relaxed supported position. The therapist must learn to effectively use his or her entire body to most effectively manipulate the spine. A diagonal stance position is usually most beneficial to create a stable base of support, and the therapist must use an athletic stance (such as a baseball player uses to hit a baseball or a football player uses to react to the direction of the ball), with the knees and hips slightly flexed, the spine in neutral, and the weight forward on the balls of the feet. The touch must be a firm

professional contact that shows the patient competence and caring. The forearms, when appropriate, should be positioned in line with the direction of the manipulation force to be applied. With application of the manipulation forces, a firm stable trunk should be created through use of self cocontraction/stabilization of the spinal and scapular muscles. The fingers/hands should be as relaxed and supple as possible for patient comfort.

For a thrust manipulation, the tissue slack of the joint and surrounding soft tissues is taken up with the primary and secondary levers. A primary lever is used to first begin the application of the force, followed by further slack taken up with use of secondary levers; the final manipulation force is through the primary lever. The application of multiple vectors or levers of force used in a spinal manipulation follows the same basic principles regardless of the technique used. Once the therapist and patient positionings are attained, the therapist should begin with application of the primary vector (force plus direction) to take up part of the tissue slack. Secondary vectors are then used to further take up tissue slack to create a firm joint barrier. As each secondary force vector is applied, the primary vector is retested to determine whether a firm joint barrier (end feel) has been reached. Once a firm joint barrier has been attained, the primary force vector (or lever) is applied with a manipulative force to create a treatment effect.

The advantage of use of multiple vectors or levers of force with a thrust manipulation is that a barrier can be attained against which to stretch a joint without a forceful end range of motion position of the targeted joint. This is thought to provide a safer technique, especially in avoiding end range rotation of the cervical spine, which has been implicated as a risk factor for injury to vertebral artery with cervical spine thrust manipulations. The use of multiple lever arms/directions of force creates a firm end feel or barrier at which point the primary technique lever is used to induce the final manipulative thrust. Many of the oscillatory techniques do not use a great deal of locking with multiple levers of motion but instead use only one direction of force to induce the motion. With the thrust techniques, creation of firm end barrier is necessary for effective manipulation of the targeted spinal segment.

Patients need to be encouraged to relax throughout the manipulation procedure. If a patient is actively resisting the premanipulation positioning, a less vigorous technique is best to try to gain greater confidence from the patient, or an isometric manipulation technique can be used. For an isometric manipulation technique or muscle energy technique, the patient is positioned at a joint barrier and then light manual pressure is applied as the patient actively resists the movement to create an isometric contraction of the agonistic muscles for the desired motion. After a 10-second hold, the tissue slack is taken up with passive or active moving of the spine further into the desired range of motion. The barrier could be a sense of tissue resistance or pain. At this new barrier or just short of the painful barrier, another 10-second agonist isometric contraction is completed. The sequence is repeated three to four times, after which the motion is reassessed. If gains are made, this treatment may be enough at that segment for the treatment session; or if joint stiffness is still evident, the segment may be further manipulated.

Before manipulation, warming of the tissues and body through exercise is advisable. Often a general warm-up is used, such as an upper body ergometer, NuStep (NuStep Inc., Ann Arbor, Michigan), elliptical machine, or treadmill. The warm-up is followed by specific exercises that target the impaired region, such as cervical or lumbar stabilization exercises or scapular theraband exercises. Beginning with exercise also emphasizes the importance of the home exercise program to the patient and allows the therapist to reassess the patient by observing movement patterns and range of motion with the exercises. Key impairment findings should be reexamined before application of the manual therapy techniques. At this point, manual therapy techniques can be applied to the impaired regions and might include, in the case of a patient with primary LBP symptoms, manipulation of the hip joints, lumbopelvic region, lumbar spine, or thoracic spine.

Immediately after the manipulation procedures, key findings should be reassessed, such as muscle tissue tone and active or passive motion testing, to determine whether the patient had a positive effect from the manipulation. Additional exercise or functional activities should be completed after the manipulation to further assess the patient's progress, to provide further education on lifting or home exercise programs, and to move into the greater and more comfortable ranges of motion created with the manual therapy procedures.

## TEACHING STRATEGIES FOR THE PSYCHOMOTOR COMPONENTS OF MANIPULATION

In the past, physical therapist educators have argued that only experienced physical therapists are qualified to learn high velocity thrust manipulation.[91] However, Cohen et al[124] showed that skilled performance of a spinal manipulation technique, as quantified with a force plate device, was no different for a group of experienced chiropractors as compared with a group of newly trained chiropractic students. However, 12 of the 15 experienced chiropractics admitted to not using the manipulation technique that was tested on a regular basis even though they were previously trained in the technique. This study suggests that with training and practice, a novice practitioner can have an equal level of skill in performance of a spinal manipulation procedure as an experienced manipulator. The key to further skill enhancement for both the novice and the experienced practitioners is further practice and feedback. Flynn, Fritz, and Wainner[125] further illustrated how well physical therapy students could do with training in manipulation by reporting on the successful clinical outcomes of final year physical therapy students who used an evidence-based approach to show successful patient outcomes with use of manipulation and therapeutic exercise for patients with symptoms of low back pain. The physical therapy students showed practice behaviors more

in line with clinical practice guidelines than past surveys of practicing physical therapists.[125]

There are three stages of learning motor skills such as manipulation. First is the cognitive stage in which the learner is new at a task and the primary concern is to understand what is to be done, how the performance is to be scored, and how best to attempt the first few trials.[126] Much cognitive activity is needed to determine appropriate strategies, but with practice, the performance rapidly improves. The second phase is the associative phase in which the individual has determined the most effective way of doing the task and begins to make more subtle adjustments in how the skill is performed.[126] Performance improvements are subtler, but gradual changes in performance make the task more effective. The last stage is the autonomous phase in which the skill has become automatic.[126] At this phase, the learner can perform the task at a high level without much thought and can concurrently perform other tasks if needed.[126] For students to develop enough confidence in manipulation technique performance to use them on a regular basis in a clinical situation after graduation, they likely need to develop the skill to at least the associative phase.

Mann, Patriquin, and Johnson[127] reported on the use of the mastery learning technique to instruct osteopathic students in the performance of a shoulder manipulation procedure. The four key components of mastery learning are: first, clear specification of desired learning outcomes; second, careful development of detailed learning materials that closely match the learning objectives; third, self-paced learning that may include independent study and group-based methods so that the student studies and practices until confident of meeting the criteria specified in the objectives; and fourth, multiple opportunities to demonstrate achievement of the learning objectives with individualized corrective feedback.[127] Ninety second year osteopathic students were given a handout and asked to view a videotape of a shoulder manipulation technique.[127] They were given 2 days to practice the shoulder manipulation procedure and then set up an appointment with an instructor to demonstrate the technique and receive feedback. No penalty was applied for students who needed corrective feedback, but after the feedback, the students were requested to demonstrate the technique correctly. Only four students were required to repeat the technique, and their errors were easily corrected after the feedback session.[127] The authors commented that student anxiety was less because students were given more than one opportunity to demonstrate the technique correctly. Students reported that they practiced on average 67 minutes, with a range of 5 minutes to 4 hours. Positive student feedback was received regarding this method of teaching; however, a retest was never performed to determine retention of the manipulative procedure nor was this learning method compared with other traditional means of teaching manipulation.[127]

Watson[128] completed a pilot study that used a similar method of instruction of a thoracic spinal manipulation technique (HVT) with physical therapy students. In this study, 23 students were divided into three groups. All students received training in a thoracic spinal manipulation technique. Group 1 (n = 8) was trained by an instructor who gave delayed (summary) verbal feedback after a practice session. Group 2 (n = 8) received training via videotape observation with no instructor feedback, and group 3 (n = 7) was trained by an instructor who gave concurrent verbal feedback while the students practiced.[128] The students were then asked to train 10 minutes per day for 1 week, after which time they were graded on performance of the technique. Next, the students were asked to refrain from practice and to return 1 week later for retention testing. No difference was seen in acquisition of the motor skill at the first testing session between the three teaching methods, but group 3 showed significantly better retention of the skill when tested 1 week later as compared with the other two groups.[128] Although Watson's study is somewhat inconclusive because of the small sample size, it provides some initial data to illustrate the importance of qualitative concurrent performance feedback in skill retention. Also of interest is that the results of the initial level of performance were the same regardless of whether the technique was demonstrated via videotape or in person but the primary factor that influenced retention was the quality and quantity of the feedback.

In the motor learning literature, practice and feedback have been recognized as the two most important factors in learning motor skills. First, a student must be motivated to learn a task. For facilitation of motivation, Schmidt[126] suggests taking the time to make the task seem important and setting goals. Next, the learner must be provided with an image of the task, which can be done with instructions, demonstrations, videos and other means. The instruction can begin to develop the student's "error detection mechanism" and the do's and don'ts of the task.[126] Further research is needed to investigate the optimal amount of instructions to give at one time, but Schmidt recommends starting with the most essential elements of the task followed by more instruction and feedback as the student starts to practice and refine the task.[126] However, for complex tasks, instructions alone are crude and inadequate. Demonstration enhances performance when compared with just verbal instruction, and a second demonstration during the practice session further enhances learning.[126]

Once the task is instructed and demonstrated, the student must practice. Variability in practice tends to allow students to learn the task more effectively and allows them to perform a new version of the task with less error than if the practice was more constant.[126] Therefore, students should be encouraged to practice manipulation techniques for multiple regions of the spine during one practice session to be challenged in discussing and manipulating the varying spinal mechanics of each region of the spine. This practice should facilitate greater retention and skill acquisition, but further research is needed in this area. The two most important variables in practice are the amount of practice attempts and the knowledge of results (i.e., feedback).

Knowledge of results (KR) refers to the information about the success in performance of the task that the performer receives after the trial has been completed, and it serves as a basis for corrections on the next trial, leading to more effective performance as the trial continues.[126] Although more practice trials tend to result in greater learning, without knowledge of success in the task, as practice continues, learning may be drastically reduced (or nonexistent) even though many practice trials are provided.[126] Students should be given basic guidelines of self-assessment measures to be used in manual therapy, such as proper body mechanics, forearm alignment, and use of a diagonal stance. Students should also seek feedback from classmates and instructors regarding depth and comfort of pressure application.

Knowledge of results can facilitate motivation to practice, provide guidance to the practice session, and assist with better goal setting, which causes the performer to set higher performing goals, but these effects may disappear as soon as KR is removed.[125] Decreasing the relative frequency of KR by increasing frequency of no KR aids long-term retention of the task.[125] Relative frequency of KR should be high in initial practice, when guidance and motivation are critical, but the instructor should systematically decrease frequency of KR as the performer becomes more proficient.[125] Therefore, initially, the instructor and classmates should provide a great deal of feedback, but as practice continues, the student needs to develop intrinsic means to monitor performance and to self correct to perform successfully in future clinical setting.

Guidance is useful for skill acquisition, but some loss of long-term learning effect occurs as a result of loss of trial and error and the self corrections that facilitate learning.[126] Guidance is, however, helpful to prevent injury with potentially dangerous motor skills like certain maneuvers in gymnastics, but the student must eventually practice the task without guidance to fully develop the skill.[126] With more complex manipulation procedures such as lumbar rotation manipulation, verbal step-by-step instructions to the class are often helpful to talk the students safely through the procedure during the first attempt. For facilitation of learning, students must be allowed to progress to further practice without verbal cueing. However, feedback on performance errors are needed to enhance the skill performance.

Knowledge of performance (KP) is the feedback instructors typically give students regarding correction of improper movement patterns rather than just outcome of movement in the environment.[126] Knowledge of performance has been studied with videotape replays, and in general, the benefit of this type of feedback is best if the instructor can cue the learner to focus on specific aspects of the task. A more general viewing can provide too much extra information that may not enhance performance.[126] KP feedback can be provided verbally during a performance by a coach or instructor who is knowledgeable of the procedure. Detailed analysis of movement patterns of skilled individuals can also facilitate training programs.[126] A skilled manual therapy instructor can observe the student's performance and provide feedback to instantly enhance the student's performance of the technique. In contrast, knowledge of results is often provided in manual therapy by the patient's response to the treatment, such as favorable reassessment results like increased range of motion.

Despite the evidence supporting the importance of feedback for motor skill learning, the quality and quantity of feedback provided to physical therapy students learning new manual therapy techniques are often lacking. In many academic laboratory sessions, the instructor demonstrates a technique and the students practice the techniques on each other as the instructor walks through the room to provide feedback. However, because the student-to-faculty ratios are typically 15:1 (standard deviation = 4.9),[129] the instructors is not able to provide feedback for most of the students for each technique. Most instructors are hopeful that the students provide each other with quality feedback. However, Petty and Cheek[130] found that even postgraduate students participating in a manual therapy residency program provided inconsistent and unreliable feedback to classmates while learning manual therapy procedures. Petty and Cheek[130] point out that one factor that likely contributes to the poor reliability commonly associated with passive intervertebral motion testing procedures is inadequate learning of the skills. The cause of the inadequate learning of manual therapy procedures may be inadequate teaching, practice, and feedback that are necessary for complex skill acquisition and retention.

Keating and Bach[131] used a bathroom scale to train a group of six postgraduate manual therapy residency students to produce a specific level of posterior-anterior force and compared this group's ability to reproduce these forces on a subject's lumbar spine with a similar group of manual therapy residents who did not participate in the bathroom scale training. The trained group was able to be more specific with force application for PA force application in the lumbar spine compared with the control group.[131] This study shows that if the therapist is given specific knowledge of results (i.e., feedback), skill level improves.[131]

Lee and Refshauge[132] used a similar force plate treatment table device to provide concurrent quantitative feedback to a group of 31 physical therapy students who were taught a grade II mobilization technique at the third lumbar vertebral level. A second group of 22 students were in the control group and were taught the same procedures in the traditional manner. After training with this device, the students' forces were compared with the "ideal forces" as applied by the expert instructor. The accuracy and consistency of force application of the experimental group was greater than that of the control group.[132] If this type of device were more readily available, mobilization/manipulation skill acquisition might be enhanced. However, this force plate device does not provide the student with feedback regarding tissue tension, resistance, or end feel. Therefore, this device cannot replace the type of qualitative feedback that a skilled clinical instructor can provide a student in a clinical setting.

Further research is needed in development of training tools to assist therapists to learn to more effectively and accurately grade passive intervertebral motion and end feel resistance. The research suggests that manual skills can be learned and retained more effectively if concurrent qualitative and quantitative feedback is provided. If an instructor must provide all the feedback, small student-to-faculty ratios are needed to provide the necessary feedback or more open laboratory practice sessions are needed with instructors present to provide quality feedback.

## REFERENCES

1. American Physical Therapy Association (APTA): Guide to physical therapist practice, ed 2, *Phys Ther* 81:9-746, 2001.

2. APTA, Manipulation Education Committee: *Manipulation education manual for physical therapist professional degree programs,* Alexandria, VA, 2004, APTA.

3. Maitland G: *Vertebral manipulation,* ed 5, London, 1986, Butterworth.

4. Paris SV: *Introduction to spinal evaluation and manipulation,* Atlanta, 1986, Institute Press.

5. Goodridge JP: Muscle energy technique: definition, explanation, methods of procedure, *J Am Osteopath Assoc* 81(4):249-254, 1981.

6. Knott M, Voss D: *Proprioceptive neuromuscular facilitation,* ed 2, New York, 1968, Harper and Row.

7. Sackett DL, Straus SE, Richardson WS, et al: *Evidence-based medicine: how to practice and teach EBM,* ed 2, Edinburgh, 2000, Churchill Livingstone.

8. Bigos S, Bowyer O, Braen G: *Acute low back problems in adults: clinical practice guideline no. 14; AHCPR publication no. 95-0642,* Rockville, MD, 1994, Agency for Health Care Policy and Research, Public Health Service, US Department of Health and Human Services; www.ahcpr.gov.

9. Department of Defense/Veterans Administration (DOD/VA): *Guidelines,* available at www.cs.amedd.army.mil/qmo/lbpfr.htm.

10. Hutchinson A, Waddell G, Feder G, et al: *Clinical guidelines for the management of acute low back pain,* London, 1996 (updates 1999, 2001), Royal College of General Practitioners; www.rcgp.org.uk.

11. Gross AR, Hoving JL, Haines TA, et al: A Cochrane review of manipulation and mobilization for mechanical neck disorders, *Spine* 29(14):1541-1548, 2004.

12. Paris SV: Spinal manipulative therapy, *Clin Orthop Related Res* 179:55-61, 1983.

13. Nansel D: Effects of cervical adjustment on lateral-flexion passive end-range asymmetry and on blood pressure, heart rate and plasma catecholamine levels, *J Manipulative Physiol Ther* 14:450-456, 1991.

14. Suter E, McMorland G: Decrease in elbow flexor inhibition after cervical spine manipulation in patients with chronic neck pain, *Clin Biomech* 17:541-544, 2002.

15. Cassidy JD, Lopes AA, Yong-Hing K: The immediate effect of manipulation versus mobilization on pain and range of motion in cervical spine: a randomized controlled trial, *J Manipulative Physiol Ther* 15:570-575, 1992.

16. Gavin D: The effect of joint manipulation techniques on active arrange of motion in the mid-thoracic spine of asymptomatic subjects, *J Manual Manipulative Ther* 7:114-122, 1999.

17. Sims-Williams H, Jayson MIV, Yong SMS, et al: Controlled trial of mobilization and manipulation for patients with low back pain in general practice, *BMJ* 11:1338-1340, 1978.

18. Frankel VH, Norkin M: *Basic biomechanics of the skeletal system,* Philadelphia, 1980, Lea & Febiger.

19. Woo S, Matthews J, Akeson WH, et al: Connective tissue response to immobility, *Arthritis Rheum* 18(3):257-264, 1975.

20. Taylor DC, Dalton JD, Seaber AV, et al: Viscoelastic properties of muscle tendon units. the biomechanical effects of stretching, *Am J Sports Med* 18(3):211-220, 1990.

21. Warren CG, Lehmann JF, Koblanski JN: Elongation of rat tail tendon: effect of load and temperature, *Arch Phys Med Rehabil* 52:465-474, 1971.

22. Warren CG, Lehmann JF, Koblanski JN: Heat and stretch procedures: an evaluation using rat tail tendon, *Arch Phys Med Rehabil* 57:122-126, 1976.

23. Nachemson AL, Evans JH: Some mechanical properties of the third human lumbar interlaminar ligament, *J Biomech* 1:211-220, 1968.

24. Tipton CM, Matthes RD, Maynard JA, et al: The influence of physical activity on ligaments and tendons, *Med Sci Sports* 7(3):165-175, 1975.

25. Cummings GS, Crutchfield CA, Barnes MR: *Orthopedic physical therapy series volume I: soft tissue changes in contractures,* ed 2, Atlanta, 1983, Stokesville Publishing Co.

26. Hertling D, Kessler RM: *Management of common musculoskeletal disorders: physical therapy principles and methods,* ed 3, Philadelphia, 1996, Lippincott Williams and Wilkins.

27. Baur PS, Parks DH, Hudson JD: Epithelial mediated wound contraction in experimental wounds: the purse-string effect, *J Trauma* 24(8):713-721, 1984.

28. Gainsbury JM: High-velocity thrust and pathophysiology of segmental dysfunction. In Glaswo EF, Twomey LT, Scull ER, et al, editors: *Aspects of manipulative therapy,* ed 2, New York, 1985, Churchill Livingstone.

29. Lewitt K: *Manipulative therapy in rehabilitation of the local motor system,* Boston, 1985, Butterworth.

30. Edmond SL: *Joint mobilization/manipulation extremity and spinal techniques,* ed 2, St Louis, 2006, Mosby.

31. Bogduk N, Engel R: The menisci of the lumbar zygapophyseal joints: a review of their anatomy and clinical significance, *Spine* 9:454-459, 1984.

32. Engel R, Bogduk N: The menisci of the lumbar zygapophyseal joints, *J Anat* 135:795-809, 1982.

33. Tullberg T, Blomberg S, Branth B, et al: Manipulation does not alter the position of the sacroiliac joint: a roentgen stereophotoprammetric analysis, *Spine* 23:1124-1128, 1998.

34. Thomas JS, France CR: Pain-related fear is associated with avoidance of spinal motion during recovery from low back pain, *Spine* 32(16):E460-E466, 2007.

35. Groen GJ, Baljet B, Drukker J: Nerve and nerve plexuses of the human vertebral column, *Am J Anat* 188:282-296, 1990.

36. McLain RF: Mechanoreceptor endings in human cervical facet joints, *Spine* 19:495-501, 1994.

37. Amonoo-Kuofi HS: The number and distribution of muscle spindles in human intrinsic postvertebral muscles, *J Anat* 135:585-599, 1982.

38. Richmond FJR, Bakker DA: Anatomical organization and sensory receptor content of soft tissues surrounding upper cervical vertebrae in the cat, *J Neurophysiol* 48:49-61, 1982.

39. McLain RF, Pickar JG: Mechanoreceptor endings in human thoracic and lumbar facet joints, *Spine* 23:168-173, 1998.

40. Wyke B: The neurology of joints: a review of general principles, *Clinics Rheum Dis* 7(1):223-239, 1981.

41. Bolton PS: The somatosensory system of the neck and its effect on the central nervous system, *J Manipulative Physiol Ther* 21:553-563, 1998.

42. Souvils T, Vicenzino B, Wright A: Neurophysiological effects of spinal manual therapy. In Boyling JD, Jull G. editors: *Grieve's modern manual therapy: the vertebral column*, Edinburgh, 2004, Churchill Livingstone.

43. Cannon JT, Prieto GJ, Lee A, et al: Evidence for opioid and non-opioid forms of stimulation produced analgesia in the rat, *Brain Res* 243:315-321, 1982.

44. Hosobuchi Y, Adams JE, Linchitz R: Pain relief by electrical stimulation of the central gray matter in human an its reversal by naloxone, *Science* 197:183-186, 1977.

45. Reynolds DV: Surgery in the rat during electrical analgesia induced by focal brain stimulations, *Science* 164:444-445, 1969.

46. Fanselow MS: The midbrain periaqueductal gray as a coordinator of action in response to fear and anxiety. In Depaulis A, Bandler R, editors: *The midbrain periaqueductal gray matter*, New York, 1991, Plenum Press.

47. Lovick TA: Interactions between descending pathways from dorsal and ventrolateral periaqueductal gray matter in rats. In Depaulis A, Bandler R, editors: *The midbrain periaqueductal gray matter*, New York, 1991, Plenum Press.

48. Morgan MM: Differences in antinociception evoked from dorsal and ventral regions of the caudal periaqueductal gray matter. In Depaulis A, Bandler R, editors: *The midbrain periaqueductal gray matter*, New York, 1991, Plenum Press.

49. Yezierski RP: Somatosensory input to the periaqueductal gray: a spinal relay to a descending control center. In Depaulis A, Bandler R, editors: *The midbrain periaqueductal gray matter*, New York, 1991, Plenum Press.

50. Wright A: Hypoalgesic post-manipulative therapy: a review of a potential neurophysiological mechanism, *Manual Ther* 1:11-16, 1995.

51. Sterling M, Jull G, Wright A: Cervical mobilization: concurrent effects on pain, sympathetic nervous system activity and motor activity, *Manual Ther* 6:72-81, 2001.

52. Terrett ACJ, Vernon H: Manipulation and pain tolerance, *Am J Phys Med* 63:217-225, 1984.

53. Dhouldt W, Willaeys T, Verbruggen LA, et al: Pain threshold in patients with rheumatoid arthritis and effect of manual therapy, *Scand J Rheumatol* 28:88-93, 1999.

54. Peterson NP, Vicenzino B, Wright A: The effects of a cervical mobilization technique on sympathetic outflow to the upper limb in normal subjects, *Physiother Theory Pract* 9:149-156, 1993.

55. Vicenzino B, Guschlag F, Collins D, et al: An investigation of the effects of spinal manual therapy on forequarter pressure and thermal pain thresholds and sympathetic nervous system activity in asymptomatic subjects. In Shakclock M, editor: *Moving in on pain*, Melbourne, 1995, Butterworth Heinneman.

56. Wright A, Vicenzino B: Cervical mobilization techniques, sympathetic nervous system effects and their relationship to analgesia. In Shacklock M, editor: *Moving in on pain*, Melbourne, 1995, Butterworth Heinneman.

57. Vernon HT, Dhami MSI, Howley TP, et al: Spinal manipulation and beta-endorphin: a controlled study of the effects of a spinal manipulation on plasma beta-endorphin levels in normal males, *J Manipulative Physiol Ther* 9(2):115-123, 1986.

58. Christian GH, Stanton GJ, Sissons D, et al: Immunoreactive ACTH, beta-endorphin, and cortisol levels in plasma following spinal manipulative therapy, *Spine* 13:141-147, 1988.

59. Sanders GE, Reinnert O, Tepe R, et al: Chiropractic adjustive manipulation on subjects with acute low back pain: visual analog scores and plasma beta-endorphin levels, *J Manipulative Physiol Ther* 13:391-395, 1990.

60. Zusman M, Edwards B, Donaghy A: Investigation of a proposed mechanism for the relief of spinal pain with passive joint movement, *J Manual Med* 4:58-61, 1989.

61. Vicenzino B, O'Callaghan J, Felicity K, et al: *No influence of nnaloxone on the initial hypalgesic effect of spinal manual therapy*, Vienna, 2000, Ninth World Congress on Pain.

62. Sykba DA, Radhakrishnana R, Rohlwing JJ, et al: Joint manipulation reduces hyperalgesia by activation of monoamine receptors by not opioid or GAGA receptors in the spinal cord, *Pain* 106:159-168, 2003.

63. McGuiness J, Vicenzino B, Wright A: The effects of a posteroanterior cervical mobilization technique on central sympathetic nervous system function, *Physiother Theory Pract* 1995.

64. Vicenzino B, Cartwright T, Collins D, et al: Cardiovascular and respiratory changes produced by lateral glide mobilization of the cervical spine, *Manual Ther* 3:67-71, 1998.

65. Vicenzino B, Collins D, Wright A: The initial effects of cervical spine manipulative physiotherapy on pain and dysfunction in lateral epicondylagia, *Pain* 68:69-74, 1996.

66. Cleland JA, Whitman JM, Fritz JM: Effectiveness of manual physical therapy to the cervical spine in the management of lateral epicondylalgia: a retrospective analysis, *JOSPT* 34:713-724, 2004.

67. Shambaugh P: Changes in electrical activity in muscles resulting from chiropractic adjustment: a pilot study, *J Manipulative Physiol Ther* 10:300-304, 1987.

68. Fisk JW: A controlled trial of manipulation in a selected group of patients with low back pain favoring one side, *N Z Med J* 90:228-291, 1979.

69. Dishman JD, Cunningham BM, Burke J: Comparison of tibial nerve H-reflex excitability after cervical and lumbar spine manipulation, *J Manipulative Physiol Ther* 25:318-325, 2002.

70. Liebler EJ, Tufano-Coors L, Douris P, et al: The effect of thoracic spine mobilization on lower trapezius strength testing, *J Manual Manipulative Ther* 9:207-212, 1986.

71. Cleland J, Selleck B, Stowell T, et al:. Short-term effects of thoracic manipulation on lower trapezius muscle strength, *JMMT* 12(2):82-90, 2004.

72. Suter E, McMorland G, Herzog W, et al: Decrease in quadriceps inhibition after sacroiliac joint manipulation in patients with anterior knee pain, *J Manipulative Physiol Ther* 22:149-153, 1999.

73. Jamison JR, McEwen AP, Thomas SJ: Chiropractic adjustment in the management of visceral conditions: a critical appraisal, *J Manipulative Physiol Ther* 15:171-180, 1992.

74. Schenk RJ, MacDiarmid A, Rousselle J: The effects of muscle energy technique on lumbar range of motion, *JMMT* 5(4):179-183, 1997.

75. Schenk RJ, Adelman K, Rousselle J: The effects of muscle energy technique on cervical range of motion, *JMMT* 2(4):149-155, 1994.

76. Beaulieu JE: Developing a stretching program, *Phys Sports Med* 9(11):59-65, 1981.

77. Levine MG, Kabat H, Knott M, et al: Relaxation of spasticity by physiological technics, *Arch Phys Med Rehabil* 35:214-223, 1954.

78. Greenman P: *Principles of manual medicine*, Baltimore, 1989, Williams and Wilkins.

79. Roston JB, Haines RW: Cracking in the metacarpophalangeal joint, *Anatomy* 81(2):166-173, 1947.

80. Unsworth A, Dowson D, Wright V: Cracking joints: a bioengineering study of cavitation in the metacarpophalangeal joint, *Ann Rheum Dis* 30:348-357, 1971.

81. Flynn TW, Fritz JM, Wainner RS, et al: The audible pop is not necessary for successful spinal high-velocity thrust manipulation in individuals with low back pain, *Arch Phys Med Rehabil* 84:1057-1060, 2003.

82. Cleland JA, Childs JD: Does the manual therapy technique matter? *Orthop Division Rev* Sep/Oct:27-28, 2005.

83. Farrell JP, Twomey LT: Acute low back pain: comparison of two conservative treatment approaches, *Med J Aust* 1:160-164, 1982.

84. Hoving JL, Koes BW, de Vet HCW, et al: Manual therapy, physical therapy, or continued care by a general practitioner for patients with neck pain: a randomized controlled trial, *Ann Intern Med* 136:713-722, 2002.

85. Jull G, Trott P, Potter H, et al: A randomized controlled trial of physiotherapy management for cervicogenic headache, *Spine* 27:1835-1843, 2002.

86. Kulig K, Landel RF, Powers CM: Using dynamic MRI: a proposed mechanism of sagittal plane motion induced by manual posterior-to-anterior mobilization, *JOSPT* 34(2):61-64, 2004.

87. Chiradejnant A, Maher CG, Latimer J, et al: Efficacy of "therapist-selected" versus "randomly selected" mobilization techniques for the treatment of low back pain: a randomized controlled trial, *Aust J Physiother* 49:223-241, 2003.

88. Haas M, Groupp E, Panzer D, et al: Efficacy of cervical endplay assessment as an indicator for spinal manipulation, *Spine* 28(11):1091-1096, 2003.

89. Ross JK, Bereznick DE, McGill SM: Determining cavitation location during lumbar and thoracic spinal manipulation: is spinal manipulation accurate and specific? *Spine* 29(13):1452-1457, 2004.

90. Childs JD, Fritz JM, Flynn TW, et al: A clinical prediction rule to identify patients with low back pain most likely to benefit from spinal manipulation: a validation study, *Ann Intern Med* 141:920-928, 2004.

91. Flynn TW: Move it and move on, *J Orthop Sports Phys Ther* 32(5): 192-193, 2002.

92. Fritz J, Whitman JM, Childs JD: Lumbar spine segmental mobility assessment: an examination of validity for determining intervention strategies in patients with low back pain, *Arch Phys Med Rehabil* 86:1745-1752, 2005.

93. Hurwitz EL, Morgenstern H, Vassilaki M, et al: Frequency and clinical predictors of adverse reactions to chiropractic care in the UCLA neck pain study, *Spine* 30(13):1477-1484, 2005.

94. Cagnie B, Vinck E, Beernaert A, et al: How common are side effects of spinal manipulation and can these side effects be predicted? *Manual Ther* 9:151-156, 2004.

95. Rivett DA: The vertebral artery and vertebrobasilar insufficiency. In Bouling JD, Jull GA, editors: *Greive's modern manual therapy, the vertebral column*, ed 3, London, 2004, Churchill Livingstone.

96. Magarey ME, Rebbeck T, Coughlan B, et al: Pre-manipulative testing of the cervical spine review, revision and new clinical guidelines, *Manual Ther* 9:95-108, 2004.

97. Daubs V, Lauretti WJ: A risk assessment of cervical manipulation versus NSAIDs for the treatment of neck pain, *J Manipulative Physiol Ther* 18(8):530-535, 1995.

98. Haldeman S, Kohlbeck FJ, McGregor M: Risk factors and precipitating neck movements causing vertebrobasilar artery dissection after cervical trauma and spinal manipulation, *Spine* 24:785-794, 1999.

99. Krespi Y, Mahmu EG, Coban O, et al: Vertebral artery dissection presenting with isolated neck pain, *J Neuroimaging* 12(2):179-182, 2002.

100. Thiel H, Rix G: Is it time to stop functional pre-manipulation testing of the cervical spine? *Manual Ther* 10:154-158, 2005.

101. DiFabio RP: Manipulation of the cervical spine: risks and benefits, *Phys Ther* 79(1):50-65, 1999.

102. Rivett DA, Milburn P: A prospective study of complications of cervical spine manipulation, *J Manual Manipulative Ther* 4:166-170, 1996.

103. Hurwitz EL, Aker PD, Adams AH, et al: Manipulation and mobilization of the cervical spine: a systematic review of the literature, *Spine* 21:1746-1760, 1996.

104. Haldeman S, Rubinstein SM: Cauda equina syndrome in patients undergoing manipulation of the lumbar spine, *Spine* 17(12):1469-1473, 1992.

105. Childs JD, Flynn TW, Fritz JM, et al: Screening for vertebrobasilar insufficiency in patients with neck pain: manual therapy decision-making in the presence of uncertainty, *JOSPT* 35(5):300-306, 2005.

106. Cote P, Kreitz BG, Cassidy JD, et al: The validity of the extension-rotation test as a clinical screening procedure before neck manipulation: a secondary analysis, *J Manipulative Physiol Ther* 19:159-164, 1996.

107. Dvorak J, Orelli F: *How dangerous is manipulation to the cervical spine? Case report and results of a survey*, Manual Med 2:1-4, 1985.

108. Haldeman S, Kohlbeck FJ, McGregor M: Unpredictability of cerebrovascular ischemia associated with cervical spine manipulation therapy: a review of sixty-four cases after cervical spine manipulation, *Spine* 27:49-55, 2002.

109. Mitchell J, Keene D, Dyson C, et al: Is cervical rotation, as used in the standard vertebrobasilar insufficiency test, associated with a measurable change in intracranial vertebral artery blood flow? *Manual Ther* 9:220-227, 2004.

110. Cote P: Screening for stroke: let's show some maturity! *J Can Chiropract Assoc* 43:72-74, 1999.

111. Grant R: Vertebral artery testing: the Australian Physiotherapy Association Protocol after 6 years, *Manual Ther* 1:149-153, 1996.

112. Kunnasmaa KTT, Thiel HW: Vertebral artery syndrome: a review of the literature, *J Orthop Med* 16:17-20, 1994.

113. Cleland JA, Childs JD, Fritz JM, et al: Development of a clinical prediction rule for guiding treatment of a subgroup of patients with neck pain: use of thoracic spine manipulation, exercise, and patient education, *Phys Ther* 87(1):9-23, 2007.

114. Bronfort G, Haas M, Evans RL, et al: Efficacy of spinal manipulation and mobilization for low back pain and neck pain: a systematic review and best evidence synthesis, *Spine J* 4(3):335-356, 2004.

115. Danish Institute for Health Technology Assessment: *Low back pain: frequency, management and prevention from a health technology perspective*, Copenhagen, Denmark, 2000,

National Board of Health; www.gacguidelines.ca/article.pl?sid=02/07/05/2022215-.

116. Assendelft WJ, Bouter LM, Knipschild PG: Complications of spinal manipulation: a comprehensive review of the literature, *J Fam Pract* 42(5):475-480, 1996.

117. Senstad O, Leboeuf-Yde C, Borchgrevink C: Frequency and characteristics of side effects of spinal manipulative therapy, *Spine* 22(4):435-441, 1997.

118. Hungin AP, Kean WF: Nonsteroidal anti-inflammatory drugs: overused or underused in osteoarthritis? *Am J Med* 110(1A): 8S-11S, 2001.

119. Tamblyn R, Berkson L, Dauphinee WD, et al: Unnecessary prescribing of NSAIDS and the management of NSAID-related gastropathy in medical practice, *Ann Intern Med* 127(6):429-438, 1997.

120. Tannenbaum H, Davis P, Russell AS, et al: An evidence-based approach to prescribing NSAIDs in musculoskeletal disease: a Canadian consensus: Canadian NSAID consensus participants, *CMAJ* 155(1):77-88, 1996.

121. Albert CM, Mittleman MA, Chae CU, et al: Triggering of sudden death from cardiac causes by vigorous exertion, *N Engl J Med* 343(19):1355-1361, 2000.

122. Shekelle, PG, Adams AH, Chassin MR, et al: Spinal manipulation for low-back pain [see comments], *Ann Intern Med* 117(7):590-598, 1992.

123. Leboeuf-Yde C, Hennius B, Rudberg E, et al: Side effects of chiropractic treatment: a prospective study, *J Manipulative Physiol Ther* 20(8):511-515, 1997.

124. Cohen E, Triano J, McGregor M, et al: Biomechanical performance of spinal manipulation therapy by newly trained vs. practicing providers: does experience transfer to unfamiliar procedures? *J Manipulative Physiol Ther* 18(6):347-352, 1995.

125. Flynn TW, Fritz JM, Wainner RS: Spinal manipulation in physical therapist professional degree education: a model for teaching and integration into clinical practice, *JOSPT* 36(8):577-587, 2006.

126. Schmidt RA: *Motor control and learning,* ed 2, Champaign, Ill, 1988, Human Kinetics Publishers, Inc.

127. Mann DD, Patriquin DA, Johnson DF: Increasing osteopathic manipulative treatment skills and confidence through mastery learning, *J AOA* 100(5):301-304, 2000.

128. Watson TA: Comparison of three teaching methods for learning spinal manipulation skill: a pilot study, *J Manual Manipulative Ther* 9(1):48-52, 2001.

129. Bryan JM, McClune LD, Romito S, et al: Spinal mobilization curricula in professional physical therapy education programs, *J Phys Ther Educ* 11(2):11-15, 1997.

130. Petty NJ, Cheek L: Accuracy of feedback during training of passive accessory intervertebral movements, *J Manual Manipulative Ther* 9(2):99-108, 2001.

131. Keating JM, Bach TM: The effect of training on physical therapists' ability to apply specified forces of palpation, *Phys Ther* 73(1):38-46, 1993.

132. Lee M, Refshauge K: Effect of feedback on learning vertebral joint mobilization skill, *Phys Ther* 70(2):97-103, 1990.

## CHAPTER 4

# Examination and Treatment of Lumbopelvic Spine Disorders

## CHAPTER OVERVIEW

This chapter covers the kinematics of the lumbar spine, pelvis, and hips; describes common lumbopelvic spine disorders with a diagnostic classification system to guide clinical decision making; and provides a detailed description of special tests, manual examination, manipulation, and exercise procedures for the lumbar spine, pelvis, and hips.

## OBJECTIVES

- Describe the significance and impact of lumbopelvic spine disorders
- Describe lumbar spine, pelvic, and hip kinematics
- Classify lumbopelvic spine disorders based on signs and symptoms
- Describe interventions for lumbar spine, pelvic, and hip disorders
- Demonstrate and interpret lumbopelvic spine and hip examination procedures
- Describe contraindications and precautions for lumbopelvic spine manipulation
- Demonstrate manipulation techniques for the lumbar spine, pelvis, and hips
- Instruct exercises for lumbopelvic spine disorders

## SIGNIFICANCE OF THE LOW BACK PAIN PROBLEM

As many as 80% of Americans have symptoms of low back pain (LBP) during their lifetime.[1] LBP is the leading cause of injury and disability for those younger than 45 years of age and the third most prevalent impairment for those 45 years or older.[2]

Lumbar spinal stenosis (LSS) is associated with substantial medical costs, with an estimated 13% to 14% of patients seeking help from a specialty physician; up to 4% of those who seek care from a general practitioner for low back pain are diagnosed with LSS.[3]

In 2001, 122,316 lumbar spinal fusion procedures were performed for degenerative conditions in the United States, compared with 32,701 operations in 1990, which calculates to 61.1 operations per 100,000 adults in 2001 compared with 19.1 operations per 100,000 adults in 1990.[4] The increase is 220%.[4] The most rapid rise in fusion rates occurred for the diagnosis of degenerative disc disease. Lumbar fusion is among the most rapidly increasing of all major surgical procedures and one of the most expensive, with $4.8 billion spent on spinal fusion

surgeries in 2001 in the United States.[4] A twentyfold regional variation of lumbar fusion rates is found in the United States among Medicare enrollees in 2002 and 2003, which is likely the result of a lack of scientific evidence to guide surgical decision making, financial incentives, and professional opinion.[5] In other words, the likelihood of patients with degenerative spinal conditions undergoing fusion procedures is more dependent on where they live than clinical presentation.

The rapid increase in surgical rates and the escalating costs for treatment of lumbar conditions have not been matched by improved outcomes and reductions in disability. On the contrary, the level of disability associated with LBP as noted with work loss, early retirement, and state benefits has escalated as cost and surgical rates have increased.[6] An evidence-based approach to management of lumbar spine disorders is needed to prevent long-term disability and to empower patients to self manage recurrent future episodes of LBP. A nonsurgical evidence-based approach to management of lumbopelvic disorders is presented. An understanding of the functional anatomy and mechanics of the lumbar spine, pelvis, and hips establishes a foundation for the nonsurgical examination and treatment of these anatomic areas.

## Lumbopelvic Kinematics: Functional Anatomy and Mechanics

Lumbar spine active range of motion has been reported as 60 degrees flexion, 25 degrees extension, 25 degrees left and right lateral flexion, and 30 degrees left and right rotation.[7] Troke et al[8] used a modified CA6000 spine motion analyzer (Orthopedic Systems Inc., Union City, Calif., and Troke/University of Brighton) to establish normative lumbar spine range of motion values for 405 subjects aged 16 to 90 years. The median range of motion for lumbar forward bending ranged from 73 degrees for the youngest age group to 40 degrees for the oldest.[8] Backward bending ranged from 29 to 6 degrees, with a decline of 79% from the youngest age group to the oldest. Lateral flexion declined from 28 to 16 degrees, and rotation stayed consistent at 7 degrees.[8] Troke et al[8] found little difference in the median range of lumbar motion between male and female subjects across a large age spectrum (Table 4-1).

The lumbopelvic region moves in coordination with the hip joints to create a lumbopelvic rhythm with forward and backward bending. In a standing position with the knees extended, forward bending is produced with hip flexion, anterior pelvic tilt, and forward bending of the lumbar spine. The relative contribution of each to the total amount of forward bending is dependent on muscle length (e.g., hamstrings), joint mobility (e.g., hips, facet joints, and sacroiliac joint [SIJs]), and neuromuscular control. For correct function of lumbopelvic rhythm, hip flexion should be greater than lumbar forward bending and should occur first with functional activities.[9]

With forward bending of the lumbar spine, the posterior annular fibers of the intervertebral disc become taut and the anterior fibers become slack and bulge anteriorly. The nucleus pulposus of the disc is compressed anteriorly, and pressure is relieved over the posterior surface.[9] Based on computed tomography (CT) scan data, forward bending increases the size of the central canal 24 mm², or 11%, and backward bending decreases the size of the canal 26 mm², or 11%.[10] The neuroforaminal area increases 13 mm² (12%) in forward bending and decreases 9 mm² (15%) in backward bending.[10] Among the 25 motion segments studied, three compressed nerve roots were relieved with forward bending and five nerve roots were compressed with backward bending[10] (Figure 4-1).

The layers of annular fibers have an alternating oblique orientation to allow for only half of the fibers to be on tension during rotation. Forward bending places tension through all the posterior annular fibers, so the combination of rotation with forward bending may result in excessive strain to the posterior annular intervertebral disc fibers.[9] Nachemson[11] measured intradiscal pressure of the L3 vertebrae in various positions and found that intervertebral disc pressure was greatest with subjects sitting and leaning forward 20 degrees with weights in the hands. The standing position had less intradiscal pressure than did the sitting position, and the supine position was the least loaded discal pressure position (Figure 4-2). Nachemson's[11] work provides a basis for clinical decision making in interpretation of the symptom behaviors in patients with discogenic symptoms. For instance, if low back and leg pain symptoms are provoked with sitting and leaning forward, the likelihood of symptoms originating from a discogenic condition is increased.

The facet joints have two principal movements: translaction (slide or glide) and distraction (gapping).[12] When upglide occurs from both sides simultaneously, the result is forward bending; likewise, when downglide occurs from both sides simultaneously, backward bending is the result.[12] Forward bending involves a flattening of the lumbar lordosis, especially at the upper lumbar levels,[13] and involves a combination of anterior sagittal rotation and superior anterior translation (i.e., upglide) of the bilateral facet joints.

When upglide occurs on one side alone with downglide on the opposite side, the result is side bending (lateral flexion). Distraction occurs with axial rotation of the lumbar spine when one facet is compressed and becomes a fulcrum and when the facet on the side of rotation is distracted[12] (Figure 4-3). Tables 4-2 and 4-3 provide a list of the segmental lumbar forward and backward bending motions reported in the literature. These finding are based on healthy young adult subjects.

| TABLE 4-1 | Maximal and Minimal Median Ranges of Lumbar Spinal Motion Across All Subjects (Overall Age Range of Subjects, 16 to 90 y) | | | | |
|---|---|---|---|---|---|
| | **MALE** | | **FEMALE** | | |
| **MOVEMENT** | **MAXIMAL (MEDIAN OF VALUES; DEG)** | **MINIMAL** | **MAXIMAL (MEDIAN OF VALUES; DEG)** | **MINIMAL** | |
| Flexion | 73 | 40 | 68 | 40 | |
| Extension | 29 | 7 | 28 | 6 | |
| Right lateral flexion | 28 | 15 | 27 | 14 | |
| Left lateral flexion | 28 | 16 | 28 | 18 | |
| Right axial rotation | 7 | 7 | 8 | 8 | |
| Left axial rotation | 7 | 7 | 6 | 6 | |

From Troke M, Moore AP, Maillardet FJ, et al: *Manual Ther* 10:198-206, 2005.

### Anterior pelvic tilt with lumbar extension

### Posterior pelvic tilt with lumbar flexion

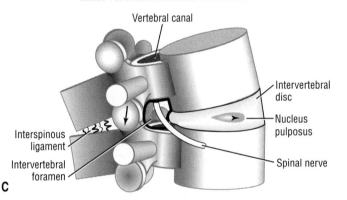

A

B

### Intervertebral lumbar extension

### Intervertebral lumbar flexion

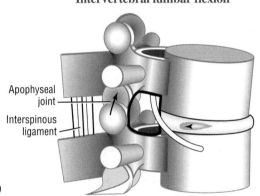

C

D

**FIGURE 4-1** Anterior and posterior tilt of pelvis and its effect on kinematics of lumbar spine. *A* and *C*, Anterior pelvic tilt extends lumbar spine and increases lordosis. *B* and *D*, Posterior pelvic tilt flexes lumbar spine and decreases lordosis. This action tends to shift nucleus pulposus posteriorly and increases diameter of intervertebral foramina. Muscle activity is shown in *blue*. From Neumann DA: *Kinesiology of the musculoskeletal system*, St Louis, 2002, Mosby.

| TABLE 4-2 | Lumbar Forward-Bending Segmental Range of Motion in Degrees | | |
|---|---|---|---|
| **LEVEL** | **PEARCY** | **PLAMONDON** | **PANJABI** |
| L1-L2 | 8.0 ± 5.0 | 5.1 ± 2.1 | 5.0 ± 1.0 |
| L2-L3 | 10.0 ± 2.0 | 8.8 ± 0.8 | 7.0 ± 1.2 |
| L3-L4 | 12.0 ± 1.0 | 11.6 ± 2.7 | 7.3 ± 1.5 |
| L4-L5 | 13.0 ± 4.0 | 13.1 ± 1.7 | 9.1 ± 2.5 |
| L5-S1 | 9.0 ± 6.0 | – | 9.0 ± 2.0 |

Adapted from Pearcy MJ, Tibrewal SB: *Spine* 9:582-587, 1984; Plamondon A, Gagnon M, Maurais G: Application of a stereoradiographic method for the study of intervertebral motion, *Spine* 13:1027-1032, 1988; and Panjabi MM, Oxland TR, Yamamoto I, et al: *J Bone Joint Surg (Am)* 76:413-424, 1994.

| TABLE 4-3 | Lumbar Backward-Bending Segmental Range of Motion in Degrees | | |
|---|---|---|---|
| **LEVEL** | **PEARCY** | **PLAMONDON** | **PANJABI** |
| L1-L2 | 5.0 ± 2.0 | 3.0 ± 3.0 | 4.1 ± 1.5 |
| L2-L3 | 3.0 ± 2.0 | 3.9 ± 2.9 | 3.3 ± 1.2 |
| L3-L4 | 1.0 ± 1.0 | 2.1 ± 0.9 | 2.6 ± 1.2 |
| L4-L5 | 2.0 ± 1.0 | 1.2 ± 1.2 | 3.6 ± 1.5 |
| L5-S1 | 5.0 ± 4.0 | – | 5.3 ± 2.0 |

Adapted from Pearcy MJ, Tibrewal SB: *Spine* 9:582-587, 1984; Plamondon A, Gagnon M, Maurais G: Application of a stereoradiographic method for the study of intervertebral motion, *Spine* 13:1027-1032, 1988; and Panjabi MM, Oxland TR, Yamamoto I, et al: *J Bone Joint Surg (Am)* 76:413-424, 1994.

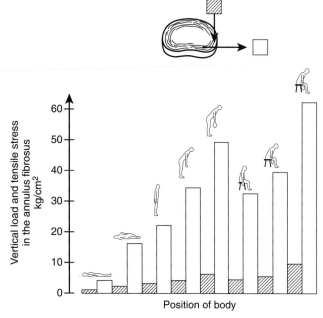

**FIGURE 4-2** Vertical load per unit of area on annulus fibrosus and tangential tensile stress in dorsal part of annulus fibrosus in L-3 disk in subject weighing 70 kg and assuming positions schematically shown. From Nachemson A: The load on lumbar disks in different positions of the body, *Clin Orthop* 45:107-122, 1966.

| TABLE 4-4 | Lumbar Axial Rotation Segmental Range of Motion with Couple Lateral Flexion in Degrees | | | |
|---|---|---|---|---|
| | **PEARCY** | | **PANJABI** | |
| **LEVEL** | **LEFT ROTATION** | **RIGHT LATERAL FLEXION** | **LEFT ROTATION** | **RIGHT LATERAL FLEXION** |
| L1-L2 | 1.0 | 3.0 | 2.3 ± 1.2 | 1.9 ± 0.8 |
| L2-L3 | 1.0 | 3.0 | 1.7 ± 0.9 | 2.2 ± 1.8 |
| L3-L4 | 2.0 | 3.0 | 2.3 ± 0.7 | 0.2 ± 1.6 |
| L4-L5 | 2.0 | 2.0 | 1.2 ± 1.0 | −2.2 ± 0.5 |
| L5-S1 | 0.0 | −1.0 | 1.0 ± 1.0 | −2.5 ± 1.8 |

Data compiled from Pearcy MJ, Tibrewal SB: *Spine* 9:582-587, 1984, and Panjabi MM, Oxland TR, Yamamoto I, et al: *J Bone Joint Surg (Am)* 76:413-424, 1994.

| TABLE 4-5 | Lumbar Lateral Flexion Segmental Range of Motion with Coupled Axial Rotation in Degrees | | | |
|---|---|---|---|---|
| | **PEARCY** | | **PANJABI** | |
| **LEVEL** | **RIGHT LATERAL FLEXION** | **LEFT ROTATION** | **RIGHT LATERAL FLEXION** | **LEFT ROTATION** |
| L1-L2 | 5.0 | 0.0 | 4.4 ± 0.5 | 0.0 ± 1.9 |
| L2-L3 | 5.0 | 1.0 | 5.8 ± 1.5 | 1.7 ± 0.6 |
| L3-L4 | 5.0 | 1.0 | 5.4 ± 1.1 | 0.9 ± 0.5 |
| L4-L5 | 3.0 | 1.0 | 5.3 ± 1.3 | 1.8 ± 1.0 |
| L5-S1 | 0.0 | 0.0 | 4.7 ± 0.9 | 1.7 ± 0.7 |

Data compiled from Pearcy MJ, Tibrewal SB: *Spine* 9:582-587, 1984, and Panjabi MM, Oxland TR, Yamamoto I, et al: *J Bone Joint Surg (Am)* 76:413-424, 1994.

Lateral flexion and axial rotation of the lumbar spine tend to occur as coupled motions, but the exact patterns of coupling direction seem to vary from one individual to another and from one lumbar spinal level to another. With rotation, a coupled lateral flexion tends to occur to the opposite side; and this pattern is more consistent for levels L1-L2 to L3-L4 in subjects without low back pain. Inconsistent findings are seen with lower lumbar spinal segments with this coupling pattern. Panjabi et al[14] found L4-L5 and L5-S1 rotation and coupled lateral flexion that occurred to the same side (Tables 4-4 and 4-5). Other findings showed that in patients with chronic low back pain with three different patterns of coupled motion may occur: either the opposite lateral flexion was coupled with axial rotation ("normal"), the same direction of lateral flexion was coupled with rotation, or no coupling lateral flexion occurred with rotation.[15] In one study, only 14% of the patients had "normal" coupling patterns of axial rotation in the opposite direction of the lateral flexion. Fifty percent showed coupled axial rotation in the same direction as the lateral flexion, and the remainder showed no rotation with lateral flexion.[15]

Legaspi and Edmond[16] completed an extensive review of the literature on studies (n = 32) that measured lumbar segmental coupled motion and concluded that no consistent coupling pattern was seen with lumbar lateral flexion or rotation. Twenty-nine percent of the studies in which lateral flexion was the first motion performed found that, for most subjects, lateral flexion and rotation were coupled to the opposite side (the classic "normal" description). However, 33% of the studies in which lateral flexion was the first motion performed found that, for most of the subjects, coupling varied depending on the spinal level.[16]

Forty-five percent of the studies in which rotation was the first motion performed found that coupling between lateral flexion and rotation was inconsistent, and another 45% of the studies found that, for most subjects, coupling varied depending on the spinal level.[16]

Based on these findings, manual therapy practitioners should not rely on classical descriptions of coupling patterns for development and implementation of spinal manipulation techniques. When restoration of rotation or lateral flexion is a goal of intervention, multiple planar manipulation techniques can be used to take up tissue slack and isolate the forces to a specific spinal level, but the primary directional impairments should be addressed with the primary lever used in performance of the manipulation techniques.

The muscles of the back can be grossly divided between the global and the local muscles.[17] The global muscle system consists of large torque-producing muscles that act on the trunk and spine without directly attaching to the vertebrae. The muscles include the rectus abdominis, external oblique, and thoracic part of the lumbar iliocostalis. The local muscle system consists of muscles that directly attach to the lumbar vertebrae and are responsible for providing segmental stability and directly controlling the lumbar segments.[17] The lumbar multifidus, psoas major, quadratus lumborum, interspinalis,

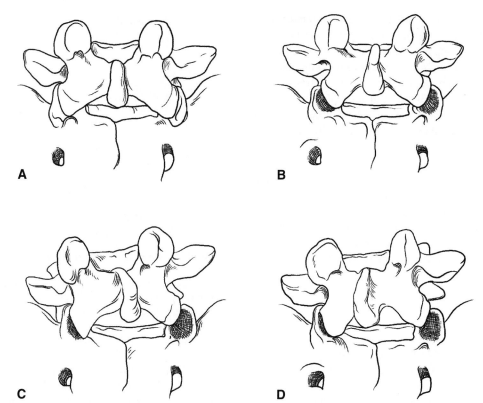

**FIGURE 4-3** Taken from videotape of fresh cadavers mounted in frame, this illustration shows hatched areas where facets are exposed. *A,* Neutral position with facets neatly coupled is shown. *B,* Forward bending is depicted and exposes some 40% of facet joint area. *C,* Side bending to left causes more upward slide on right facet than did forward bending. Further, angular distraction of lower pole of left facet is shown. Note also upper vertebrae in side bending left also rotated to that side. *D,* Right rotation is shown, in which right facet has distracted and left facet has compressed and slid somewhat forward with vertebrae tilting into left side bending. From Paris SV: Anatomy as related to function and pain, *Orthop Clin North Am* 14(3):475-489, 1983.

intertransversarii, lumbar portions of the iliocostalis and longissimus, transversus abdominis, diaphragm, and posterior fibers of the internal oblique all form part of the local muscle system.[18] The local muscles, transversus abdominis, and lumbosacral multifidus tend to play a large role in the successful rehabilitation of spinal instability disorders.

The lumbar mulfidus muscle is bipennate in both origin and insertion. It arises from a tendinous slip from the mamillary process just lateral and inferior to the facet joint.[12] From this point, it passes upwards and medially to gain a muscle origin from the upper third of the facet adjacent to its origin.[12] Two sets of these muscles then are joined together with further muscle tissue that ends in a tendinous slip that inserts into the posterior inferior aspect of the spinous process[12] (Figure 4-4). The fascicles of the lumbar multifidus are well positioned to act as posterior sagittal rotators on the vertebrae of their origin, and the length of the spinous process provides a great mechanical advantage.[19] The multifidus is not well positioned to contribute to the posterior translation component of extension, and the multifidus has a short lever arm to assist with vertebral axial rotation. The muscles best suited for axial rotation are the oblique abdominal muscles, but they also at the same time produce a flexion moment.[19] The erector spinae and the multifidus have been suggested to be active during rotation to counter this flexion moment.[19] Although the multifidus has been said to be a

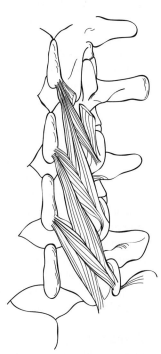

**FIGURE 4-4** Multifidus complex, which is difficult to illustrate, has both bipennate origin and bipennate insertion. Fiber orientation is shown. From Paris SV: Anatomy as related to function and pain, *Orthop Clin North Am* 14(3):475-489, 1983.

lateral flexor of the lumbar vertebral column, it attaches too close to the axis of the movement to contribute significantly to lateral flexion.[19] Any apparent lateral flexion produced by the multifidus causes a combination of extension combined with slight contralateral axial rotation, which may be part of the reason for the more consistent upper lumbar coupled contralateral rotation motion with lateral flexion.[19] The multifidus contributes to the control of lumbar segmental motion by maintaining segmental equilibrium and development of intersegmental stiffness.[17]

Most of the structures of the lumbar spine are innervated by at least two, and usually three, segmental nerves.[12] This multiple segmental innervation may explain the variability of referred pain and pain perception reported by patients with lumbopelvic disorders.[12] Clinically, the result is that clinicians cannot diagnose a specific anatomic structure as the primary cause of the patient's symptoms purely on the patient's reports of pain location.

## Pelvic Mechanics

Analysis of motion of the pelvis is difficult to measure with functional radiography because of the oblique orientation of the sacroiliac joints and the lack of definitive horizontal or vertical landmarks to use for motion measurement purposes. Strruresson, Selvik, and Uden[20] inserted four steel balls into the posterior aspect of the pelvis on 21 women and four men volunteers to study the motion of the pelvis with roentgen stereophotogrammetric analysis.[20] The x-ray tubes were oriented at oblique angles to the subject to capture radiographs of the subject in multiple positions. The pelvic motion measured with this technique was a mean of 0.5 mm translation and 1 to 2 degrees rotation.[20] The mean errors for rotation and translation were 0.1 to 0.2 degrees and 0.1 mm, respectively.[20]

The typical mean values of sacroiliac motion fall within the range of 0.2 to 2 degrees for anterior and posterior rotation and the range of 1 to 2 mm for translation.[21] Movements of the sacroiliac joint are primarily in the sagittal plane and primarily occur as a result of compression force of the articular cartilage and slight movement of the joint surfaces.[21] Terms commonly used to describe the motion of sacroiliac joints include *nutation, counternutation*, and *anterior/posterior rotation*. Nutation (meaning "to nod") is defined as the anterior tilt of the base (top) of the sacrum relative to the ilium and is also called sacral flexion.[21] Counternutation or sacral extension is the reverse motion, defined as the posterior tilt of the base of the sacrum relative to the ilium (Figure 4-5).

Anterior rotation refers to the forward movement of the iliac crest and the backward movement of the ischial tuberosity in relation to the sacrum. Posterior rotation is the backward movement of the iliac crest and the forward movement of the ischial tuberosity in relation to the sacrum. Anterior rotation of the ilium tends to occur with end range hip extension, and posterior rotation tends to occur with end range hip flexion. The iliac crest of the ilium tends to move superiorly as it rotates anteriorly and move inferiorly as it rotates posteriorly.

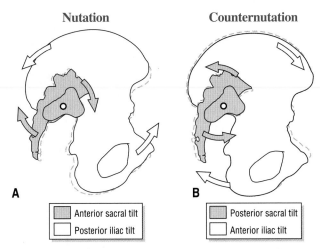

**FIGURE 4-5** Kinematics at sacroiliac joint. **A**, Nutation. **B**, Counternutation. Sacral rotations are indicated in *gray*; iliac rotations in *white*. Axis rotation for sagittal plane movement is indicated with *small circle*. From Neumann DA: *Kinesiology of the musculoskeletal system*, St Louis, 2002, Mosby.

In a young person, the joint surfaces of the SIJ are relatively flat; but with increasing age, they develop a series of peaks and troughs that interdigitate with each other.[22] These anatomic changes increase the joint's resistance to shearing movements by a mechanism termed "form closure."[23] In theory, if two opposing peaks catch on each other, the joint could become "locked" or "displaced" and require manipulation to restore the normal motion and position of the pelvis. Valid clinical measures for detection and measurement of the presence of a displaced SIJ have yet to be developed.

Sacroiliac joint stability can be enhanced by muscle action. Transversus abdominus contractions have been shown to enhance SIJ stability,[24] and in theory, tension generated by the gluteal muscles on one side of the body can work synergistically through the thoracolumbar fascia and the contralateral latissimus dorsi to press the joint surfaces closer together and increase stability by a mechanism termed "force closure."[23] Therefore, training of the gluteal, the contralateral latissimus dorsi, and the transversus abdominis muscles can form a muscular sling to enhance stability of the SIJ when hypermobility is suspected.

## Hip Mechanics

Normal lumbopelvic rhythm includes a coordinated movement of the hip, pelvis, and lumbar spine. Typical lumbopelvic rhythm consists of about 40 degrees of forward bending of the lumbar spine and 70 degrees of flexion of the hips.[21] Limited flexion of the hips, such as with tight hamstrings or a tight hip joint capsule, requires greater flexion of the thoracic and lumbar spines. Excessive hip flexion as a result of excessive length of the hamstrings requires less lumbar and thoracic forward bending for full forward bending.[21]

The hip joint allows osteokinematic motions of flexion (120 degrees), extension (20 degrees), abduction (40 degrees), adduction (25 degrees), internal rotation (35 degrees), and external rotation (45 degrees).[21] These motions may be initiated as femur on pelvis or pelvis on femur movements. The hip joint is formed by the head of the femur and the deep socket of the acetabulum of the ilium to create the classic ball-in-socket joint. The deep socket is surrounded by an extensive set of capsular ligaments, and many large forceful muscles provide the forces needed to propel and stabilize the body.[21] The arthrokinematics tend to follow the concave-convex rules, so that if the motion is initiated with the femur on the pelvis, the gliding movement at the joint tends to be in the opposite direction of the femur movement (e.g., anterior glide of femoral head with hip extension). If the motion is initiated as the pelvis moves on the fixed femur (concave on convex), the gliding motion at the joint is in the same direction of the pelvic movement.

In a sitting position with the hips flexed about 90 degrees, an anterior pelvic tilt includes flexion of the hip joint and backward bending of the lumbar spine. A posterior pelvic tilt performed in a sitting position includes a relative extension motion of the hip joint and forward bending (straightening) of the lumbar spine.[21] With a single leg weight-bearing position, abduction and adduction of the hip joint can occur with frontal plane movements of the pelvis. Horizontal plane rotation of the pelvis occurs with internal and external rotation of the hips with the leg in a weight-bearing position.

The hip joint mobility (accessory motion) and muscle length and strength of the muscles that cross the hip joint must be evaluated and treated in patients with lumbopelvic disorders. The hamstrings, hip flexors, piriformis, and iliotibial band are muscles that typically guard and tighten with dysfunctions in the region. The gluteal muscles (especially the gluteus medius), multifidus, and transversus abdominis are commonly weak with hip and lumbopelvic dysfunctions.

## DIAGNOSIS AND TREATMENT OF LUMBOPELVIC DISORDERS

Evidence-based treatment guidelines for acute LBP have been endorsed by at least 11 countries, and a recent review of the available guidelines found consensus in several areas.[25] Regarding diagnosis, agreement exists that diagnostic triage is indicated to differentiate nonspecific LBP, radicular syndrome, and specific pathological conditions. In addition, the history taking and physical examination must strive to identify red flags and screen the neurological system. Radiographic examinations should not be used for the initial diagnosis of acute low back pain conditions in the absence of red flags, and psychosocial factors should be assessed and considered as a component of a conservative approach.[25]

The guidelines also provide common recommendations for treatment for acute low back pain, including reassuring the patient of a favorable prognosis, advising the patient to stay active, and prescribing medication if necessary, starting with paracetamol (acetaminophin), then considering nonsteroidal antiinflammatory agents, and lastly considering muscle relax-

ants or opioids.[25] Discouragement of bed rest and consideration of spinal manipulation for pain relief were also recommended by most of the guidelines.[25]

A European guideline provided the following recommendations for the treatment of chronic low back pain: cognitive behavior therapy, supervised exercise therapy, brief educational interventions, and multidisciplinary (biopsychosocial) treatment, with short-term use of nonsteroidal antiinflammatory drugs and weak opioids.[26] Additional treatments to be considered include back schools and short courses of manipulation and mobilization, noradrenergic or noradrenergic-seratoninergic antidepressants, and muscle relaxants.[26] Passive treatments, such as therapeutic ultrasound and diathermy, and invasive surgical procedures are not recommended for nonspecific low back pain.[26] A significant note is that the recommendations of most evidence-based treatment guidelines for both acute and chronic low back pain include patient education, manipulation, and exercise, the primary interventions provided by physical therapists.

Lumbopelvic disorders are not a homogeneous group of conditions, and subgrouping or classification of patients with back pain has been shown to enhance treatment outcomes.[27,28] Classification of lumbopelvic disorders should adequately define the primary signs and symptoms and guide therapeutic interventions. Once red flags have been screened, and the patient has been determined through use of medical screening procedures to be an appropriate candidate for physical therapy, further information should be gathered to arrive at a diagnosis and impairment or treatment classification for the condition.

The low back pain treatment-based classification system was first described by Delitto, Erhard, and Bowling[29] and was based on the available evidence, common practice, and expert opinion for treatment of patients with low back pain. The classification categories are named by the primary intervention to be provided, and determination of the subgroup into which the patient is categorized is based on sets of signs and symptoms from the examination. Over time, the classification system has been modified based on results of clinical research studies to develop clinical prediction rules for manipulation[30] and stabilization[31] and based on results of reliability studies[32] and randomized controlled clinical trials.[28] The specific exercise category is based on a McKenzie[33] approach for treatment of "derangements," with use of repeated lumbar movements, that has been refined and tested by Werneke and Hart[34,35] and Long and Donelson.[36]

The treatment-based classification system avoids the pitfalls of attempts to identify the pathoanatomic cause of the patient's symptoms. Although clinicians often theorize the primary anatomic structure at fault, studies estimate that the true pathoanatomic structure causing low back pain can be identified in less than 15% of the cases.[37] Lumbar spinal stenosis is perhaps the one main exception in which strong correlation between the pathoanatomic findings on imaging findings and a specific treatment approach seems to provide favorable treatment outcomes.[38]

Evidence is found of improved outcomes with patients whose treatment approach is matched versus unmatched in use of the treatment-based classification for the conservative management of acute low back pain.[27] Patients who underwent matched treatments had greater short-term and long-term reductions in disability than those who underwent unmatched treatments.[27] Earlier research by Fritz, Delitto, and Erhard[39] showed significantly better outcomes from 4 weeks of classification-based physical therapy treatment compared with guideline-based treatment, which consisted of low-stress aerobic exercise and advice to remain active. Box 4-1 outlines the primary categories used in the treatment-based classification system for low back pain. In this text, the names of the categories have been modified to highlight the primary impairments to be addressed in the category (i.e., impairment-based classifications), and the treatment-based name of the classification is provided in parentheses in Box 4-1.

## Lumbar Hypomobility (Manipulation)

The strongest research support for the safe and effective use of manipulation (especially thrust techniques) is in the treatment of patients with acute low back pain (LBP). Numerous independent agencies have conducted systematic reviews of the literature to develop clinical practice guidelines based on the strength of the evidence and have concluded that spinal manipulation is a safe effective intervention for the management of acute LBP.[6,40-42] Spinal manipulation received the highest level of evidence awarded any intervention for the treatment of LBP in the 1994 Agency for Health Care Policy and Research (AHCPR) Guidelines, which were the first clinical practice guidelines to recommend the use of manipulation in the care of acute LBP.[40]

The level of research evidence to support the use of manipulation by physical therapists for the treatment of acute LBP has been further strengthened by the development, refinement, and validation of the clinical prediction rule for manipulation for acute low back pain. Childs et al[28] published a randomized controlled trial that validated the clinical prediction rule for use of manipulation for acute LBP. The clinical prediction rule was developed by Flynn et al[30] and is a set of five criteria that was determined to predict successful outcomes from a lumbopelvic manipulation when at least four of the five criteria were met in the patient examination findings. See Box 4-2 for an outline of clinical prediction rule (CPR) for manipulation for acute low back pain.

The study from Childs et al[28] examined 131 patients (18 to 60 years of age) with acute LBP who were referred to a physical therapist. Patients were randomly assigned to receive physical therapy that included two sessions of high-velocity thrust spinal manipulation plus an exercise program (manipulation + exercise group) or an exercise program without spinal manipulation (exercise-only group).[28] During the first two sessions, patients in the manipulation + exercise group received high-velocity thrust manipulation and range of motion exercise. Patients in the exercise-only group were treated with a low-stress aerobic and lumbar spine–strengthening program.

| BOX 4-1 | Outline of an Impairment-Based (Treatment-Based) Classification System for Low Back Pain |
|---|---|

Lumbar and leg pain that centralizes with repeated movements (specific exercise)
  Extension syndrome
    Symptoms centralize with lumbar backward bending
    Symptoms peripheralize with lumbar forward bending
  Flexion syndrome
    Symptoms centralize with lumbar forward bending
    Symptoms peripheralize with lumbar backward bending
    Imaging evidence of lumbar spinal stenosis
    Older age (>50 y)
  Lateral shift
    Visible frontal plane deviation of the shoulders relative to the pelvis
    Symptoms centralize with side glide and backward bending
Lumbar hypomobility (manipulation)
  Hypomobility with passive accessory intervertebral motion testing
  Low back and leg pain that does not travel beyond the knee
  Low fear avoidance beliefs (FABQ work subscale <19)
  Recent onset of back pain (<16 d)
  Adequate hip rotation motion (at least one hip >35 degrees IR)
Lumbopelvic instability (stabilization)
  Hypermobility with posterior-anterior segmental mobility testing
  Younger age group (<41 y)
  Greater general flexibility (SLR > 90 degrees)
  Positive prone instability test
  For patients who are postpartum
    Positive posterior pelvic pain provocation (P4) and ASLR and modified Trendelenburg's tests
    Pain provocation with palpation of the long dorsal sacroiliac ligament or pubic symphysis
Lumbar radiculopathy that does not centralize with repeated movements (traction)
  No lumbar movements centralize symptoms
  No directional preference noted with history or clinical examination to alleviate lower leg pain
  Peripheralization of leg pain with lumbar backward bending
  Positive SLR for lower leg pain at <45 degrees hip flexion
  Positive crossed SLR test at <45 degrees hip flexion
  Lower extremity neurologic signs (weakness, numbness, DTR)
  Poor tolerance to weight-bearing postures (i.e., sitting or standing)
  Symptoms alleviated with traction

*FABQ,* Fear Avoidance Beliefs Questionnaire; *IR,* internal rotation; *SLR,* straight leg raise; *ASLR,* active straight leg raise; *DTR,* deep tendon reflexes.

| BOX 4-2 | Clinical Prediction Rule for Improvement with Lumbopelvic Manipulation for Acute Low Back Pain[30] |
|---|---|

Duration of symptoms <16 d
At least one hip with >35 degrees of internal rotation
Hypomobility with lumbar PAIVM testing
FABQ work subscale score <19
No symptoms distal to the knee

Patients in both groups attended physical therapy twice during the first week and then once a week for the next 3 weeks, for a total of 5 sessions.[28]

The patients with positive results for the clinical prediction rule for manipulation and who received the manipulation intervention (manipulation + exercise group) had dramatic improvements in pain and disability after 1 week and 4 weeks and sustained that improvement at the 6-month follow-up examination.[28] The patients with positive results for the clinical prediction rule (at least four of five findings) who received the thrust spinal manipulation had a 92% chance of a successful outcome at the end of 1 week.[28] At the 6-month follow-up examination, patients who fit the clinical prediction rule but did not receive spinal manipulation showed significantly greater use of medication and healthcare services and more lost time from work because of back pain than did the manipulation group.[28] Most of the subjects (72%) showed meaningful clinical improvements with lumbar spinal manipulation, which supports the rationale that patients with acute onset low back pain without signs of nerve root compression are excellent candidates for a trial of manipulation.[43]

Further analysis of this study reveals that the number needed to treat with spinal manipulation to prevent one additional patient from a worsening in disability at 1 week was 9.9 (95% confidence interval [CI], 4.9-65.3); this number persisted at 4 weeks.[5] The patients with LBP who were provided with exercise only were eight times more likely to have a worsening in disability after 1 week than were patients who received manipulation.[5] Only 10 patients need to be treated with manipulation to prevent one patient from a worsening in disability after 1 week.[5]

Clinical practice can be further guided by identification of the patients whose conditions will not respond or may even worsen with manipulation. Fritz et al[43] further analyzed the data from the CPR validation study and found six variables related to the inability of patients to respond favorably to the manipulation intervention; these factors are listed in Box 4-3. These six variables explained 63% of the poor outcomes with the lumbopelvic manipulation outcome. If a patient has several of these variables during an initial examination, the likelihood of improvement with manipulation may be minimal.[43]

Although a supine lumbopelvic thrust manipulation technique was used in the studies by Flynn et al[30] and Childs et al[28]

| **BOX 4-3** | Factors Related to the Inability to Respond to Lumbopelvic Manipulation (based on data from Fritz et al[43]) |
|---|---|

Longer duration of symptoms
Symptoms in the buttock or leg
Absence of lumbar hypomobility (with PAIVM testing)
Less hip total rotation range of motion
Less discrepancy in the left to right hip medial rotation
   range of motion
Negative Gaenslen sign

to develop and validate the clinical prediction rule, Cleland et al[44] showed excellent results of treatment with a different lumbar thrust manipulation technique (side-lying lumbar rotation) in a case series of 12 patients who fit the lumbar manipulation clinical prediction rule. This study suggests that selection of correct patient characteristics is likely more important than selection of correct technique for successful outcomes with lumbar thrust manipulation.

The clinical prediction rule can be used to predict which patients are likely to have a dramatic response to lumbopelvic manipulation. Many patients have one or two components of the clinical prediction rule for manipulation combined with other findings that must be assessed to develop an appropriate plan of care. In these cases, use of an impairment-based approach can yield successful outcomes as long as reliable and valid examination procedures are used to identify the impairments. The direction, location, and force used for spinal manipulation in the plan of care are based on detection of lumbopelvic hypomobility with active and passive mobility and end feel testing. For instance, if left lower trunk rotation is limited with active range of motion testing combined with posterior to anterior passive accessory intervertebral movement (PAIVM) motion restriction at the L4L5 spinal segment and passive intervertebral joint motion (PIVM) testing limitation of the left rotation at the same spinal segment, a left rotation manipulation targeting the L4L5 spinal segment is used. After the manipulation, the active and passive motion is reassessed to determine whether a positive change occurred with the intervention, such as better freedom of motion or less pain with movement. An exercise program that includes lumbar mobility exercises enhances the clinical outcomes after the manipulation (Box 4-4). As symptoms subside and mobility improves, the patient may also benefit from progression of lumbar stabilization and conditioning exercises.

Psychosocial issues, such as fear avoidance beliefs, must also be considered because of evidence that spinal stabilization exercise programs are more effective than manipulation with high Fear Avoidance Beliefs Questionnaire (FABQ) scores.[31]

## Lumbar Spine Instability (Stabilization)

Clinical instability is defined by Panjabi[45] as the inability of the spine under physiological loads to maintain its pattern of displacement so that no neurological damage or irritation, no development of deformity, and no incapacitating pain occur. The total range of motion of a spinal segment may be divided into the neutral zone and the elastic zone.[45,46] Motion that occurs in and around the neutral mid position of the spine is produced against minimal passive resistance (i.e., neutral zone), and motion that occurs near the end range of spinal motion is produced against increased passive resistance (i.e., elastic zone).[45,47] Clinical instability is believed to be a result of increase in the size of the neutral zone and reduction in the passive resistance to motion created in the elastic zone.

Panjabi[45] conceptualized the components of spinal stability into three functionally integrated subsystems of the spinal stabilizing system. According to Panjabi,[45] the stabilizing system

**BOX 4-4** | Lumbopelvic Mobility Exercises*

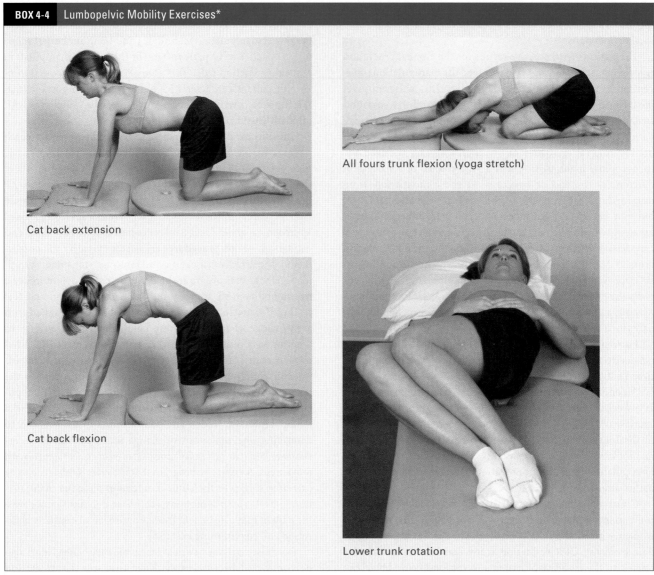

Cat back extension

All fours trunk flexion (yoga stretch)

Cat back flexion

Lower trunk rotation

*After lumbopelvic manipulation, lumbopelvic mobility exercises are useful to maintain the mobility gained with the manual therapy techniques.

of the spine consists of the passive, active, and neural control subsystems.

The passive subsystem consists of the vertebral bodies, facet joints and joint capsules, spinal ligaments, and passive tension from spinal muscles and tendons. The passive subsystem provides significant stabilization of the elastic zone and limits the size of the neutral zone. Also, the components of the passive subsystem act as transducers and provide the neural control subsystem with information about vertebral position and motion.

The active subsystem, which consists of spinal muscles and tendons, generates the forces needed to stabilize the spine in response to changing loads. The active subsystem is primarily responsible for controlling the motion that occurs within the neutral zone and contributes to maintaining the size of the neutral zone. The spinal muscles also act as transducers that provide the neural control subsystem with information about the forces generated by each muscle.

Through peripheral nerves and the central nervous system, the neural control subsystem receives information from the transducers of the passive and active subsystems about vertebral position, vertebral motion, and forces generated by spinal muscles. With the information, the neural control subsystem determines the requirements for spinal stability and acts on the spinal muscles to produce the required forces.

Clinical spinal instability occurs when the neutral zone increases relative to the total range of motion, the stabilizing subsystems are unable to compensate for this increase, and the quality of motion in the neutral zone becomes poor and uncontrolled.[45,46,48] Degeneration and mechanical injury of the spinal stabilization components are the primary causes of increases in neutral zone size.[45] Factors that contribute to degeneration or mechanical injury of the stabilizing components are poor posture, repetitive occupational trauma, acute trauma, and weakness of the local lumbar musculature.[45,49-51]

Because poor quality of motion is a key aspect of clinical instability, the presence of aberrant motions during active movement has been suggested by several authors to be a cardinal sign of clinical instability.[52-54] Aberrant motions are described as either sudden accelerations or decelerations of movement or motions that occur outside the intended plane of movement.[52,54,55] Other signs and symptoms of clinical instability are general tenderness of the lumbar region, referred pain in the buttock or thigh area, paraspinal muscle guarding, and pain with sustained postures.[26,49,52,54,56-58] Also, passive intervertebral motion and joint play testing may reveal hypermobility and decreased passive restraints to motion at end range of passive intervertebral motion (i.e., a loose end feel).[59] Imaging studies may show alterations of the components of the passive subsystem, such as ligament damage, osteophytes, vertebral fractures, disc degeneration, vertebral displacement, and vertebral displacement.[45,48,50,60-62]

Objective criteria have been established in the analysis of end range flexion and extension radiographs for diagnosis of spine instability.[52,54,57,61,63,64] However, radiographs do not yield information about the quantity or quality of motion that occurs in the neutral zone (i.e., mid range), which limits the value of radiographic evidence in the diagnosis of clinical instabilities.[52,61] Video fluoroscopy shows some promise as a means for analysis of the quality of spine motion at mid range, but its use is still experimental for this purpose.[65] Teyhan et al[65] developed a kinematic model with digit fluoroscopy to illustrate aberrant rates of attainment of angular and linear displacement around the mid range postures with patients with clinical signs of instability; these patients tend to have a combination of altered segmental structural integrity, segmental stiffness, and altered neuromuscular control during lumbar spine movements. Passive intervertebral motion and joint play testing have diagnostic value with assessment of neutral zone size, but the tests have poor interrater reliability and only assess passive motion.[47,66] Because a definitive diagnostic tool for instability has not been established, clinical instability continues to be diagnosed based on clinical findings, including history, subjective symptoms, visual analysis of active motion quality, and manual examination methods.[59]

Hicks et al[31] developed a clinical prediction rule (Box 4-5) to predict the likelihood of success with use of a lumbar stabilization exercise program for patients with low back pain. If a patient has three or more of the four variables, the positive likelihood ratio of success is 4.0 (95% CI, 1.6-10.0) that the patient will respond favorably to a spinal stabilization exercise program.[31] Of the four variables, age was the single most significant factor to predict success.[31]

The study from Hicks et al[31] involved 8 weeks of physical therapy with instruction and monitoring of a spinal stabilization exercise program. Patients underwent reassessment after 8 weeks, and if the Oswestry score improved by 50%, the treatments were considered a success.[31] If 6 points of improvement were seen to 49% improvement, conditions were considered improved; with a less than 6-point reduction on the Oswestry Disability Questionnaire (ODQ), the treatments were consid-

| BOX 4-5 | Significant Predictors (CPR) of Lumbar Stabilization Exercise Program Success and Failure[31,65] | |
|---|---|---|
| | **Variables** | **Accuracy statistics** |
| Predictors of success | Positive prone instability test | If two of the four variables are present: |
| | Aberrant motion present | Sensitivity: 0.83 (0.61-0.94) |
| | Age <41 y | Specificity: 0.56 (0.40-0.71) |
| | SLR >91 | |
| Predictors of failure | Negative prone instability test | If two of the four variables are present: |
| | Hypomobility with PAIVM testing | Sensitivity: 0.85 (0.70-0.93) |
| | Aberrant motion absent | Specificity: 0.87 (0.62-0.96) |
| | FABQ score ≤9 (activity scale) | |

ered a failure. The study found 18 successes, 15 failures, and 21 improved.[31] The characteristics of each group were analyzed to determine clinical findings at the initial evaluation that could predict success or failure.

The four variables that were found to predict failure of a spinal stabilization exercise program were negative prone instability test results, absent aberrant movements, FABQ physical activity subscale score less than 9, and no hypermobility with lumbar PAIVM testing.[31] An interesting note is that patients with higher fear avoidance belief scores had conditions that responded more favorably to the stabilization exercise program. These results are contrary to the findings of previous clinical trials regarding interventions such as spinal manipulation in which high FABQ work subscale scores were associated with a lower chance of success.[28,30] This finding reinforces the importance of an active exercise-based approach for patients with high levels of fear of activity.

Bergmark[17] divided the muscles of the trunk into two groups: local and global systems. The global muscle group includes the larger more superficial muscles, such as the erector spinae, rectus abdominus, and internal/external obliques. The primary functions of the global muscles are to transfer loads between the thoracic cage and the pelvis and to change the position of the thoracic cage in relation to the pelvis.[17] The local muscle system includes the deeper smaller muscles with direct attachments into the vertebrae. The local system is used to control the spinal curvature and to give sagittal and lateral stiffness to maintain mechanical stability of the spine.[17] Examples of the local muscles include the transverses abdominus (because of its attachment into the lumbar fascia) and the lumbar multifidi and intertransverse muscles. The quadratus lumborum is classified into both systems, with the lateral portion functioning as a global muscle and the medial portion that attaches to the lumbar transverse processes as a local muscle that stabilizes the lumbar spine in a lateral direction.[17]

In patients with clinical spinal instability, an imbalance tends to exist between the function of the global and local muscles. The global muscles tend to be strong and overactive and in a state of muscle holding. The local muscles are weak, atrophied, and delayed in response times and coordination. The primary purpose of the early phases of a lumbopelvic stabilization exercise program is to facilitate the control, strength, and coordination of the local muscles and inhibit the action of the global muscles. Manual physical therapy techniques directed to the thoracic spine may be used to inhibit the increased tone of the erector spinae (global muscles system). Motor relearning principles are used to facilitate a therapeutic exercise program designed to train the local muscle system.

Electromyogram (EMG) study results have shown a delay in firing of the local lumbopelvic muscles in patients with a history of LBP compared with paired healthy subjects when active upper extremity motions are performed.[67] The results of a fine-wire EMG study show that both deep and superficial fibers of the multidus muscle are controlled differentially during movements of the arm that challenge the stability of the spine, with the superficial fibers of the multifidus acting to control spine orientation and the deep fibers controlling intersegmental motion.[68] The multifidus muscles are active in anticipation of arm movements and are active earlier for shoulder flexion than extension motions. This direction-specific activity is matched to the direction of reactive forces caused by limb movement and linked to the control of spine orientation and the displacement of the center of mass.[68] In contrast to the superficial fibers, the EMG onset of deep multifidus and transversus abdominis (TrA) fibers was not altered by movement direction.[68] These deeper muscles are not affected by which direction the arm is moved. They are active through the activity regardless of direction of arm movements. Because the deep fibers are independent of reactive force direction, they may therefore control intersegmental motion and stability.[68]

Evidence also exists of severe fat infiltration in the lumbar multifidus muscle in subjects with a history of LBP.[69] Fat infiltration seems to be a late stage of muscular degeneration and can be measured in a noninvasive manner with magnetic resonance imaging (MRI). The results of this study provide the first convincing evidence from a large population sample that fat infiltration in the lumbar multifidus muscles (LMM) is strongly associated with LBP in adults.[69] Therefore, these patients lack the dynamic intersegmental stability provided by the multifidus.

Hides, Jull, and Richardson[70] followed a control group and a group that received a spinal stabilization exercise program after a first-time episode of low back pain. At the 10-week follow-up examination, atrophy was noted of the lumbar multifidus at the side and spinal level of the patient's primary pain symptom. Both groups had a return to a good functional level, but significantly higher recurrence rates of low back pain episodes were noted in the control group that did not receive a spinal stabilization exercise program at the 2-year to 3-year follow-up exam-

ination.[70] During the 2-year to 3-year period after the first-time episode of low back pain, the patients in the control group who did not receive the exercise program instruction were 5.9 times more likely to have recurrences of LBP than were patients in the specific exercise group and 12.4 times more likely to have a recurrence in the first year.[70] These studies support the concept that permanent motor control and physiologic muscle changes can occur after injury to the lumbar spine and that specific skilled physical therapy intervention is needed to normalize muscle function and prevent recurrence of future low back pain episodes. Recovery of local muscle function appears to be a key factor in full recovery and future prevention of low back pain episodes.

Hodges and Richardson[67] studied 15 patients with low back pain and 15 matched control subjects who performed rapid shoulder flexion, abduction, and extension while standing in response to a visual stimulus. Electromyographic activity of the abdominal muscles, lumbar multifidus, and the contralateral deltoid was evaluated with fine-wire and surface electrodes.[67] The results of this study showed that shoulder movement in each direction resulted in contraction of trunk muscles before or shortly after the deltoid contraction in control subjects.[67] The transversus abdominis was usually the first active muscle and was not influenced by movement direction, which supports the hypothesized role of this muscle in spinal stiffness generation.[67] Contraction of the transversus abdominis was significantly delayed in patients with low back pain with all shoulder movements.[67] The delayed onset of contraction of the transversus abdominis indicates a deficit of motor control and is hypothesized to result in inefficient muscular stabilization of the spine.[67]

Hodges and Richardson[71] also showed with another fine-wire EMG study that the TrA fires in anticipation of lower extremity movements regardless of the direction of the movements, which supports the hypothesis that the TrA functions as a primary spinal stabilizer muscle. The lower fibers of the TrA with their horizontal orientation may contribute to the enhancement of the stability of the spine, either through their role in the production of intraabdominal pressure or via an increase in the tension in the thoracolumbar fascia through which these muscles are attached to the lumbar vertebrae and enhance the stiffness and stability of the spine.[71] MRI study results have confirmed that during the abdominal "drawing in" action, the transversus abdominis contracts bilaterally to form a musculofascial band that appears to tighten like a corset and improves stabilization of the lumbopelvic region.[72] The transversus abdominis muscle has also been shown to reduce sacroiliac laxity and is believed to play a significant role to enhance stability of the pelvis when functioning properly.[24]

Two randomized controlled trials of different subgroups of patients with LBP reported improvements in pain and function with exercise interventions that involved inward movement (drawing in maneuver) of the lower abdomen.[67,73] Inclusion criterion for subjects in the O'Sullivan, Twomey, and Allison[73] clinical trial was radiographic evidence of spondylolysis or spondylolisthesis. Forty-four patients with these conditions were assigned randomly to two treatment groups. The first group underwent a 10-week specific exercise treatment program that involved the specific training of the deep abdominal muscles, with coactivation of the lumbar multifidus.[73] The activation of these muscles was incorporated into previously aggravating static postures and functional tasks. The control group underwent treatment as directed by the treating practitioner. After the intervention, the specific exercise group showed a statistically significant reduction in pain intensity and functional disability levels, which was maintained at a 30-month follow-up examintion.[73] The control group showed no significant change in these parameters after intervention or at follow-up examination.[73] A specific exercise treatment approach appears to be more effective than other commonly prescribed conservative treatment programs in patients with chronically symptomatic spondylolysis or spondylolisthesis.

A patient is best taught a spinal stabilization exercise program with a motor learning approach that starts with the cognitive phase of learning in which a great deal of mental concentration is needed to attain the proper muscle contraction and controlled motion.[74] Much cognitive activity is necessary to use appropriate muscle control strategies initially, but with practice, the performance rapidly improves. As the patient continues to practice and feedback is provided, the patient can move into the associative phase of motor learning in which the quality of the motion and the ease of performance improve. Less mental energy is necessary. For the final phase of motor learning, autonomous new situations and challenges need to be incorporated into the training program to make the motor control more skillful, natural, and automatic in performance. At this phase, the learner can perform the task at a high level without much thought and can concurrently perform other tasks if needed.[74] Once this phase is reached, retention of the skill is enhanced and good long-term clinical outcomes are realized.

One of the goals of the early phase of a lumbopelvic stabilization exercise program is isolation of contraction of the transversus abdominis (TrA). An EMG study has confirmed that the "inward movement of the lower abdominal wall" in the supine position is the most effective way to isolate a TrA contraction in isolation of the more superficial abdominal muscles (rectus abdominis, internal oblique, and external oblique).[75] In contrast, a posterior pelvic tilt and abdominal bracing procedure showed greater activity in the internal oblique muscle.[75] More lumbopelvic motion was recorded with posterior pelvic tilt, and a negative correlation was noted between movement of the spine and TrA activity.[75] In other words, greater TrA activity is produced when spinal motion is minimized.

Boxes 4-6, 4-7, and 4-8 illustrate a three-phase program for spinal stabilization. The first phase focuses on isolation of the transversus abdominis muscle and challenging the neutral position in supported non–weight-bearing postures. Phase II continues to build on the stabilization of the neutral spine position by challenging the patient in multiple positions and with multiple extremity motions. Phase III is further progression of the program with incorporation of more dynamic controlled spine motions with upper and lower extremity motions in func-

tional movement patterns. Incorporation of functional tasks and sporting activities can be added in this phase, with reinforcement of control with the local spinal stabilizers with the functional movements.

## Lumbar and Leg Pain That Centralizes (Specific Exercise)

McKenzie[33] describes seven types of derangements based on symptom location, response to the repeated movement examination, and presence of deformity (lateral shift or kyphotic lumbar posture). The McKenzie approach to treatment of the derangements emphasizes that the direction of repeated movements should be governed by the centralization/peripheralization phenomena and that no repeated exercise movement or advise on positioning should be performed that causes the pain reference to peripheralize.

The clinical phenomenon known as centralization occurs during repeated lumbar movements or postures when the most distal extent of the referred or radicular pain recedes toward the lumbar midline.[76] Peripheralization is the spreading laterally or distally of the symptoms from the lumbar spine toward the foot with repeated lumbar movements or postures. McKenzie has speculated that the direction of bending that centralizes the pain precisely corresponds with the direction in which disc nuclear content has migrated to generate referred symptoms by mechanically stimulating the annulus or nerve root.[33]

In a study published by Donelson et al,[76] the repeated lumbar movements of flexion, extension, side gliding, extension in lying, flexion in lying, and flexion/rotation with overpressure in hook lying were used to make a mechanical diagnosis by a physical therapist; each patient was then given a discogram test for determination of the symptomatic disc and a CT scan for assessment of the disc integrity. This study found a high incidence rate of positive discogram results in centralizers (74%) and peripheralizers (69%). In the patients with positive discogram results, the difference between the incidence rates of discs with a competent annulus that occurred in centralizers (91%) was significantly greater than what occurred in peripheralizers (54%).[76] Donelson et al[76] concluded that most centralizers in this population of patients with chronic low back pain have discogenic pain with a functionally competent annulus and that peripheralizers also tend to have discogenic pain but with a higher incidence rate of outer annulus disruption.

Although a high percentage of these patients with chronic low back pain had positive discogenic findings, a significant number of patients was still found without positive discogram results and symptoms that either centralized (26%) or peripheralized (31%), which means that the discogenic theory cannot explain all these cases and the repeated movement examination and treatment concepts potentially affect more anatomic structures than just the intervertebral disc. However, when the disc is the source of the pain, the repeated movement treatment concepts tend to be more effective when the annular fibers remain intact.

Werneke and Hart[34] reported on the repeated movement examination findings of 223 patients with LBP and followed up

**BOX 4-6** | Lumbopelvic Spinal Stabilization Phase I

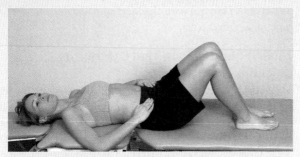

Drawing in maneuver is used to isolate TrA in hook-lying position, and tactile cues just medial to ASIS can facilitate isometric contractions. Work toward 10-second holds for 10 repetitions at least three times per day and then progress to TrA isometrics in multiple positions throughout the day

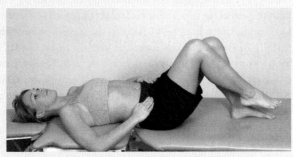

Hook-lying marching motion with TrA contraction to control lumbopelvic spine position in neutral. Preset and sustain TrA contraction throughout leg movements

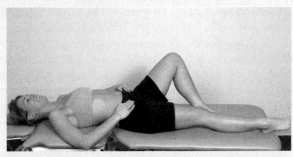

Bent knee fall out with TrA contraction to control lumbopelvic spine position in neutral. Preset and sustain TrA contraction throughout leg movements

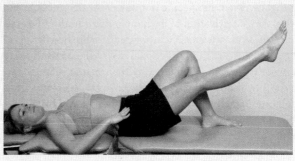

Straight leg raise with TrA contraction to control lumbopelvic spine position in neutral. Preset and sustain TrA contraction throughout leg movements

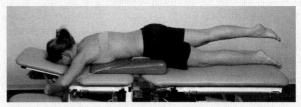

Prone over a pillow hip extension with TrA contraction to control lumbopelvic spine position in neutral. Preset and sustain TrA contraction throughout leg movements. The airbag biofeedback device can be used to provide feedback on steadiness with trunk stabilization during this exercise

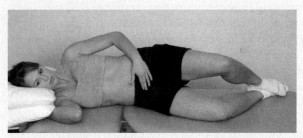

Side-lying "clamshell" hip abduction with external rotation with TrA contraction to control lumbopelvic spine position in neutral. Preset and sustain TrA contraction throughout leg movements. Patient must be cued to ensure pelvis does not rotate as hip moves

**BOX 4-7** | **Lumbopelvic Spinal Stabilization Phase II**

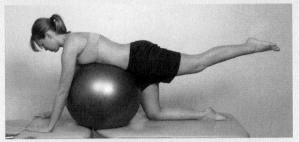

All fours position over a physioball leg lift with TrA contraction to control lumbopelvic spine position in neutral. Preset and sustain TrA contraction throughout leg movements

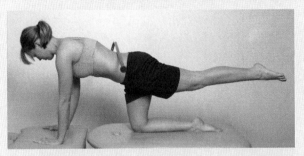

All fours position leg lift with TrA contraction to control lumbopelvic spine position in neutral. Preset and sustain TrA contraction throughout leg movements. A cane can be positioned on the lumbar spine to provide feedback regarding how well patient maintains stabile lumbopelvic position

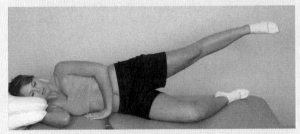

Side-lying hip abduction with TrA contraction to control lumbopelvic spine position in neutral. Preset and sustain TrA contraction throughout leg movements. Patient must be cued to ensure pelvis does not rotate as hip moves

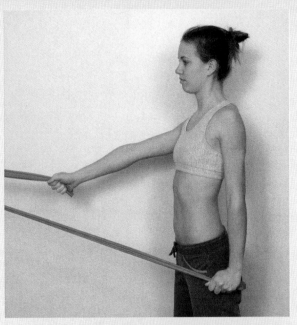

Theraband shoulder extension with diagonal stance and lumbopelvic stabilization

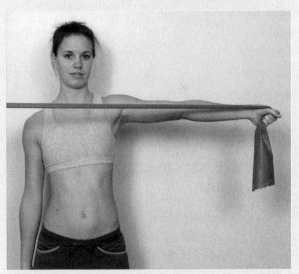

Theraband shoulder horizontal abduction with athletic stance and lumbopelvic stabilization

*Continued*

**BOX 4-7** **Lumbopelvic Spinal Stabilization Phase II**—cont'd

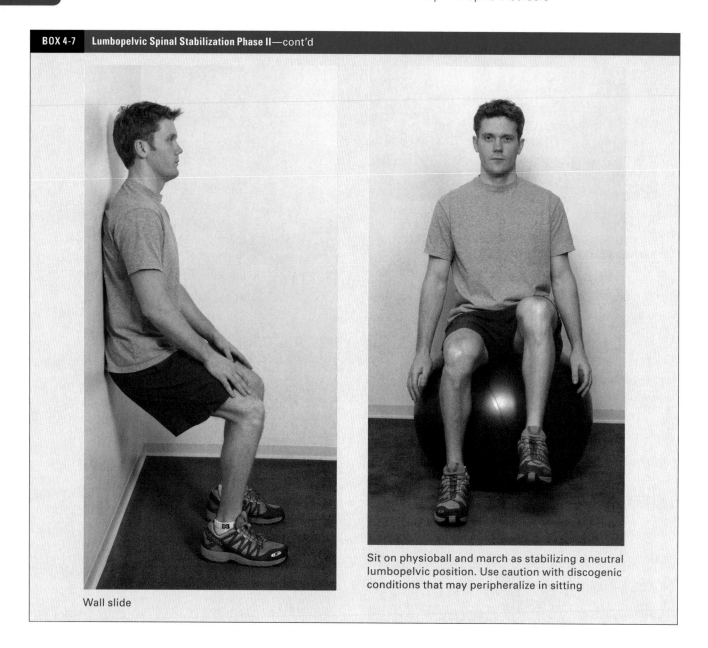

Wall slide

Sit on physioball and march as stabilizing a neutral lumbopelvic position. Use caution with discogenic conditions that may peripheralize in sitting

BOX 4-7   Lumbopelvic Spinal Stabilization Phase II—cont'd

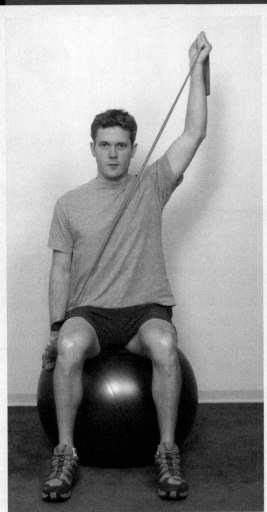

Theraband diagonal shoulder flexion as patient stabilizes a neutral lumbopelvic position. Use caution with discogenic conditions that may peripheralize in sitting

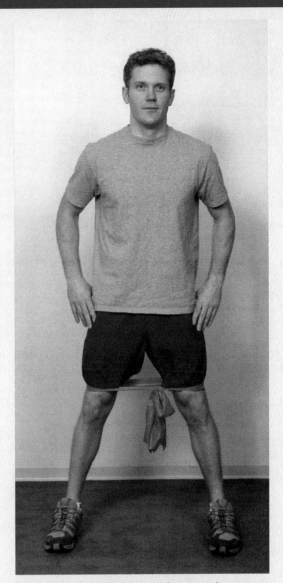

Theraband resisted side stepping as patient stabilizes a neutral lumbopelvic position. Continue in both directions until fatigue is noted in hip abductor muscles

**BOX 4-8**   Lumbopelvic Spinal Stabilization Phase III

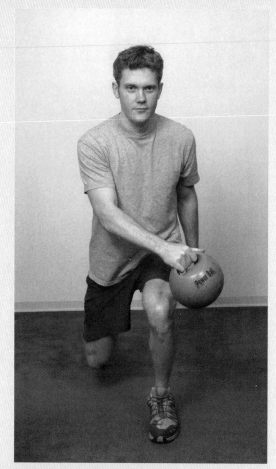

Forward lunge with weighted ball reach to knee. Spinal movement is a controlled manner into rotation and forward bending as arm reaches to knee, but a hinging flexion motion is emphasized at hips to facilitate bending that occurs with this motion

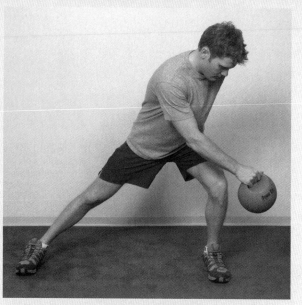

Lateral lunge with weighted ball reach to knee. Spinal movement is a controlled manner into rotation and forward bending as arm reaches to knee, but a hinging flexion motion is emphasized at hips to facilitate bending that occurs with this motion

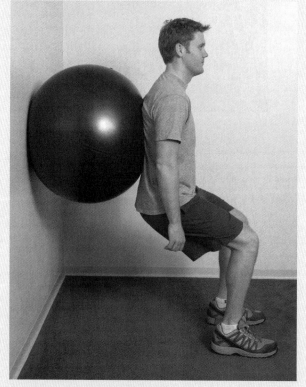

Wall slide squat with physioball

**BOX 4-8    Lumbopelvic Spinal Stabilization Phase III—cont'd**

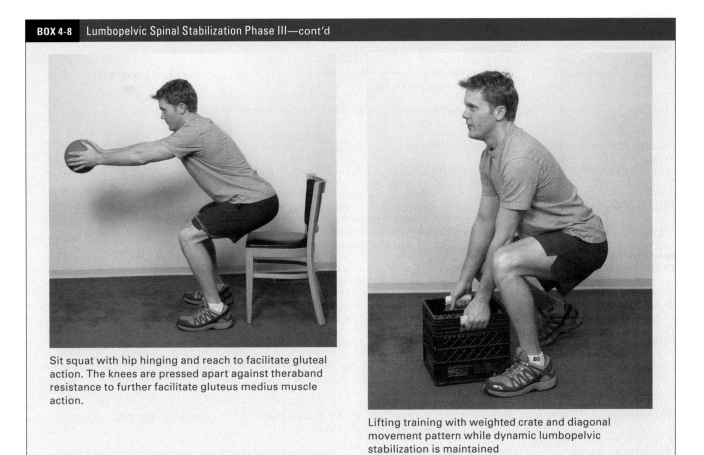

Sit squat with hip hinging and reach to facilitate gluteal action. The knees are pressed apart against theraband resistance to further facilitate gluteus medius muscle action.

Lifting training with weighted crate and diagonal movement pattern while dynamic lumbopelvic stabilization is maintained

with these patients 1 year after the initial examination. Classification in the noncentralization group at intake was a predictor of those who did not return to work, who continued to report pain symptoms, who had extended activity interference or downtime at home, and who continued to use healthcare resources at the 1-year follow-up examination.[34] Centralization appears to identify a subgroup of spinal patients who have a good prognosis for response to conservative treatment.[77]

Regardless of validity of the pathoanatomic explanation for the McKenzie repeated movement examination and treatment regime, these treatment principles can improve patient outcomes. In a study by Long and Donelson,[36] the McKenzie approach with exercise prescription based on directional preference showed better outcomes than comparison groups that performed exercises away from an identified directional preference.

According to a recent systematic review, McKenzie therapy results in a greater decrease in pain and disability in the short term than other standard therapies, such as medications and modalities, for patients with low back pain; but there has yet to be a clinical trial that compared McKenzie treatment with placebo or no treatment or with manipulation.[78] Miller et al[79] compared clinical outcomes of patients with chronic low back pain who were treated with the McKenzie repeated movement approach with outcomes of patients treated with spinal stabili-

zation exercises and found improvements in pain and function with both groups but no significant difference between the two groups.

Riddle and Rothstein[80] evaluated the reliability of the McKenzie examination system when used by novice practitioners and found poor interrater reliability for the placement of patients into one of the three syndromes (Kappa = 0.26); they reported the primary source of error was in the therapist's ability to judge centralization versus peripheralization in the patients examined. In contrast, Fritz et al[32] reported excellent interrater reliability for physical therapists (Kappa = 0.823) and physical therapist students (Kappa = 0.763) in interpretation of videotaped repeated movement examinations of patients with low back pain. The videotape examination eliminated the variability in patient response at different points in time and allowed the testers to focus on interpretation of the examination procedures. This study also illustrates that newly trained student therapists can attain acceptable levels of reliability without undergoing extensive training regimes. Table 4-6 provides an outline of the McKenzie repeated movement examination scheme. Box 4-9 outlines the extension progression used in the McKenzie approach when extension centralizes the patient's symptoms.

In summary, a subgroup of patients with low back pain seems to show a directional preference for specific exercises;

| TABLE 4-6 | Test Movements Used in a McKenzie AROM Examination |
|---|---|
| **MOVEMENT** | **DEFINITION** |
| Side bending in standing | Patient is standing; examiner asks patient to bend in frontal plane to right or left as far as possible, then return to starting position. |
| Flexion in standing | Patient is standing; examiner asks patient to bend forward as far as possible without flexing knees, then return to starting position. |
| Repeated flexion in standing | Flexion in standing movement is repeated 10 times. |
| Extension in standing | Patient is standing; examiner asks patient to bend backwards as far as possible without flexing knees, then return to starting position. |
| Repeated extension in standing | Extension in standing movement is repeated 10 times. |
| Sustained extension in standing | Extension in standing movement is maintained for 30 seconds before returning to starting position. |
| Pelvic translocation in standing | Patient is standing; examiner passively shifts patient's pelvis in frontal plane while stabilizing shoulders, then returns patient to starting position. |
| Extension in prone | Patient is prone; examiner asks patient to press up by placing hands on examining surface and extending elbows while keeping pelvis flat on the surface, then return to starting position. |
| Sustained extension in prone | Extension in prone movement is maintained for 30 seconds before returning to stating position. |
| Sustained extension with pelvic translocation in prone | Patient is prone; examiner passively shifts patient's pelvis in frontal plane. Patient is asked to prop up on elbows with pelvis flat on examining surface. This position is maintained for 30 seconds before returning to stating position. |
| Repeated flexion in sitting | Patient is sitting; examiner asks patient to bend forward as far as possible, then return to starting position. This movement is repeated 10 times. |
| Flexion in quadruped | Patient is in quadruped position; examiner asks patient to rock backwards approximating heels to buttocks, then return to starting position. |
| Repeated flexion in quadruped | Flexion in quadruped movement is repeated 10 times. |

From Fritz JM, Delitto A, Vignovic M, et al: *Arch Phys Med Rehabil* 81:57-61, 2000.
   *AROM*, Active range of motion.

incorporation of these exercises in the treatment approach tends to yield positive clinical outcomes. Once symptomatic improvement is achieved, these patients may benefit from general conditioning, mobility, and strengthening (stabilization) programs to restore function and prevent future episodes of low back pain. Patients with leg pain that peripheralizes tend to have a poorer prognosis for conservative management; these patients may be candidates for activity modification, stabilization exercise, and spinal traction. Speculation exists that the patients with a directional preference toward lumbar extension (repeated backward bending) may have a symptomatic intervertebral disc with an intact annulus and that patients with a directional preference toward spinal flexion may have underlying spinal stenosis.

## Lumbar Spinal Stenosis (Flexion Syndrome)

Lumbar spinal stenosis is a common degenerative condition in the elderly and is associated with narrowing of the spinal canal or nerve root canals caused by degenerative arthritic changes of the facet joints and intervertebral discs; it is often associated with chronic low back pain and leg symptoms. The leg symptoms are thought to result from compression on the vertebral venous plexus from multilevel stenosis that creates venous pooling and congestion and leads to ischemic pain and fatigue in the lower extremities during walking.[81] Spinal extension is commonly limited. Sitting or assuming a spinal flexion (forward bent) position often alleviates the leg symptoms. This clinical syndrome is termed neurogenic claudication and has been defined as pain, paresthesias, and cramping of the lower extremities brought on by walking and relieved by sitting.[81]

Pain in the legs brought on by walking and relieved by sitting in the elderly can be the result of several other conditions, such as osteoarthritis of the hips or knees, or vascular or intermittent claudication from peripheral vascular disease, that must be screened before a diagnosis of spinal stenosis can be made.[81] The spinal canal is further narrowed in a lordotic posture and tends to widen in a more flexed posture, which explains the postural dependency exhibited by patients with spinal stenosis with neurogenic claudication.

The two-stage treadmill test is a clinical procedure that can be used to assist in the differentiation between neurogenic and

**BOX 4-9** McKenzie Prone Extension Exercise Sequence

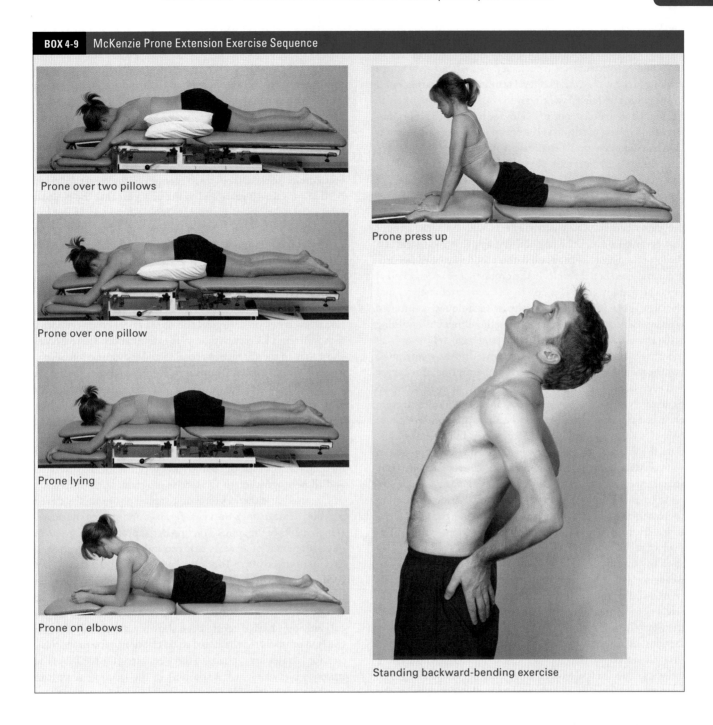

Prone over two pillows

Prone over one pillow

Prone lying

Prone on elbows

Prone press up

Standing backward-bending exercise

vascular claudication. The neurogenic claudication should be more affected by the position of the spine during the lower extremity exertion. The vascular claudication should only be affected by the level of lower extremity exertion and the demands of blood flow to the lower extremity muscles.

The two-stage treadmill test is performed with the patient walking on a level treadmill for up to 10 minutes, followed by a 10-minute rest period in sitting and then another bout of walking on the treadmill set at a 15-degree incline for up to 10 minutes. The speed is set at 1.0 miles per hour and then adjusted to a comfortable pace for the patient. The patient is asked to report

any symptoms increased beyond the baseline level and given the opportunity to stop the test before 10 minutes if symptoms become intense. A positive test result for neurogenic claudication is demonstration of a greater tolerance for walking in the inclined position, which places the lumbar spine in a more flexed (forward bent) position.

Fritz et al[81] found a high specificity (92.3%) for correlation with lumbar spinal stenosis for patients with positive test results for the two-stage treadmill test, but the sensitivity was low (50%). Fritz et al[81] also found that the most accurate diagnosis of spinal stenosis occurred with variables based on time to onset of symptoms and recovery time, which identified 20 of 26 stenotic subjects (sensitivity, 76.9%) and correctly classified 18 of 19 nonstenotic subjects (specificity, 94.7%). Subjects with a prolonged recovery time after level walking and an earlier onset of symptoms with level walking were 14.5 times more likely to be stenotic than nonstenotic (likelihood ratio, 14.51).[81] In addition, the ranking of sitting as the best posture showed a significant association with the stenosis diagnosis.[81]

A flexion-based exercise physical therapy program has been shown to result in positive outcomes in the conservative management of lumbar spinal stenosis in older adults.[38] Whitman et al[38] compared the long-term effects of two physical therapy programs and showed positive effects with both the groups that received 6 weeks of physical therapy that consisted of a flexion-based exercise program with a progressive walking program and even better results in the group that received manual physical therapy interventions to the hip, lumbopelvic, and thoracic spine (thrust and nonthrust techniques) combined with a progressive exercise and unweighted treadmill walking program. At 6 weeks, 1 year, and long-term follow-up (29 months) examinations, both groups showed positive outcomes, but the manual physical therapy group perception of recovery was even better (79% versus 41% at 6 weeks) at each follow-up period.[38] Nearly 25% of the patients in this clinical trial were classified as having severe spinal stenosis at multiple levels, and 55% of the patients had bilateral leg pain.[38] These results illustrate the importance of exhausting a nonsurgical approach in spite of MRI and radiographic evidence of severe degenerative spinal changes. The study also shows the importance of combining manual physical therapy with an active exercise program to maximize outcomes for patients with more chronic conditions. The manual physical therapy interventions in the Whitman et al[38] study were provided by physical therapists with specialty training in manual therapy (Fellows of the American Academy of Orthopaedic Manual Physical Therapists [AAOMPT]), and the specific interventions and exercises were selected to address the specific impairment findings in mobility, flexibility, and strength throughout the spine and lower extremities. Special attention should be paid to the hip joint in this patient population for signs of joint mobility limitation, muscle length limitations (especially hip flexors), and signs of weakness (commonly the gluteus medius). Correction of the hip dysfunctions with manual therapy techniques, stretching, and specific exercise programs can assist in positive clinical outcomes.[82]

## Lumbar Radiculopathy That Does Not Centralize (Traction)

The clinical decisions of how to manage patients with leg pain that does not centralize with repeated movements and does not fit the hypomobility or instability classifications create a clinical challenge for physical therapists and physicians. Saal and Saal[83] showed excellent clinical outcomes in 90% of the patients who met the typical criteria for surgery of a herniated nucleus pulposus (HNP), including straight leg raise (SLR) less than 60 degrees, computed tomography scan results that showed a

herniated nucleus pulposis, and positive electromyographic results that showed evidence of radiculopathy. These patients underwent treatment with an active stabilization and conditioning exercise and ergonomic program and attained excellent results with avoidance of surgery.[83]

Likewise, Weber[84] randomly divided 126 patients into two groups of patients who met similar criteria for lumbar laminectomy surgery for HNP, with one group receiving the surgery and the other group treated nonsurgically with an exercise and ergonomic "back school" treatment program. Weber followed both groups for 10 years and found at 1 year that the patients who received surgical treatment showed a better result than the nonsurgical group.[84] At the 4-year and 10-year follow-up examinations, no significant difference was found between the surgical and nonsurgical groups.[84]

In a more recent study that compared surgical and nonsurgical management of lumbar disc protrusion with radiculopathy, Thomas et al[85] found no difference in pain, disability, or functional levels between surgical and nonsurgical groups at both a 6-month and a 12-month follow-up examination. These studies show that, in the absence of bowel/bladder dysfunction or progressive motor deficits, nonsurgical interventions should be exhausted before surgery is considered in treatment of lumbar HNP and that nonsurgical care should include physical therapy with an emphasis on an active exercise and conditioning program.

Lumbar traction is another commonly used treatment method for this type of condition that can assist in pain relief and allow progression to an exercise program. Lumbar traction can be used in either a prone or a supine position. The flexed position tends to open the neuroforamin and stretch the posterior elements of the spine. Traction in the prone position with a normal amount of lordosis tends to unload the intervertebral disc more effectively.[86] The typical protocol for traction is use of a force equal to 50% of the patient's body weight and use of an intermittent force pattern of 20 to 30 seconds on and 10 to 15 seconds off, for a total duration of 15 minutes.[86] Positive clinical outcomes have recently been shown with use of a lumbar traction protocol that included static traction in the prone position for 12 minutes applied at a force equal to 40% to 60% of the patient's body weight.[87] Variations in the traction setup can also be made to provide a unilateral pull and to vary the patient position into side bending or flexion/extension to begin the traction in a position of patient comfort. With subsequent treatments, the traction position is gradually brought back into a more neutral spine position based on the patient's response to the treatment. Boxes 4-10, 4-11, and 4-12 provide further guidelines on the use of lumbar traction. Box 4-13 provides examples of lumbar traction patient setups.

Compared with the other treatment-based classifications, the subgroup of patients who receive traction has not been studied extensively. A systematic review found a lack of quality studies and studies that were somewhat inconclusive regarding the effectiveness of lumbar traction.[88] Historically, lumbar traction tends to be used in conditions that do not respond well to other manual therapy or exercise-based approaches. This group

| BOX 4-10 | Proposed Theoretical Effects of Spinal Traction |
|---|---|

Widens the intervertebral foramina
Temporarily reduces the size of a disc herniation/protrusion
Creates a negative pressure in the disc to "suck back" a protrusion as a result of tauting of the spinal ligaments pushing in on a disc protrusion
Neurophysiological effects of pain inhibition
Straightens the spinal curve
Mobilizes the facet joints (nonspecific)
Stretches spinal muscles

| BOX 4-11 | Indications for Spinal Traction |
|---|---|

Spinal nerve root impingement (deep tendon reflexes, numbness, weakness, +SLR test)
Peripheralization of leg pain with lumbar backward bending
Positive crossed straight leg raise test (<45 degrees)
Lower extremity pain that centralizes with lumbar traction

| BOX 4-12 | Contraindications and Precautions of Spinal Traction |
|---|---|

Movement is contraindicated
Acute strains/inflammation
Hypermobility/instability
Rheumatoid arthritis
Respiratory problems
Compromised structural integrity
   Malignant disease
   Tumor
   Osteoporosis
   Infection
Current pregnancy
Uncontrolled hypertension
Aortic aneurysm
Severe hemorrhoids
Cardiovascular disease
Abdominal hernia
Hiatal hernia, for lumbar mechanical traction

| BOX 4-13 | Lumbar Traction |
|---|---|

Prone lumbar traction set up with portable hydraulic lumbar traction device

Supine lumbar traction set up with portable hydraulic lumbar traction device

of patients may also proceed to surgical interventions, most commonly lumbar discectomy/laminectomy.

Fritz et al[87] reported preliminary data to support favorable outcomes in a subgroup of patients with lumbar radiculopathy (leg pain with signs of nerve root compression) who had peripheralization of symptoms with lumbar extension or had a positive crossed straight leg raise test (<45 degrees). Patients with low back and leg pain and signs of nerve root compression (positive straight leg raise or lower extremity neurologic signs) were randomly assigned to one of two treatment groups: lumbar extension exercise protocol for 6 weeks or lumbar traction for 2 weeks combined with the lumbar extension exercise protocol.[87] At the 2-week follow-up examination, the lumbar traction group showed improvements in disability and fear avoidance beliefs, but no between-group differences were seen at the 6-week follow-up period.[87] However, further analysis of the subject baseline examination results revealed that the subgroup of patients with symptoms that peripheralized with extension or with positive crossed straight leg raise test showed significantly better outcomes at 2 and 6 weeks if they received the lumbar traction.[87]

Positional distraction is an alternative to lumbar traction that can be performed both in the clinic and at the patient's home. Box 4-14 shows a positional distraction demonstration. Advantages of positional distraction are that it can isolate the spinal level to maximally open the effected neuroforamen, it is inexpensive (a bolster can be made at home by tightly rolling a pillow in a sheet), and it is under the control of the patient.[89] Creighton[90] showed with radiographic evidence that positional distraction that combines isolated lumbar flexion, lateral flexion away from the targeted neuroforamen, and rotation toward the affected side focused to a spinal segment via manual therapy techniques can maximally open a targeted neuroforamen. Once the patient is placed in positional distraction, he or she should be monitored to ensure patient comfort. For the intervention to be effective, the patient should report relief of leg pain shortly after placement in the position. The treatment sessions typically last 10 to 20 minutes, and the patient can perform the procedure at home three to six times per day. Positional distraction allows frequent intermittent unloading of the effected nerve root, which is believed to have positive clinical

**BOX 4-14**   Positional Distraction

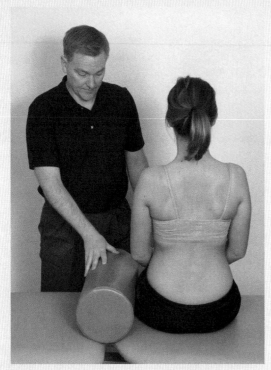

Patient sits next to bolster with bolster on side opposite targeted nerve root and neuroforamen

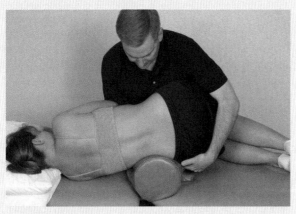

Patient lies over bolster with targeted neuroforamen on top side, and therapist adjusts bolster to create a fulcrum point to side bend targeted spinal segment

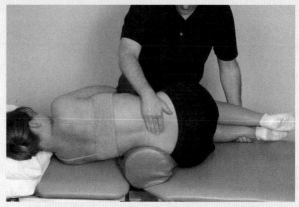

Both hips are flexed to induce forward bending at targeted segment

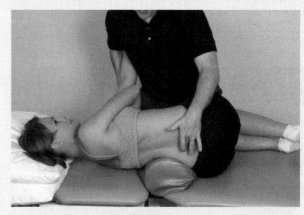

Patient's bottom arm is pulled upward to induce lumbar rotation at targeted segment

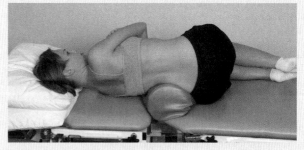

Patient rests in positional distraction that combines forward bending, left side bending, and right rotation isolated to targeted spinal segment to maximally open neuroforamen and relieve nerve root compression

effects. The patient gradually progresses into an exercise program as the intensity of leg symptoms subsides.

## Postsurgical Lumbar Rehabilitation

A systematic review of the literature regarding postoperative lumbar intervertebral disc surgery management concluded that strong evidence exists for intensive exercise programs to enhance functional status and faster return to work and that no evidence exists that these programs increase the reoperation rates.[91] No studies investigated whether active rehabilitation programs should start immediately after surgery or start 4 to 6 weeks later.[91]

The clinical assumption after lumbar disc surgery is that functional instability results from the surgery and that the patient needs to be progressed into a spinal stabilization and conditioning program. A thorough examination should be conducted of the surrounding structures, including thoracic spine, pelvis, and hips, to determine impairments that could hinder a full recovery; if identified, these impairments should be addressed in the plan of care. The patient should be cautioned on sitting greater than 15 to 20 minutes at a time for the first 6 to 12 weeks after lumbar disc surgery to avoid unnecessary loading of the intervertebral disc structures. The patient needs to be guided through progression of a lumbar stabilization exercise program (see Boxes 4-6, 4-7, and 4-8 for phases I to III of a lumbar stabilization program). A walking program is also advisable in most circumstances.

## Sacroiliac Joint Dysfunctions

Laslett et al[92] used a standard of three of five positive sacroiliac joint (SIJ) provocation tests to make the diagnosis of a painful SIJ; this diagnosis was tested against the gold standard of a double SIJ anesthetic and cortisone injection. The five tests were anterior superior iliac spine (ASIS) distraction, thigh thrust, Gaenslen's test, ASIS compression, and sacral thrust. Based on the results in testing 43 patients with chronic low back and leg symptoms with mean duration of symptoms of 32 months (standard deviation [SD], 39 months), the results of the study were reported as sensitivity of 0.91 (95% CI, 0.62-0.98), specificity of 0.78 (95% CI, 0.61-0.89), positive likelihood ratio of 4.16 (95% CI, 2.16-8.39), and negative likelihood ratio of 0.12 (95% CI, 0.02-0.49). Nine of these patients showed centralization or peripheralization of symptoms with repeated movement testing, and a second subset of data was analyzed once these patients were removed from the dataset. Based on the remaining 34 patients, the sensitivity was reported as 0.91 (95% CI, 0.62-0.98), the specificity as 0.87 (95% CI, 0.68-0.96), and the negative likelihood ratio as 0.11 (95% CI, 0.02-0.44). Exclusion of patients whose pain centralized or peripheralized with repeated lumbar active movement testing increased the positive likelihood ratio for identifying symptomatic SIJ from 4.16 (95% CI, 2.16-8.39) to 6.97 (95% CI, 2.70-20.27). With this clinical reasoning, the combination of three or more positive provocation SIJ test results and no centralization or peripheralization is 3 to 20 times more likely in patients with positive diagnostic SIJ injection results than in patients with negative injection results. The SIJ provocation tests used in this study were found in a previous study by Laslett and Williams[93] to have good to excellent reliability (Kappa = 0.52-0.88).

There appears to be a subgroup of patients with chronic lumbopelvic pain with symptoms that originate from the sacroiliac joint. In addition, the SIJ is a likely source of symptoms in female subjects during and after pregnancy because of the hypermobility that results from the release of the hormone relaxin.

Lee[94] describes the function of the pelvis as the transference of loads from the trunk to the lower extremities and from the lower extremities to the trunk. The active straight raise test has been shown to be an effective means to differentiate SIJ symptoms (posterior pelvic pain) that occur from lack of stability of

the pelvis either from the anterior (transversus abdominis) or posterior (multifidus) musculature.[95] Evidence shows that training the TrA muscle can enhance the functional stability of the pelvis and sacroiliac joints.[24]

In addition, much clinical speculation exists that a hypermobile SIJ can displace and can be detected clinically as hypomobility and altered positioning of the ilium and sacrum. Unfortunately, studies that have assessed the reliability of palpation examination procedures designed to detect pelvic position and mobility have shown poor reliability.[96] In clinical situations, therapists rarely use passive joint mobility examinations in isolation. Rather, they combine the results of the single assessment with those of other examination procedures. Cibulka and Koldehoff[97] showed excellent interrater reliability in assessing the sacroiliac joint (Kappa = 0.88) by using a cluster of four examination procedures and requiring that three of the four results be positive to diagnose a sacroiliac dysfunction. Cibulka and colleagues[5,97] used tests for position, mobility, and provocation of SIJ impairments. However, Potter and Rothstein[96] showed poor reliability when studying each of those same four examination procedures in isolation. Cibulka's study seems to more closely emulate how therapists actually assess patients in the clinic. Riddle and Freburger[98] attempted to reproduce Cibulka's study of the sacroiliac joint. They used the same four clinical examinations; however, they used multiple pairs of testers and multiple clinical sites and showed poor reliability, with Kappa scores ranging from 0.11 to 0.23.[98] The reliability of manual examination procedures is enhanced with careful attention to the training process and standardization of the examination procedures.

For clinical management purposes, classification is helpful of sacroiliac conditions into three categories: sprain, hypermobility, and displacement.[89] Sacroiliac sprain may be caused by a direct or indirect trauma to the joint. The signs and symptoms tend to include pain and inflammation well localized over the SIJ, ipsilateral muscle guarding of the thoracolumbar erector spinae, and positive pain provocation test results. The treatment should include support with an SIJ belt, relative rest to avoid activities that strain the involved structures, and manual therapy and exercise to treat any surrounding dysfunctions of the lumbar spine and hip.

Sacroiliac hypermobility tends to be caused by repetitive minor trauma, childbirth strains, or a history of trauma. The signs and symptoms are a dull ache on assuming a fixed posture with occasional radiation to the posterior thigh, periodic episodes of sharper or more acute pain associated with displacement of the SIJ, hypermobility with passive mobility assessments, and positive pain provocation test results.[89] These patients often present with a positive active straight leg test indicative of poor ability to stabilize the lumbopelvic region. Treatment of a hypermobile SIJ includes use of a sacroiliac (SI) belt to be worn 24 hours per day for up to 6 to 12 weeks and treatment of surrounding joint dysfunctions and muscle imbalances with use of exercise and manual therapy.[99] The SI belt can be weaned as the patient gains proper control of the local lumbopelvic muscles and becomes less symptomatic (see Box 4-15

**BOX 4-15** | Sacroiliac Binder

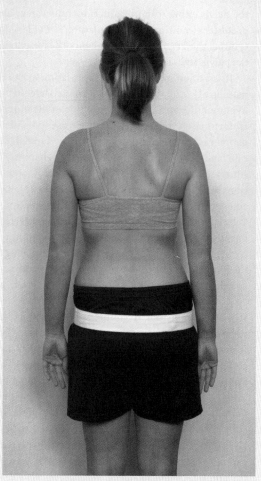

Sacroiliac belt should be worn at level of PSISs to attempt to bind and support pelvis

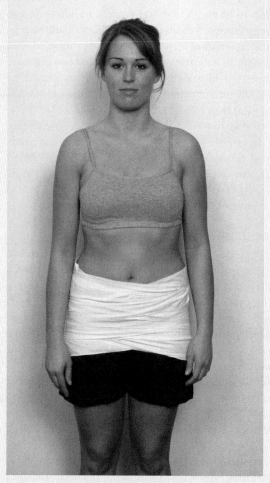

Skultetus maternity binder can provide more comprehensive stabilization of pelvis when instability of pelvis is suspected

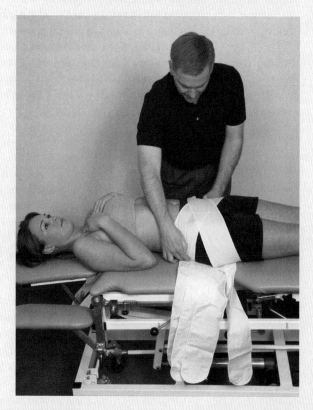

Skultetus maternity binder should be applied in supine position

for SIJ stabilization binders). An exercise program that focuses on specific stabilizing exercises that target the multifidus and transversus abdominis muscles has been show to attain positive outcomes in patients with pelvic girdle pain after pregnancy.[99]

Sacroiliac displacement is thought be caused by a hypermobile joint overriding an articular prominence or by severe trauma to the joint.[89] Signs and symptoms include a lowered iliac crest (on sitting and standing), restricted passive motion, and positive provocation test results. If the lower iliac crest is the symptomatic SIJ with provocation testing and limited mobility assessment, the symptomatic SIJ is considered to be displaced in posterior rotation. If the higher iliac crest side is the symptomatic and restricted side, this SIJ is consider to be displaced in anterior rotation. Treatment should include manipulation reduction followed by treatment as outlined for a hypermobile SIJ once it is reduced.

Sacroiliac joint dysfunctions tend to occur more commonly in females for the following reasons: smaller joint surfaces in the female SIJ, flatter and smoother joint surfaces, and SIJ mechanical disadvantage in the female because the axis of the hip is further from the line of gravity, which places more torque on the SIJ from a longer lever arm.[100] In addition, hormonal changes, childbirth strains, and intercourse strains can also contribute to development of SIJ dysfunctions in women.

O'Sullivan and Beales proposed a classification for pelvic girdle pain disorders based on an examination to include palpation and provocation tests of the SIJ and surrounding ligamentous and myofascial structures, active straight leg raise tests in supine and prone positions, careful analysis of pain-provoking and pain-relieving activities and postures, and tests for specific muscle function for pelvic floor, abdominal wall, back muscles, iliopsoas, quadratus lumborum, gluteal, and piriformis muscles. O'Sullivan and Beales[101] describe two types of "peripherally mediated pelvic girdle pain disorders": reduced force closure and excessive force closure.

Reduced force closure is characterized by sensitized painful sacroiliac joint and surrounding connective tissues with signs of hypermobility and poor motor control of the lumbopelvic and hip muscles. The maladaptive motor control leads to impaired load transfer through the pelvis acting as a mechanism for ongoing strain and pain at the SIJ. Hormonal influences may be a contributing factor to this condition. These patients have positive active straight leg raise (ASLR) test results with poor motor control patterns of force closure of the pelvis involving poor control of the local lumbopelvic muscles (pelvic floor, TrA, mulfiifdus, inlopsosas, and gluteal muscles) and excessive activation of the more global spinal muscles.[101] Pain is seen with weight-bearing postures, such as sitting, standing, and walking, and loaded activities that induce rotation pelvic strain coupled with spine and hip loading activities.[101] The pain may be relieved with an SIJ belt, training optimal alignment of the spine and pelvis, and retraining of the local lumbopelvic muscles with inhibition of the thoracopelvic muscles. These disorders may gain temporary relief with manual therapy techniques, but for long-term improvements, comprehensive stabilization exercise program is necessary.[99,101]

Excessive force closure is associated with excessive, abnormal, and sustained loading of sensitized pelvic structures by excessive activation of the local and global lumbopelvic muscle systems. This patient group has positive SIJ provocation test results and localized pain of the SIJ and surrounding ligamentous and myofascial tissues.[101] These patients do not have positive ASLR test results (no feeling of heaviness), and SIJ belts and manual pelvic compression tend to make the symptoms worse.[101-103] The patients commonly hold habitual erect lordotic lumbopelvic postures associated with high levels of cocontraction across various muscles such as the abdominal wall, pelvic floor, piriformis, and local spinal muscles.[101] These patients often have had extensive physical therapy and are preoccupied with concern with "pelvic alignment" and beliefs of being "unstable" or "displaced."[101] Often these patients have been engaged in intensive stabilization exercise programs and are commonly anxious and under high levels of stress.[101] Management of this disorder focuses on reducing force closure across the pelvic structures with targeted relaxation strategies, breathing control, muscle inhibitory techniques, enhancement of passive/relaxed spinal postures, pacing strategies, hydrotherapy, cessation of stabilization exercise training, and focus on cardiovascular exercise.[101]

With management of SIJ and pelvic pain conditions, manual therapy and exercise interventions should address the surrounding impairments such as hip stiffness, tightness of the hip flexors or iliotibial bands (ITBs), or thoracolumbar hypomobility. Most patients ultimately need to be progressed into a lumbopelvic stabilization exercise program. Assessment and treatment of pelvic floor muscle function may also facilitate a positive clinical outcome.

The stabilization exercise program must be progressed with caution to avoid straining the painful pelvic structures by forcing hip motions into directions that provoke symptoms. For instance, if anterior rotation motions of the pelvis provoke a patient's symptoms, the prone hip extension exercise should not be prescribed until the patient can perform this exercise pain free and with good control. Instead, hip flexion stabilization exercises (such as marching with stabilization) should be used early in the program, and the multifidus muscles can be trained with static stabilization postures that are challenged in the standing position, such as shoulder extension theraband exercises.

## Chronic Low Back Pain

The treatment-based classification system has been shown to be most effective in management of patients between 18 and 60 years of age with acute LBP. With patients who do not fit neatly into one of these categories, further assessment of movement impairments is warranted, including assessment of extremity movement effect on the spine motion and symptoms, assessment of muscle length and strength (i.e., muscle imbalances), and evaluation of spinal impairments superior and inferior to the primary pain symptoms.

The longer a patient has LBP, the more deconditioned the patient seems to become and the more secondary impairments

---

**BOX 4-16    Factors That Compound Complex Chronic Back Pain**

Psychosocial components of chronic pain
    Elevated fear avoidance beliefs
    Depression
    Anxiety disorders
Underlying pathology
    Rheumatoid arthritis, osteoarthritis, ankylosing spondylitis, fibromyalgia
Movement impairments
Muscle imbalances
Multiple joint impairments
Deconditioning

---

seem to develop (Box 4-16). In addition, patients with greater psychosocial issues and fear avoidance beliefs are more likely to have chronic back pain conditions develop.[104] O'Sullivan[105] has outlined a classification system that categorizes patients with more complex chronic spine conditions and that takes into account the complexity of the more chronic low back pain conditions.

O'Sullivan[105] outlined three main groups of patients with chronic disabling lumbopelvic pain with regard to motor control impairments. The first group of patients has movement impairment and motor dysfunction that is secondary or adaptive to an underlying pathologic process, such as inflammatory pain disorder, neurogenic pain, neuropathic or centrally mediated pain disorder, or severe structural disorder. The second group consists of patients in whom psychological or social factors are the underlying perpetuating factors behind the disorder, which results in altered central processing, amplification of pain, and resultant disordered movement and motor dysfunction. In these two groups, attempts to simply normalize the motor dysfunction and movement impairment in isolation without dealing with the other factors of the multifactorial disorders are likely to fail.

The third group consists of patients in whom maladaptive movement and motor patterns result in chronic abnormal tissue loading and ongoing pain and distress.[105] This third group can be subgrouped into movement impairment and control impairment classifications. The movement impairment classification is associated with a loss of normal physiologic lumbopelvic mobility in the direction of pain. These patients have abnormally high levels of muscle guarding and cocontraction of lumbopelvic muscles that cause abnormally high levels of compressive loading across articulations, excessive stability, and movement restriction that results in muscle strain and fatigue. These conditions are commonly accompanied by fear of movement and faulty cognitive coping strategies and beliefs regarding the pain disorder.[105] Management is based on a cognitive behavioral model that aims to reduce fear of movement and reduce muscle tone with education and facilitating graduated movement exposure into the painful range in a relaxed and normal manner.

The control impairment classification is not associated with impairment in mobility of the symptomatic spinal segment in the direction of pain provocation but instead presents with deficits in motor control with the inability to effectively control the neutral zone of the motion segment or fix the spinal segment at an end range provocative position.[105] This condition appears to result in pain from recurrent end range strain and nonphysiological spinal segment movement and loading.[105] The patients adopt postures and movement patterns that are maladaptive and provocative and represent a mechanism for ongoing pain and disability.

Janda[106] describes the pathogenesis of spinal syndromes as originating from imbalances in muscle function between the phasic and postural muscles. Based on clinical and electromyographic observations, the postural muscles have a tendency to develop tightness, hypertonia, and shortening when in dysfunction. The following muscles are included as predominately postural muscles: triceps, rectus femoris, thigh adductors, hamstrings, iliopsoas, tensor fasciae latae, some trunk erectors, quadratus lumborum, sternal portion of the pectoralis major, upper part of the trapezius, levator scapulae, and upper extremity flexors.[106]

The muscles with a predominately phasic function show a tendency for hypotonia, inhibition, and weakening; are less readily activated in most movement patterns; and atrophy more easily and to a greater extent when in dysfunction. Janda[106] states that imbalance between these two muscle systems creates imbalances across joints and leads to pain and degeneration. Motor performance is evaluated with assessment of the sequence of activation of the certain movement patterns. For instance, with prone hip extension, the opposite side multifidus should fire first and strongest in comparison with the ipsilateral mutifidus and erector spinae. If the erector spinae fires first and strongest, tightness and guarding of the erector spinae (postural) and weakness of the multifidus (phasic) could occur.

Goldby et al[107] conducted a randomized controlled trial (RCT) for patients with chronic low back pain and compared manual physical therapy, stabilization exercise, and education. The long-term and short-term follow-up results for measures of pain and disability showed improvements in all three treatment groups, but the greatest amount of improvement was noted in the spinal stabilization exercise group. In patients with chronic low back pain and higher initial pain rating scores (>50), the patients in the manual physical therapy group had better outcomes than the education-only group, which shows that mobilization/manipulation can assist in pain reduction with patients with chronic low back pain and high pain scores.[107] An active program of spinal stabilization exercises is an effective approach for most patients with chronic low back pain, but manual therapy techniques can be used to reduce pain and assist in transitioning patients into an active exercise program. Further research is needed to determine whether subgroups of patients with chronic low back pain would respond best to manual therapy, exercise, education, or a combination of the three approaches.

High FABQ scores about work with patients with acute LBP can be used to predict which patients are likely to develop more chronic disability and longer term absences from work at a 4-week follow-up examination, after controlling for initial levels of pain intensity, physical impairment, disability, and the type of therapy received.[108] In another study with a 12-month follow-up period, LBP history and pain intensity, rather than high FABQ scores, were found to be the most important predictors of chronic pain.[109]

Fritz and George[110] studied a group of patients with acute work-related LBP and showed that FABQ work subscale scores greater than 34 were associated with an increased risk of not returning to work (positive likelihood ratio, 3.33; 95% CI, 1.65-6.77) and that work subscale scores of less than 29 were associated with a decreased risk of not returning to work (negative likelihood ratio, 0.08, 95% CI, 0.01-0.54).

Patient education based on a fear avoidance model encourages confrontation of the feared activities and consists of educating the patient that pain is a common condition, rather than a serious disease that needs careful protection.[111] FABQ activity subscale scores that exceed 15/24 are considered high.[1] George, Bialosky, and Fritz[112] describe a case report with a progressively graded monitored specific exercise and education approach for successful treatment of a patient with low back pain and high FABQ scores. Pain levels were monitored throughout the treatment sessions but did not influence the treatment sessions exercise quota. At a 6-month follow-up examination, the patient had partial return of fear avoidance beliefs but only minimal increase in perception of disability.[112]

Evidence also shows that for most patients with LBP, the level of disability can be reduced with a conditioning program. The best outcomes can be produced by first providing the intervention based on subgrouping, but once improvements are noted in function and perception of disability, a strengthening and conditioning program is indicated. The stabilization program should start with guidance, with a good deal of feedback for training in isolation of the local muscles, especially transverses abdominus and multifidus muscles, in a supported position, such as prone or supine hook lying, and with a stabilizer airbag biofeedback pressure gauge device (see Box 4-6). The second phase should include addition of exercises in less stable positions, such as quadruped and standing, that further challenge maintenance of a neutral spine position (see Box 4-7). The final phase includes more dynamic movement patterns in functional planes that require control of movement of the spine combined with extremity movements in a controlled manner. For example, lunge exercises require controlled dynamic stabilization in a functional movement pattern. Use of a weighted medicine ball assists in guiding the movement pattern, and the reaching theoretically facilitates the hip gluteal muscles to eccentrically assist in control of the movement pattern (see Box 4-8). Work-specific and sport-specific activities can also be incorporated in the phase III dynamic stabilization program, which might include lifting training or balance or throwing activities.

In coordination with the progression of a stabilization exercise program, muscle imbalances should be addressed through mobility and stretching exercises (Box 4-17), strengthening exercise, and use of myofascial techniques to target myofascial tightness or weakness noted in the examination of both the trunk and the lower extremities. Manipulation should be incorporated with overall management of the spinal disorder to address the impairments found in the patient examination. In chronic LBP conditions, often the manipulation is directed to enhance thoracic and hip mobility as the patient is gradually progressed into a lumbar spinal stabilization and conditioning program.

The patient's signs and symptoms change through the course of physical therapy treatment, both between and within treatment sessions, and so does the classification and the focus of the treatment. For instance, a patient may have signs and symptoms for both manipulation and stabilization with lower lumbar hypomobility and upper lumbar hypermobility. Direct manipulation techniques focused at the lower lumbar spine with a follow up with both range of motion and spinal stabilization exercises are appropriate. The patient must be reassessed frequently throughout the treatment session to assess the effect of the manipulation and the need for further manual treatment. Once a change for the positive of enhanced mobility, reduced muscle tone, and reduced pain is achieved, the emphasis of the treatment should shift to stabilization exercises and general conditioning for all the classification groups.

**BOX 4-17**    Lower Extremity Stretching Exercises and Myofascial Techniques

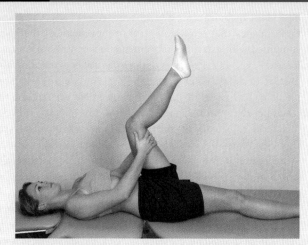

Hamstring stretch

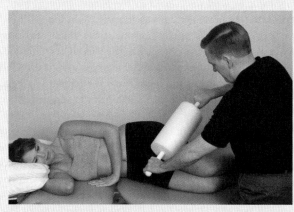

Myofascial rolling technique to loosen iliotibial band

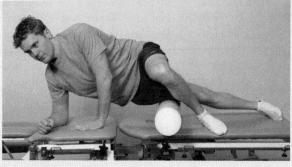

Self-myofascial rolling technique to loosen iliotibial band

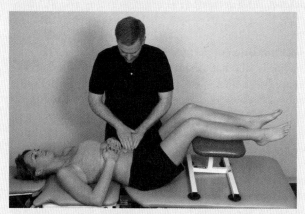

Psoas release: slowly sink into lower abdomen and sustain pressure on psoas until tension subsides in tight guarded muscle

## SELECTED SPECIAL TESTS FOR LUMBOPELVIC EXAMINATION

### Palpation for a Lower Lumbar Step  DVD

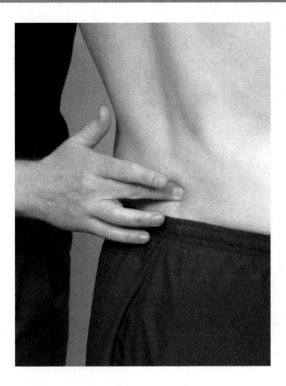

| | |
|---|---|
| **PATIENT POSITION** | The patient stands, with good posture and arms relaxed at the sides. |
| **THERAPIST POSITION** | The therapist stands to the side and slightly behind the patient. |
| **PROCEDURE** | The pad of the long finger is used to palpate the spinous process of each lumbar vertebra. The fingers of the other hand are spread across the patient's upper chest to provide gentle countersupport to the patient's chest. |
| **NOTES** | Note the presence of a step between adjacent vertebrae. A palpable step is suspected to be a sign of lumbar instability and can be accompanied by a band of paraspinal muscle guarding across the lumbar vertebrae. A positive finding should be followed up with further instability and mobility testing for detection of other signs of instability. |

## Lumbar Posterior Shear Test

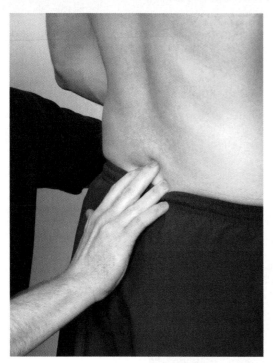

Finger placement for lumbar anterior/posterior shear test

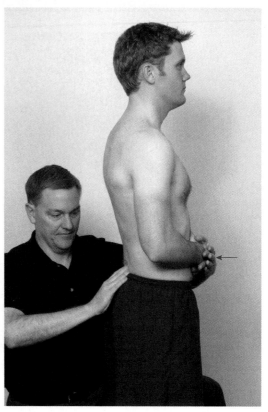

Hand placement for lumbar anterior/posterior shear test

| | |
|---|---|
| **PURPOSE** | The test is used to assess for instability of lumbar segments L1-L2 through L5-S1. |
| **PATIENT POSITION** | The patient stands with hands folded across the abdomen. |
| **THERAPIST POSITION** | The therapist kneels to the side and slightly behind the patient. |
| **HAND PLACEMENT** | **Left hand:** The left hand is placed on the patient's hands. |
| | **Right hand:** The pad of the long finger is used to palpate the specified spinous process; the index and fourth fingers are used to block the transverse processes of the inferior vertebra; and the heel (thenar/hypothenar eminences) of the hand is used to block the sacrum. |
| **PROCEDURE** | The pad of the long finger on the right hand is used to palpate the spinous process of L5. The heel of the right hand blocks the sacrum. The left hand is used to give an anterior to posterior force through the patient's hands and forearms. The pad of the long finger on the right hand is used to palpate for posterior translation of the specified lumbar segment. The procedure is repeated with palpation of the spinous processes of L4, L3, L2, and L1. The amount of posterior translation at each segment is compared, and positive test results include provocation of familiar symptoms or detection of excessive anterior to posterior mobility. |
| **NOTES** | Patient relaxation (of abdominal muscles) is vital for proper performance of this technique. Excessive posterior translation at a segment may indicate instability at that segment. This technique should be used in conjunction with other tests to confirm the signs and symptoms of lumbar instability. Reliability testing for this procedure has been reported at a Kappa value of 0.35.[113] Fritz, Piva, and Childs[114] tested 49 patients with low back pain and found intertester reliability of 64% agreement and a Kappa value of 0.27 (0.14, 0.41). |

## Prone Instability Test

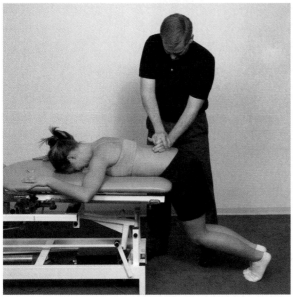

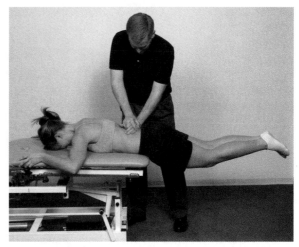

Prone instability test position

Prone instability test start position

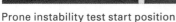

| | |
|---|---|
| **PURPOSE** | The test is used to assess for instability of lumbar segments L1-L2 through L5-S1. |
| **PATIENT POSITION** | The patient lies prone with the body on the examining table, the legs over the edge of the table, and the feet resting on the floor. |
| **THERAPIST POSITION** | The therapist stands at the side of the patient's lumbar spine. |
| **HAND PLACEMENT** | **Left hand:** The ulnar aspect of the hypothenar eminence (just distal to the pisiform) is placed at the targeted spinous process, with the wrist extended and the forearm perpendicular to the angle of the contour of the lumbar spine.<br><br>**Right hand:** The second and third digits are interlaced across the radial aspect of the left hand to support the position of the left hand. |
| **PROCEDURE** | The examiner applies a posterior to anterior pressure to each targeted lumbar vertebrae. If provocation of pain is reported, the patient lifts the feet off the floor and the pressure is reapplied at the symptomatic vertebrae. Test results are positive if the pain is present in the first position but is not reproduced to the same severity when pressure is reapplied to the symptomatic vertebra with the second position (i.e., feet lifted off the floor). |
| **NOTES** | This technique should be used in conjunction with other tests to confirm the signs and symptoms of lumbar instability. This test is reliable, with a Kappa value of 0.87.[113] This test also was included in the clinical prediction rule developed by Hicks for patients with favorable responses to spinal stabilization exercise programs.[31] Therefore, positive test results were correlated with patients with favorable responses, and negative test results were correlated with patients without favorable responses to spinal stabilization exercise programs.[31] This test was one of four variables identified and reported in Box 4-5 in the clinical prediction rule for spinal stabilization exercise program success and failure. Fritz, Piva, and Childs[114] tested 49 patients with low back pain and found intertester reliability of 85% agreement and a Kappa value of 0.69 (0.59, 0.79) for the prone instability test. |

## Femoral Nerve Tension Test (Ely's Test)

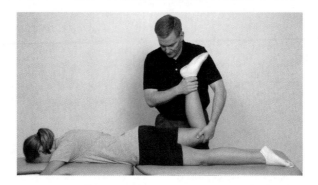

| | |
|---|---|
| **PURPOSE** | The test is used to assess for irritation of the femoral nerve. |
| **PATIENT POSITION** | The patient is prone. |
| **THERAPIST POSITION** | The therapist stands at the edge of the table. |
| **HAND PLACEMENT** | **Cranial hand:** The cranial hand supports the lower leg of the test lower extremity. |
| | **Caudal hand:** The caudal hand supports the thigh of the test lower extremity. |
| **PROCEDURE** | The therapist passively flexes the test leg knee to 90 degrees and then lifts the hip into full extension. Positive test results are found with provocation of anterior thigh pain with the stretch position. |
| **NOTES** | This test position can be considered both a muscle length test for the rectus femoris muscle and a nerve tension test for the femoral nerve. The results of this test should be correlated with other neurological examination procedures to diagnose involvement of the femoral nerve. |

## Iliotibial Band Length Tests

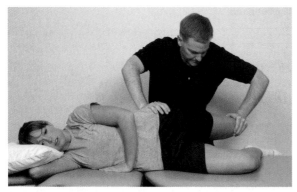

Ober test position

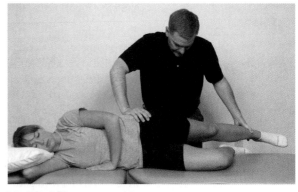

Modified Ober test position

## Iliotibial Band Length Tests—cont'd

| | |
|---|---|
| **PURPOSE** | This test assesses the length of the iliotibial band. |
| **PATIENT POSITION** | The patient is in a side-lying position, with the test leg on top and the body positioned near the back edge of the table. |
| **THERAPIST POSITION** | The therapist stands along the side of the table behind the patient. |
| **HAND PLACEMENT** | **Cranial hand:** This hand is placed on the lateral aspect of the iliac crest. |
| | **Caudal hand:** This hand supports the test leg at the knee. |
| **PROCEDURE** | **Modified Ober:** With the test leg fully extended, the therapist lifts the top leg into a fully abducted position in 10 degrees of extension; with this leg-to-trunk alignment maintained, the test leg is lowered toward the floor. The pelvis must be stabilized throughout the procedure. Hip adduction of 10 degrees is considered normal ITB length. |
| | **Ober:** With the knee flexed to 90 degrees, the therapist lifts the top leg into a fully abducted position with the hip in 10 degrees of extension. With this leg-to-trunk alignment maintained, the test leg is lowered toward the floor. The pelvis must be stabilized throughout the procedure. Hip adduction of 10 degrees is considered normal ITB length. |
| **NOTES** | The therapist can use the anterior aspect of his hip and pelvis to support the foot of the test leg during the Ober test. Use of a second examiner to measure the degree of hip adduction with an inclinometer improves the reliability of this test. Reese and Bandy[115] reported intraexaminer reliability for the Ober test as a Kappa value of 0.90 and for the modified Ober test as a Kappa value of 0.91. |

## The Slump Test[116]

| | |
|---|---|
| **PURPOSE** | This test is used to determine irritability and extensibility of the central spinal canal and dural tissues. |
| **PATIENT POSITION** | The patient sits back on the edge of the treatment table with the posterior knee crease at the edge of the side or foot of the table. |
| **THERAPIST POSITION** | The therapist stands at the side of the patient. |
| **HAND PLACEMENT** | **Left hand:** The left hand is positioned across the upper back, neck, and head. |
| | **Right hand:** The right hand holds one of the patient's feet. |
| **PROCEDURE** | 1. The patient begins in an erect sitting position and is asked about any symptoms. |

2. The patient is asked to slump the back through the full range of thoracic and lumbar flexion and at the same time prevent the head and neck from flexing. Once this position is achieved, gentle overpressure is applied to the upper thoracic area to stretch the thoracic and lumbar spines into full flexion.

3. As thoracic/lumbar flexion is maintained, the patient is asked to fully flex the neck, bringing the chin to the sternum. The therapist applies gentle overpressure to the fully flexed spine.

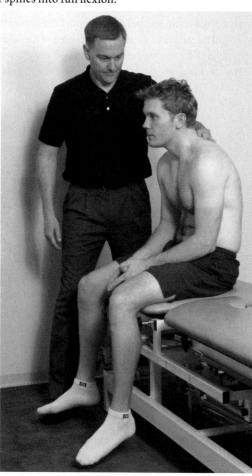
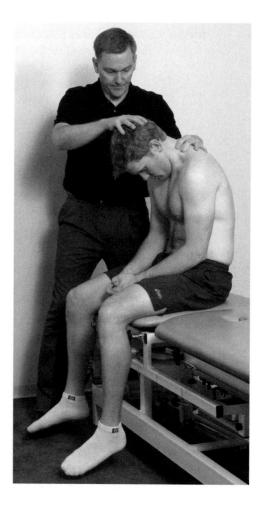

## The Slump Test—cont'd

4. As overpressure is maintained to the fully flexed spine, the patient is asked to extend one knee. The range and pain response are noted.

5. With this position maintained, active ankle dorsiflexion is added to the knee extension and the pain response is noted.

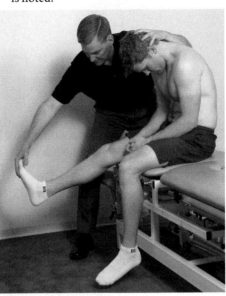

6. With the leg and thoracic/lumbar positions maintained with therapist overpressure, the patient is asked to move the neck into a neutral position. The patient is asked to report any change in symptoms and is asked to fully extend the knee, if the patient was unable to fully extend the knee when the entire spine was held in flexion. The range of knee extension and pain response are noted in this new position.

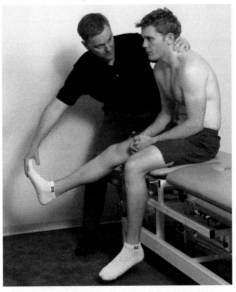

**NOTES**   This test should be performed on patients with cervical, thoracic, or lumbar symptoms. Positive test results are seen when lower extremity symptoms are reproduced and knee extension is limited in the slump sit position and when symptoms are alleviated and knee range of motion is improved with a return of the neck to a neutral position. Treatment includes treatment of joint and soft tissue restrictions throughout the spine and use of the slump sit position to perform active and passive range of motion and sustain stretch (if less irritable) exercises to improve nerve and dural tissue mobility.

## Straight Leg Raise

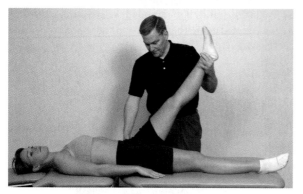

Straight leg raise test position

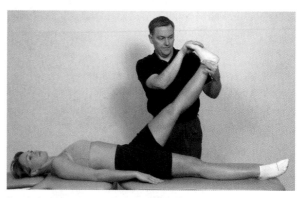

Straight leg raise with ankle dorsiflexion

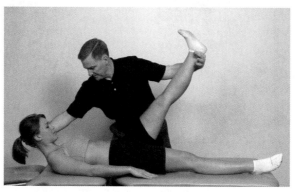

Straight leg raise with neck flexion

| | |
|---|---|
| **PURPOSE** | This test is used to determine whether the cause of leg symptoms is a lumbar herniated disc compressing a lumbar nerve root in the lower lumbar spine. |
| **PATIENT POSITION** | The patient lies supine on a treatment table. |
| **THERAPIST POSITION** | The therapist stands on the side to be tested. |
| **HAND PLACEMENT** | **Cranial hand:** This hand palpates the patient's pelvis to monitor pelvic motion during the test or supports the test leg at the posterior knee. |
| | **Caudal hand:** This hand supports the foot and ankle of the leg to be tested. |
| **PROCEDURE** | The patient's hip is slowly flexed as the knee is maintained in full extension. The patient is asked to respond to the movement, and the degree of hip flexion that is attained when symptoms are reported is recorded, with inquiries about the location and nature of the symptoms. For differentiation of a muscle length restriction of the hamstring from neural irritation, three cycles of a 10-second isometric hamstring contraction are applied, followed by attempts to further flex the hip. If greater than 15-degree hip flexion is attained with this maneuver, a muscle tightness component likely exists to the initial finding. Further neural tension sensitizing maneuvers can be applied with either adding hip adduction to the SLR movement or adding ankle dorsiflexion before raising the leg. In addition, passive neck flexion can be added to increase dural tension during the SLR test. |

## Straight Leg Raise—cont'd

| | |
|---|---|
| **NOTES** | If symptoms are reported with less range of motion during the retest with the addition of the sensitizing maneuvers, a neural irritation is likely contributing to the report of the leg symptoms. A positive straight leg raise for reproduction of lower leg pain at 30 degrees of hip flexion or less has been more strongly correlated with herniated disc of the lower lumbar spine.[117] The contralateral leg should also be tested, and if the SLR of the contralateral leg causes symptoms on the involved leg (positive cross SLR), a herniated disc as the cause of the leg pain (i.e., nerve root irritation) is suspected.[117] Deville et al[118] pooled the results of 11 studies on the straight leg raise test for detection of a lumbar disc herniation at surgery and calculated pooled sensitivity of 0.91 (0.82, 0.94), specificity of 0.26 (0.16, 0.38), positive likelihood ratio of 1.2, and negative likelihood ratio of 3.5. The pooled specificity for the cross straight leg test was 0.29 (0.24-0.34), the pooled specificity was 0.88 (0.86-0.90), the predictive value of a positive test was 0.92, and the negative predictive value was 0.22.[118] |

## Modified Straight Leg Raise Test

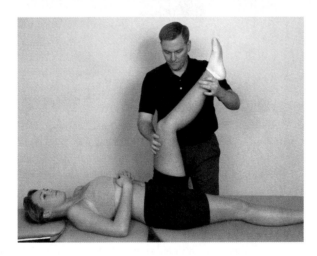

| | |
|---|---|
| **PURPOSE** | This test is used to test the length of the hamstring muscles. |
| **PATIENT POSITION** | The patient is positioned supine with the opposite leg extended. |
| **THERAPIST POSITION** | The therapist stands at the edge of the table. |
| **HAND PLACEMENT** | **Cranial hand:** The cranial hand supports the test leg at the anterior distal femur. |
| | **Caudal hand:** The caudal hand supports the test leg at the posterior aspect of the ankle. |
| **PROCEDURE** | The therapist first flexes the test leg hip to 90 degrees with the knee fully flexed and then slowly extends the patient's knee to end range of motion. A neutral lumbopelvic spine position should be maintained. |
| **NOTES** | Normal hamstring length is considered a −10-degree angle of the knee extension with the hip in 90 degrees of flexion. Reliability is enhanced if a goniometer is used to measure the knee angle with the test position. This test position can be used as a sustained stretch position for the patient, or a hold/relax stretch can be applied to attempt to lengthen the hamstring muscles. In the presence of sciatic nerve root irritation, provocation of leg pain may occur with this test position. Bandy, Irion, and Briggler[119] reported intraclass correlation coefficient (ICC) levels of 0.97 for intratester reliability in testing hamstring length on 20 subjects with this method. |

## Active Straight Leg Raise Test                                                    DVD

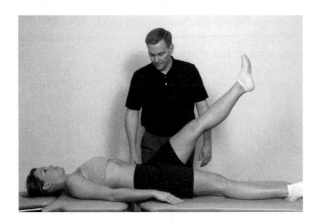

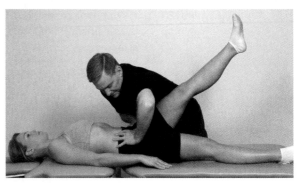

Active straight leg raise with anterior pelvic compression

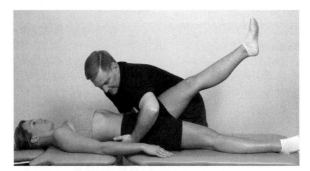

Active straight leg raise with posterior pelvic compression

---

|  |  |
|---|---|
| **PURPOSE** | This test assesses the ability of the lumbopelvic region to accept the load applied from the lower extremities. When the test results are positive, the assumption is that a lack of motor control exists for dynamic stabilization of the pelvis. |
| **PATIENT POSITION** | The patient is positioned supine with the legs straight on a treatment table. |
| **THERAPIST POSITION** | The therapist stands at the side of the patient. |
| **PROCEDURE** | The therapist asks the patient to slowly and actively raise a straight leg off the treatment table 20 centimeters (8 inches), pause, and then slowly lower the leg to the table. The movement is repeated on each side. The therapist observes the patient's ability to stabilize at the lumbopelvic region during the active leg raising and lowering and asks the patient to rate the level of difficulty in raising the leg and pain provocation with the ASLR. If the patient admits to difficulty in raising the leg or symptoms are provoked with the ASLR, the ASLR is repeated with the therapist providing compression of the anterior pelvis at the level of the pubic symphysis to simulate action of the anterior pelvic floor muscles and the transversus abdominis. If symptoms are relieved or the ease of leg raising is improved with pelvic compression, the test results are positive. The ASLR is repeated with compressive |

## Active Straight Leg Raise Test—cont'd

forces applied at the posterior pelvis at the level of the posterior superior sacroiliac spine (PSIS) to simulate action of the sacral multifidus. If symptoms are relieved or ease of leg raising is improved with posterior compression, the test results are positive.

**NOTES**   Positive test results with anterior pelvic compression are an indication of a lack of dynamic stability provided by the anterior pelvic floor and transversus abdominis muscles. Positive test results with posterior pelvic compression are an indication of a lack of dynamic stability provided by the lumbopelvic multifidus muscles. Mens et al[95] reported that test-retest reliability of the ASLR test in identification of women with posterior pelvic pain since pregnancy had a Pearson's correlation coefficient of 0.87. The sensitivity of the test was 0.87, and the specificity was 0.94.[95]

## Prone Transversus Abdominis Test

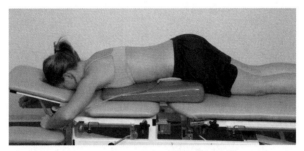

Biofeedback pressure bag is positioned under lower abdomen for prone transversus abdominis test

**PURPOSE**   The purpose of this test is to assess the ability to isolate transversus abdominis muscle control in the absence of overdominance of the global abdominal muscles.

**PATIENT POSITION**   The patient lies prone with the arms at the side, and the pressure biofeedback unit is placed under the abdomen with the navel in the center of the bag and the distal edge of the bag in line with the right and left anterior superior iliac spines. If the patient does not tolerate the prone position well, a firm foam wedge can be positioned under the pelvis.

**THERAPIST POSITION**   The therapist stands at the side of the patient with hands at the sides of the patient's lower trunk to facilitate the drawing in maneuver.

**PROCEDURE**   The pressure pad is inflated to 70 mm Hg. The patient is instructed to breathe in and out and then, without breathing in, slowly draw in the abdomen to lift the abdomen off the bag, keeping the spine position steady. Once the contraction has been achieved, the patient should return to relaxed normal breathing. A successful performance of the test reduces the pressure by 6 to 10 mm Hg, which indicates that the patient can perform an isolated transversus abdominus contraction. Normal strength is achieved when the patient can sustain up to 10 repetitions of 10-second holds of an isolated drawing in maneuver.[120]

**NOTES**   The therapist must ensure that the patient is not just tilting the pelvis or flexing the spine to attain the change in pressure. The drawing in maneuver is the foundation of successful lumbopelvic stabilization training, and the pressure biofeedback device can be used to facilitate progression of a stabilization exercise program.

## Supine Hook-Lying Lumbopelvic Control Test

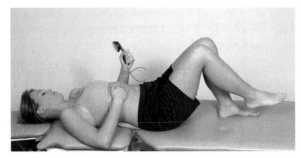

Hook-lying lumbopelvic control with lower extremity marching motion

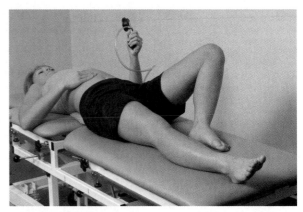

Hook-lying lumbopelvic control with lower extremity bent knee fall out motion

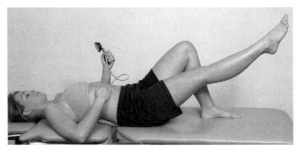

Hook-lying lumbopelvic control with lower extremity straight leg raise motion

| | |
|---|---|
| **PURPOSE** | This test assesses the ability of the transervsus abdominis to control lumbopelvic motion while imparting lower extremity motions to challenge the system. |
| **PATIENT POSITION** | The patient is in the supine hook-lying position with a pressure bag positioned at the lumbosacral region (bottom edge at S2). |
| **THERAPIST POSITION** | The therapist stands beside the patient to provide instructions and to palpate the transversus abdominus just medial to the ASIS for tactile feedback. |
| **PROCEDURE** | The pressure feedback bag is inflated to 40 mm Hg, and the patient is instructed to contract and hold the transversus abdominis muscle by performing the "drawing in" abdominal maneuver.[120] The pressure gauge either increases 2 to 3 mm Hg with the contraction or stays the same. The patient should practice 10-second isometric holds in this position. For further testing of the ability to stabilize the lumbopelvic spine, leg motions can be induced as the patient attempts to maintain the pressure gauge reading steady throughout the movement. The leg movements that can be used (in order of difficulty) include a heel slide, a 3-inch march, a bent-knee fall out (hip abduction with external rotation), and a straight leg raise (8 to 10 inches). |
| **NOTES** | If the patient is unable to stabilize the lumbopelvic spine with leg movements, the home program should focus on isolated sustained (10-second) isometric holds of the TrA. Once the patient can master this maneuver, a gradual progression of leg movements can be superimposed on the stable neutral lumbopelvic position as the TrA contraction is maintained (see Box 4-6 for further progression of lumbopelvic stabilization exercises). |

## Prone Hip Extension Neuromuscular Control Test

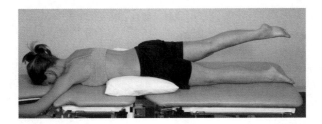

| | |
|---|---|
| **PURPOSE** | This test is used to assess the strength, control, and firing pattern of the lumbopelvic stabilizers and hip extensor muscles during active hip extension. |
| **PATIENT POSITION** | The patient is prone with a pillow positioned under the pelvis for maintenance of a neutral spine position. |
| **THERAPIST POSITION** | The therapist stands at the side of the table to observe and palpate muscle firing action with the test. |
| **PROCEDURE** | The patient is instructed to lift a straight leg 8 to 10 inches off the table. The therapist observes for the patient's ability to maintain a neutral spine position during this test and for the muscle firing pattern, which should progress as ipsilateral gluteus maximus/hamstrings, contralateral multifidus, ipsilateral multifidus, contralateral erector spinae, and ipsilateral erector spinae. Pain provocation is also noted and may occur with poor ability to stabilize the lumbopelvic spine during this test. |
| **NOTES** | When a patient has a poor ability to stabilize the lumbopelvic region with this maneuver, a pattern of overdominance of the global erector spinae muscles and delayed or poor firing of the deep local muscles (multifidus and transversus abdominus) is common. With delayed firing and weakness of the gluteus maximus, reduction in the degree of hip extension and compensation with an anterior pelvic tilt of the pelvis, hyperlordosis, and increased pressure on the lumbar segments of the spine are often found.[121] With training of the local muscles, the patient can often begin to perform this test with better control and less pain. The abdominal drawing in maneuver can be used to limit excessive anterior pelvic tilt and reduce the overactivity of the erector spinae muscle, which enhances the control of prone hip extension.[122] |

## Hip Abductor Neuromuscular Control Test

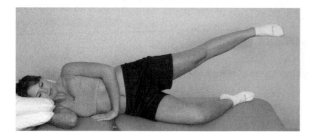

Active hip abduction neuromuscular control test

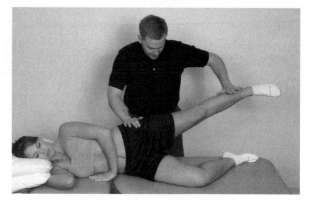

Resisted hip abduction with isolation of gluteus medius muscle strength

| | |
|---|---|
| **PURPOSE** | The purpose of this test is to assess muscle firing pattern, strength, and control of hip abductors and lumbopelvic stabilizers. |
| **PATIENT POSITION** | The patient lies in a side-lying position with the bottom hip and knee flexed at 30 degrees and the top leg extended and aligned with the plane of the trunk. |
| **THERAPIST POSITION** | The therapist stands at the edge of the table behind the patient. |
| **PROCEDURE** | The patient is instructed to actively lift the top leg approximately 24 inches off the table while keeping the leg in line with the trunk. The therapist observes the quality of the movement. A leg that is flexed at the hip joint as it abducts is a sign of weakness of the gluteus medius and overdominance or compensation with the tensor fascia lata. The patient may also have an inability to stabilize the pelvis in this position, which could be an indication of poor control of local trunk stabilizers. A gluteus medius muscle isometric (brake) strength test should also be performed with positioning of the hip at 35 degrees of abduction, 10 degrees of extension, and 10 degrees of external rotation and application of a brake test into adduction. The patient should be able to hold this position with a moderate level of force to show normal strength of the gluteus medius. |
| **NOTES** | Trendelenburg's test results are also likely to be positive when a patient has weakness of the gluteus medius. The Trendelenburg's test is performed with the patient standing and balancing on one leg and flexing the non–weight-bearing hip to 90 degrees. The non–weight-bearing side of the pelvis should remain level or slightly elevated compared with the weight-bearing side of the pelvis. If the non–weight-bearing side of the pelvis drops below horizontal or the patient attempts to compensate for the weakness by side bending the trunk over the weight-bearing extremity, the test results are considered positive. Normal gluteus medius strength and control is required for lumbopelvic dynamic stability and proper lower extremity function. Overactivation of the tensor fascia lata muscle (TFL) to compensate for weakness of the gluteus medius often results in tightness of the iliotibial band, which can contribute to lumbopelvic, hip, and knee impairments. |

## Gillet Marching Test

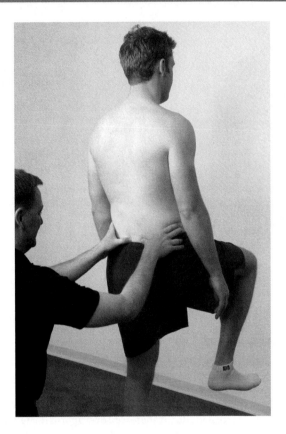

| | |
|---|---|
| **PURPOSE** | This test is used to assess for displacement/hypomobility of the sacroiliac joint. |
| **PATIENT POSITION** | The patient stands or sits on a firm level treatment table and faces away from the therapist. |
| **THERAPIST POSITION** | The therapist kneels or sits on a low stool behind the patient with eyes level with the patient's PSIS. |
| **PROCEDURE** | The therapist uses the thumb to palpate the PSIS on the side to be tested; the other thumb is on the spinous process of S1. The patient is instructed to fully flex one hip as if marching. The therapist should observe for the ipsilateral PSIS to move caudally as the hip is flexed. An alternative technique is palpation of both PSISs with the thumbs for comparison of relative movement of one PSIS with the other PSIS. |
| **NOTES** | Test results are considered positive for sacroiliac displacement if the PSIS does not move caudally with hip flexion. The therapist should observe for a Trendelenburg's sign while the patient is standing on one leg and should be aware that this test assesses for displacement, and not necessarily for hypermobility. The test is best performed in the seated position when the patient has balance or strength deficits that limit the ability to balance on one leg. Although the test is described as a SIJ mobility assessment, false-positive findings could be produced with limited L5-S1 mobility. Therefore, L5-S1 passive intervertebral motion should be assessed before a SIJ dysfunction is diagnosed. When compared with a reference standard of anesthetic blocks of the SIJ in a patient population with low back pain, the Gillet test has shown a sensitivity of 0.43, a specificity of 0.68, a negative likelihood ratio (−LR) of 0.84, and a positive likelihood ratio (+LR) of 1.3.[123] Flynn et al[30] found a Kappa value of 0.59 for intertester reliability in an examination of 71 patients with low back pain. |

## Distraction Provocation (ASIS Gap) Sacroiliac Joint Test    **DVD**

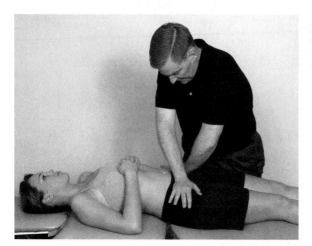

ASIS gap test

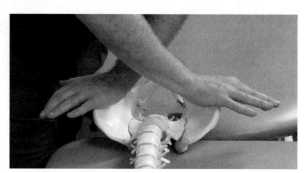

ASIS gap test hand placement

| | |
|---|---|
| **PURPOSE** | This test assesses the level of reactivity of the sacroiliac joint and provokes SIJ pain. |
| **PATIENT POSITION** | The patient is supine with the head on a pillow. |
| **THERAPIST POSITION** | The therapist stands next to the patient. |
| **PROCEDURE** | The therapist crosses arms and contacts the medial aspect of each ASIS with the soft spot of each palm. A gentle force is applied to gap the ASIS pushing in a posterior lateral direction and the force is gradually increased over approximately 10 seconds. The patient should report any pain provoked by the test. If no discomfort is reported, an impulse is given at the end of the application of the force. Again, the patient is instructed to report any pain provoked by the test. |
| **NOTES** | The test results are positive if the test provokes pain at the sacroiliac joint or symphysis pubis. The test results are not considered positive if pain is provoked at the ASIS as a result of therapist hand placement. This technique can be performed over the patient's clothing. Laslett and Williams[93] reported a Kappa value of 0.69 for interexaminer reliability for assessment of 51 patients with low back pain with and without radiation into the lower extremities. |

## ASIS Compression Provocation Sacroiliac Joint Test    (DVD)

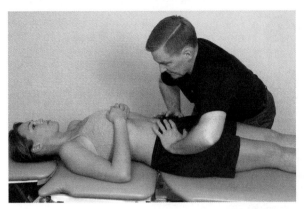

ASIS compression test

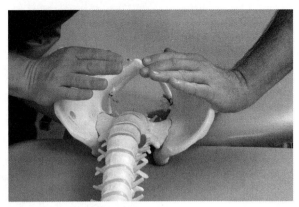

ASIS compression test hand placement

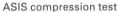

| | |
|---|---|
| **PURPOSE** | This test is used to assess the level of reactivity of the sacroiliac joint and provoke SIJ pain. |
| **PATIENT POSITION** | The patient is supine with the head on a pillow. |
| **THERAPIST POSITION** | The therapist stands next to the patient with a diagonal stance and leans over to place the chest directly over the patient's pelvis. |
| **PROCEDURE** | The therapist contacts the lateral aspect of each ASIS with the soft spot of each palm. A gentle force is applied to compress the ASISs toward midline and the force is gradually increased over approximately 10 seconds. The patient should report any pain provoked by the test. If no discomfort is reported, an impulse is given at the end of the application of the force. Again, the patient is instructed to report any pain provoked by the test. |
| **NOTES** | The test results are positive if the test provokes pain at the sacroiliac joint or symphysis pubis. The test results are not considered positive if pain is provoked at the ASIS as a result of therapist hand placement. This technique can be performed over the patient's clothing. An alternative method is application of a compressive force toward midline on one ASIS with the patient in a side-lying position. Russell, Maksymowych, and LeClercq[124] reported a sensitivity of 0.70, a specificity of 0.90, a +LR of 7.0, and a −LR of 0.33 for identification of patients with ankylosing spondylitis (AS) with reference standard of radiographically confirmed AS. Occasionally, this test may alleviate symptoms, which may be an indication of involvement of the symphysis pubis. |

## Gaenslen's Provocation Sacroiliac Joint Test

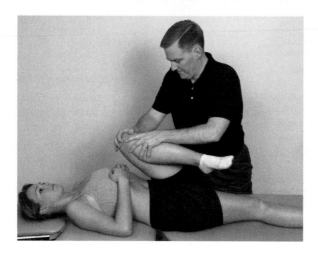

| | |
|---|---|
| **PURPOSE** | Gaenslen's provocation sacroiliac joint test is used to assess the level of reactivity of the sacroiliac joint and provoke SIJ pain. |
| **PATIENT POSITION** | The patient is supine with the head on a pillow and both legs extended. |
| **THERAPIST POSITION** | The therapist stands with a diagonal stance next to the patient. |
| **PROCEDURE** | The therapist fully flexes the patient's hip and brings the patient's knee toward the chest on the side being tested while the opposite hip remains in extension. Overpressure is applied at the end range of hip flexion. |
| **NOTES** | The test results are positive if the test provokes pain at the sacroiliac joint region. For assurance that the opposite hip remains in full extension, the leg can be extended over the edge of the table. Dreyfuss et al[123] reported a sensitivity of 0.71, a specificity of 0.26, a +LR of 1.0, and a −LR of 1.12 for Gaenslen's test with the reference standard of intraarticular injection anesthetic block of the SIJ. |

## Patrick Test (FABER Test) DVD

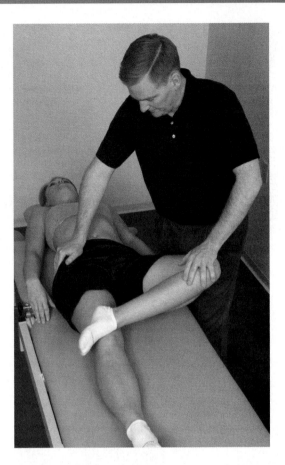

| | |
|---|---|
| **PURPOSE** | This test is both a provocation test for the SIJ and hip joint pain and a general mobility screen of the hip joint. |
| **PATIENT POSITION** | The patient is supine with one leg extended and the test leg crossed over the extended leg just above the knee. The test leg hip is flexed, abducted, and externally rotated (FABER position). |
| **HAND PLACEMENT** | **Cranial hand:** This hand is used to stabilize the opposite side of pelvis at the ASIS. |
| | **Caudal hand:** This hand is placed on the medial aspect of the knee joint of the test leg. |
| **PROCEDURE** | The therapist applies gentle overpressure of the hip into flexion, abduction, and external rotation by pressing the test leg knee down toward the table and applying a stabilizing force at the opposite ASIS. |
| **NOTES** | Positive test results are reached with reproduction of buttock or groin pain, which could be an indication of irritation of either the SIJ or hip joint. The test leg tibia should attain a horizontal position to be considered at full range of motion. More importantly, significant difference in mobility between sides should be noted. Interexaminer reliability has been reported as a Kappa value of 0.62 by Dreyfuss et al[123] and a Kappa value of 0.60 by Flynn et al.[30] |

## Sacroiliac Joint Posterior Gapping Test and Thigh Thrust Provocation Test    (DVD)

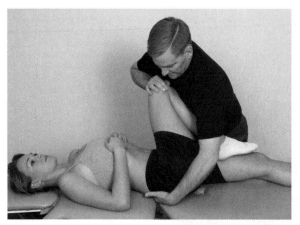

Palpation of opposite side SIJ gapping with knee to opposite chest movement

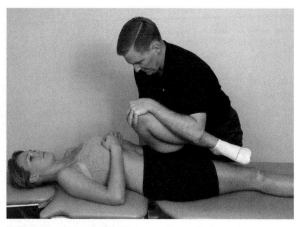

Palpation of same side SIJ gapping with knee to opposite chest movement

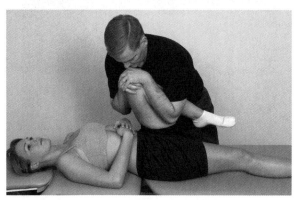

Thigh thrust overpressure for SIJ pain provocation test

| | |
|---|---|
| **PURPOSE** | This test evaluates the mobility of the sacroiliac joint to gap and to provoke SIJ pain. |
| **PATIENT POSITION** | The patient is supine with the head on a pillow. |
| **THERAPIST POSITION** | The therapist stands next to the patient. |
| **HAND PLACEMENT** | **Caudal hand:** The pads of the index and long fingers are used to palpate the medial aspect of the PSIS. |
| | **Cranial hand:** This hand is used to grasp the patient's knee on the side to be tested. |
| **PROCEDURE** | The therapist stands on the patient's left side and flexes the patient's right hip and knee to approximately 90 degrees. The patient's hip is adducted so that the right side of the pelvis comes off of the table. The pads of the index and long fingers are used to palpate the medial edge of the patient's right PSIS. The patient's pelvis is rolled back onto the left hand, and the patient's right hip is flexed and adducted toward the left shoulder. The therapist palpates for the right PSIS to move laterally and the sacroiliac joint to gap. The amount of gapping and pain provocation are noted. |

## Sacroiliac Joint Posterior Gapping Test and Thigh Thrust Provocation Test—cont'd

The procedure is repeated to assess the left sacroiliac joint. The amount of movement/pain provocation is noted and compared with the right side.

**NOTES**   The test results are considered positive if the joint does not gap or if the patient's symptoms are reproduced at the SIJ. The motion should be graded as normal, hypomobile (decreased movement), or hypermobile (increased movement). The thigh thrust test uses similar hand placement and patient position, but instead of palpation of SIJ mobility, posteriorly directed force through the femur at varying angles of abduction/adduction are used to attempt to reproduce posterior buttock pain. Dreyfuss et al[123] reported a sensitivity of 0.36, a specificity of 0.50, a +LR of 0.7, and a −LR of 1.28 for the thigh thrust test with an intraarticular injection anesthetic block of the SIJ used as a reference standard. This test has also been called the posterior pelvic pain provocation test (P4).[99]

## Sacral Thrust Provocation Sacroiliac Joint Test

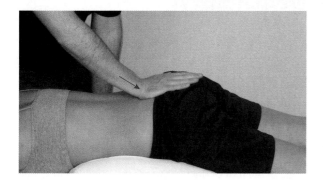
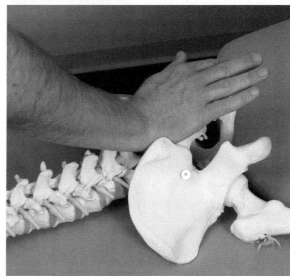

Sacral thrust provocation SIJ test hand placement

**PURPOSE**   This test assesses the level of reactivity of the sacroiliac joint and provokes SIJ pain.

**PATIENT POSITION**   The patient is prone with pillow supporting the pelvis.

**THERAPIST POSITION**   The therapist stands with a diagonal stance next to the patient.

**PROCEDURE**   The therapist contacts the base of the sacrum and gradually increases a posterior-to-anterior force over approximately 10 seconds. The patient is instructed to report pain provocation. If no discomfort is reported, an impulse is given at the end of the application of the force and pain provocation is assessed.

**NOTES**   The test results are positive if the test provokes pain at the sacroiliac joints. This technique can be performed over the patient's clothing. An alternative method is use of a second hand to reinforce the primary contact and assist in force application. Laslett and Williams[93] reported an interrater reliability of Kappa value of 0.56 with testing of 51 patients with low back pain with and without leg pain.

## Thomas Test

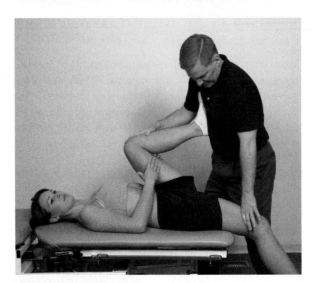

Thomas test end position

---

| | |
|---|---|
| **PURPOSE** | The Thomas test is used to assess the length of the hip flexor muscles. |
| **PATIENT POSITION** | The patient is supine at the foot of the table. |
| **THERAPIST POSITION** | The therapist stands at the foot of the table. |
| **HAND PLACEMENT** | The hands and chest are used to control both of the patient's legs during the procedure. |
| **PROCEDURE** | The patient starts sitting at the edge of the foot of the treatment table. The therapist supports the patient and guides the patient into a supine position with both knees and hips fully flexed. The therapist holds one leg in full flexion and guides the test leg down into hip extension. The thigh should come parallel with the table to attain full normal hip flexor muscle length. The therapist then uses the leg to flex the test leg knee up to 90 degrees. If the hip flexes when knee flexion is added, the rectus femoris muscle is tight. |
| **NOTES** | Hip abduction in the test position is an indication of iliotibial band tightness. The test position can be used to provide a hold/relax stretch technique or a sustained stretch for the hip flexors. Wang et al[125] reported ICC of 0.97 for Thomas test intratester reliability on 10 subjects. |

# Hip Passive Rotation Range of Motion Test (Supine)

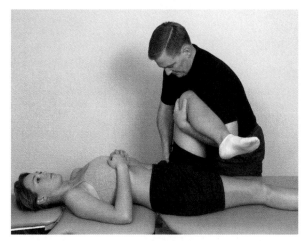

Hip external rotation passive range of motion test

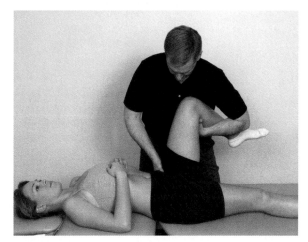

Hip internal rotation passive range of motion test

| | |
|---|---|
| **PURPOSE** | The test assesses passive range of motion of the hip joint. |
| **PATIENT POSITION** | The patient is supine with the opposite leg extended and the test leg supported by the therapist. |
| **THERAPIST POSITION** | The therapist stands with a diagonal stance at the edge of table. |
| **HAND PLACEMENT** | **Cranial hand:** The thumb and fingers are placed at the ASIS to monitor and prevent pelvic motion. |
| | **Caudal hand:** The forearm is placed under the patient's lower leg, and the hand is under the knee to support the knee and hip at 90 degrees of flexion. |
| **PROCEDURE** | The therapist palpates and stabilizes the pelvis with the cranial hand and uses the caudal arm to induce hip rotation. Overpressure can be given at end range of motion to assess tissue end feel and to assess for pain provocation. |
| **NOTES** | A goniometer can be used to measure the amount of passive rotation attained with this test. The advantage of this test position is that the therapist can limit pelvic motion that may tend to compensate for limited hip motion and the therapist can get a sense of hip joint end feel. |

## Hip Passive Rotation Range of Motion Test (Prone)

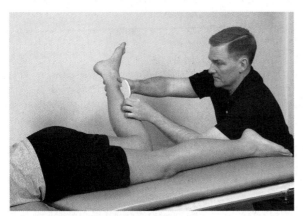

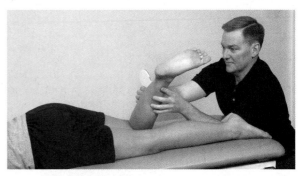

Use of inclinometer to measure prone hip external rotation

Use of inclinometer to measure prone hip internal rotation

| | |
|---|---|
| **PURPOSE** | The purpose of this test is to measure hip rotation range of motion in the prone position. |
| **PATIENT POSITION** | The patient is prone with the test leg (right) knee flexed at 90 degrees and the opposite leg extended. |
| **THERAPIST POSITION** | The therapist kneels at the foot of the treatment table. |
| **HAND PLACEMENT** | **Inclinometer hand:** This hand holds the gravity inclinometer at the distal one third of the tibia on the lateral side of the tibia to measure external rotation and is placed on the medial aspect of the tibia to measure internal rotation.<br><br>**Other hand:** The other hand is placed on the tibia on the opposite side of the inclinometer to guide hip motion. |
| **PROCEDURE** | The therapist guides the tibia medially to test hip external rotation and laterally to test hip internal rotation. The angle measured on the inclinometer is read at the end range of motion and is recorded in degrees. |
| **NOTES** | The pelvis should remain flat on the table during the hip motion. The pelvis rising from the table is an indication that the end range of hip motion has been attained. Hip internal rotation of 35 degrees or greater was one of the components of the CPR for manipulation success for treatment of acute low back pain, and Flynn et al[30] used this method of measurement in developing the CPR. Bullock-Saxton and Bullock[126] reported a Kappa value of 0.99 for external rotation and a Kappa value of 0.98 for internal rotation for intertester reliability with use of an inclinometer to measure these hip motions. The measurements could also be considered muscle length tests of the hip rotators. |

# ACCESSORY MOTION TESTING AND MANIPULATION OF THE HIP JOINT

## Hip Long Axis Distraction Test and Manipulation        (DVD)

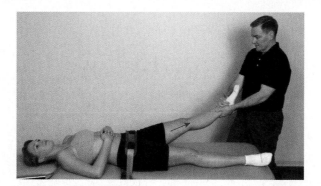

|  |  |
|---|---|
| **PURPOSE** | This test is used to test the capsular mobility of the hip joint and to mobilize a stiff joint capsule. |
| **PATIENT POSITION** | The patient is supine with the pelvis stabilized by a belt or second examiner. |
| **THERAPIST POSITION** | The therapist stands with a diagonal stance at the foot of the table. |
| **HAND PLACEMENT** | Both hands are wrapped around the distal tibia just proximal to the ankle joint. |
| **PROCEDURE** | The therapist positions the patient's test leg hip in a loose packed position of 30 degrees abduction and 30 degrees flexion. The therapist slowly applies a force to the hip by pulling the leg toward the body in the plane of the test leg. The amount of joint play at one joint is compared with the other hip joint. |
| **NOTES** | If muscle holding is seen at the hip joint, the pelvis tends to move as soon as distraction forces are applied to the leg and the patient may have difficulty relaxing the leg. In osteoarthritic hip joints, this procedure often alleviates the patient's hip area pain. When limitations in hip joint mobility are noted, this procedure can be turned into a joint manipulation by sustaining end range forces or applying a thrust impulse at the end of the available range of motion. |

## Inferior Glide Accessory Hip Motion Test and Manipulation   DVD

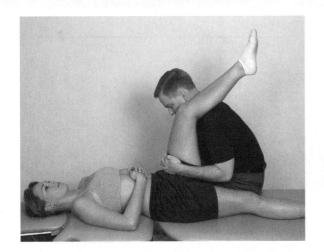

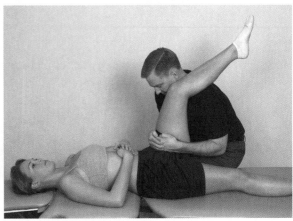

Inferior lateral glide accessory hip motion test

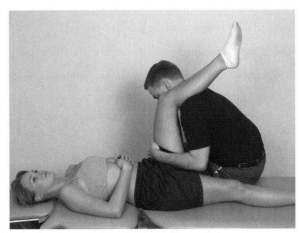

Inferior medial glide accessory hip motion test

| | |
|---|---|
| **PURPOSE** | This test is used to evaluate the capsular mobility of the hip joint and to mobilize a stiff joint capsule. |
| **PATIENT POSITION** | The patient is supine with the test leg resting on the therapist's shoulder. |
| **THERAPIST POSITION** | The therapist sits on the edge of the table with the patient's test leg resting on a shoulder. |
| **HAND PLACEMENT** | The therapist's overlaps the hands at the anterior aspect of the proximal thigh with the fifth digits of both hands at the crease formed by the flexed hip position. |
| **PROCEDURE** | An inferiorly directed force is applied through the femur to produce an inferior glide. The therapist shifts the hands laterally and the body and forearms medially to produce an inferior medial glide. The therapist shifts the hands medially and the forearms and body laterally to produce an inferior lateral glide. The amount of joint play at one joint is compared with the other hip joint. |
| **NOTES** | If muscle holding or capsular tightness is present at the hip joint, the pelvis tends to move as soon as gliding forces are applied to the leg and the patient may have difficulty relaxing the leg. In osteoarthritic hip joints, this procedure often alleviates the patient's hip area pain. When limitations in hip joint mobility are noted, this procedure can be turned into a joint manipulation by sustaining end range forces or applying a thrust impulse at the end of the available range of motion. |

# PASSIVE INTERVERTEBRAL MOTION TECHNIQUES

## Lumbar Forward-Bending Passive Intervertebral Motion Test: Side Lying with Bilateral Leg Flexion

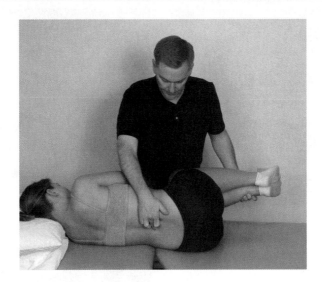

| | |
|---|---|
| **PURPOSE** | This test is used to evaluate the passive forward-bending motion of lumbar segments L5-S1 through T12-L1. |
| **PATIENT POSITION** | The patient is in a side-lying position facing the therapist and near the edge of the table with hips and knees flexed. |
| **THERAPIST POSITION** | The therapist stands in front of the patient with feet parallel to the table and weight on the balls of the feet. |
| **HAND PLACEMENT** | **Caudal hand:** This hand supports the patient's lower leg just proximal to the ankle. |
| | **Cranial hand:** The pad of the long finger is used to palpate the interspinous space of the lumbar segment. |
| **PROCEDURE** | The patient's legs are positioned together in approximately 90 degrees of hip and knee flexion. The tibial tuberosity of the patient's lower leg should rest on the therapist's anterior hip. The caudal hand is used to support the lower leg just proximal to the ankle. With the hip, slight counterpressure is applied through the patient's lower leg. The therapist induces lumbar forward bending by shifting body weight toward the patient's head while flexing the patient's hips. The top leg continues to rest on top of the lower leg throughout the procedure. The hip is flexed with small amplitude motions, and the pad of the long finger on the cranial hand is used to palpate the interspinous space of the targeted lumbar segment. The therapist palpates for the interspinous space to gap during lumbar forward bending as the inferior vertebra's spinous process of the spinal segment moves inferiorly in relationship to the superior vertebra's spinous process. The amount of passive forward-bending motion available at each lumbar segment is noted and compared. |
| **NOTES** | Assessment of PIVM begins at L5-S1 and proceeds cranially. As the assessment proceeds cranially, the amount of hip flexion is increased, but how far the hip is returned toward extension with each successive segment is reduced. In patients with wide hips and a narrow waist, a towel roll can be placed under the patient's waist to prevent lateral flexion in the lumbar spine. |

## Lumbar Forward-Bending Passive Intervertebral Motion Test: Side Lying with Single Leg Flexion

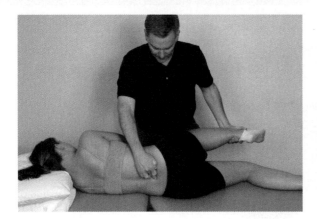

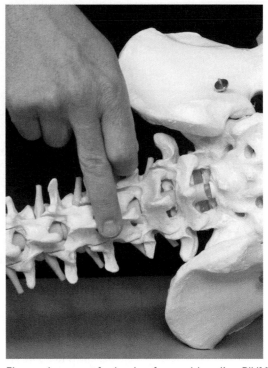

Finger placement for lumbar forward-bending PIVM test

| | |
|---|---|
| **PURPOSE** | This test is used to evaluate the passive forward-bending motion of lumbar segments L5-S1 through T12-L1. |
| **PATIENT POSITION** | The patient is in a side-lying position facing the therapist. |
| **THERAPIST POSITION** | The therapist stands next to the patient with feet parallel to the table, hips and knees flexed approximately 30 degrees, and weight on the forefeet. |
| **HAND PLACEMENT** | **Caudal hand:** The caudal hand supports the patient's top leg just proximal to the ankle. |
| | **Cranial hand:** The pad of the long finger (third digit) is used to palpate the interspinous space of the lumbar segment. |
| **PROCEDURE** | The patient's bottom leg is positioned in approximately 30 degrees of hip and knee flexion. The patient's top leg is positioned in approximately 90 degrees of hip and knee flexion. The tibial tuberosity of the patient's top leg should rest on the therapist's anterior hip. The caudal hand is used to support the top leg just proximal to the ankle. With the anterior hip, slight counterpressure is applied through the patient's upper leg to prevent the patient's pelvis from rotating. The therapist induces lumbar forward bending by shifting the body weight towards the patient's head while flexing the patient's hip. The hip is flexed with small amplitude motions, and the pad of the long finger on the cranial hand is used to palpate the interspinous space of the targeted lumbar segment. The therapist palpates for the interspinous space to gap during lumbar forward bending as the inferior vertebra's spinous process of the spinal segment moves inferiorly in relationship to the superior vertebra's |

## Lumbar Forward-Bending Passive Intervertebral Motion Test: Side Lying with Single Leg Flexion—cont'd

spinous process. The amount of passive forward-bending motion available at each lumbar segment is noted and compared.

NOTES      The assessment of PIVM begins at L5-S1 and proceeds cranially. As the assessment proceeds cranially, the amount of hip flexion is increased, but how far the hip is returned toward extension with each successive segment is reduced. This technique can be performed with the patient's top hip adducted (due to the height of the therapist), but the patient's pelvis/trunk should not be allowed to rotate. In patients with wide hips and a narrow waist, a towel roll can be placed under the patient's waist to prevent lateral flexion in the lumbar spine.

## Modification for Lumbar Backward-Bending Passive Intervertebral Motion Test

The same therapist and patient positionings can be modified to assess PIVM lumbar backward bending by moving the patient's hips toward extension from the 90-degree hip flexion start position. The palpation begins at L5-S1 and proceeds cranially as the legs are moved further toward extension. In most patients, full lumbar extension can be reached before the hips are moved into a neutral flexion/extension position.

## Lumbar Side-Bending (Lateral Flexion) Passive Intervertebral Motion Test in Prone Position

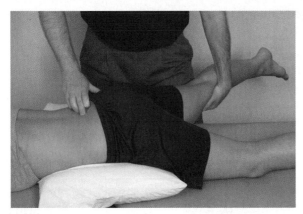

Lumbar side-bending PIVM, prone lying with hip abduction

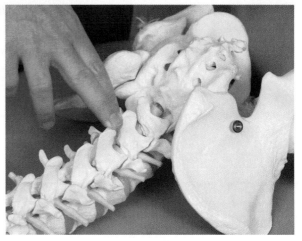

Hand placement for lumbar side-bending PIVM

| | |
|---|---|
| **PURPOSE** | This test evaluates the passive side-bending (lateral flexion) motion in the lumbar segments L5-S1 through T12-L1. |
| **PATIENT POSITION** | The patient is prone with a pillow under the abdomen and pelvis. |
| **THERAPIST POSITION** | The therapist stands next to the patient. |
| **HAND PLACEMENT** | **Caudal hand:** The caudal hand supports the patient's right leg at the knee while avoiding compression of the patient's patella. |
| | **Cranial hand:** The pad of the long finger is used to palpate the lateral aspect of the interspinous space of the lumbar segment. |
| **PROCEDURE** | The therapist stands on the patient's right side and induces lumbar side bending to the right by abducting the patient's right hip with the caudal hand. The hip is abducted, and the pad of the long finger on the cranial hand is used to palpate the right lateral aspect of the interspinous space of the specified lumbar segment. The therapist palpates for the interspinous space to close down into the palpating finger by palpating the lateral edge of the inferior spinous process in relation to the lateral edge of the superior spinous process. The amount of passive side-bending motion available at each segment is noted and compared. Lumbar side bending to the left is induced with the therapist standing on the patient's left side and repeating the procedure abducting the left hip. The amount of passive side-bending motion available at each segment and in each direction is noted and compared. |
| **NOTES** | Assessment of PIVM begins at L5-S1 and proceeds cranially. As the assessment proceeds cranially, the amount of hip abduction is increased, but the range through which the hip is adducted with each successive segment is decreased. With support of the patient's leg, hip extension (keeping the hip slightly flexed is best) and compression of the patella should be avoided. This technique can also be performed with the patient's knee slightly flexed. However, the therapist should avoid excessive knee flexion with tightness of the rectus femoris muscle. |

## Prone Lumbar Side-Bending PIVM Test with a Mobilization Table       DVD

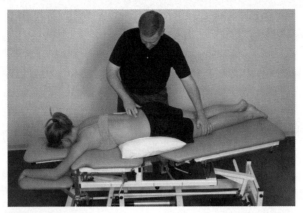

Use of mobilization table to assess prone side-bending
PIVM

This technique can be modified with use of a mobilization table. The cranial palpating hand remains the same, but the spinal side-bending motion is induced by moving the lower half of the table laterally, with the patient's legs resting on the table.

## Lumbar Side-Bending (Lateral Flexion) Passive Intervertebral Motion Test: Side Lying with Rocking the Pelvis

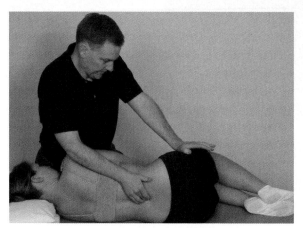

Lumbar side-bending left PIVM, side lying with rocking the pelvis

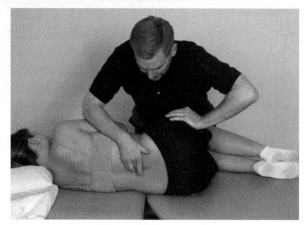

Lumbar side-bending right PIVM, side lying with rocking the pelvis

| | |
|---|---|
| **PURPOSE** | This test is used to evaluate the passive side-bending motion in the lumbar segments L5-S1 through T12-L1. |
| **PATIENT POSITION** | The patient is in a side-lying position facing the therapist with the hips and knees flexed to 90 degrees. |
| **THERAPIST POSITION** | The therapist stands with a diagonal stance in front of the patient and facing the patient's pelvis. |
| **HAND PLACEMENT** | **Caudal hand:** The palm of the hand is placed on the patient's greater trochanter. |
| | **Cranial hand:** The pad of the long finger is used to palpate the lateral aspect of the interspinous space of the lumbar segment. |
| **PROCEDURE** | With the patient in a left side-lying position, both legs are positioned in 90 degrees of hip and knee flexion. The superior aspect of the greater trochanter is contacted with the heel of the caudal hand. Lumbar side bending to the left is induced with the caudal hand pushing the patient's greater trochanter caudally. The pad of the long finger on the cranial hand is used to palpate the left lateral aspect of the interspinous space of the specified lumbar segment. The therapist palpates for the interspinous space to close down into the palpating finger on the concavity formed with the side-bend motion. The amount of passive side-bending motion available at each segment is noted and compared. |
| | Lumbar side bending to the right is induced with the caudal hand pushing the patient's greater trochanter cranially. The pad of the long finger on the cranial hand is used to palpate the right lateral aspect of the interspinous space of the specified lumbar segment. The therapist palpates for the interspinous process to close down into the palpating finger. The amount of passive side-bending motion available at each segment for both directions is noted and compared. |
| **NOTES** | Assessment of PIVM begins at L5-S1 and proceeds cranially. The forearm should be positioned parallel to the direction of the force applied through the greater trochanter. The procedure can be performed with the patient in a right side-lying position, with caudal movement of the pelvis inducing right side bending and cranial movement of the pelvis inducing left side bending. Assessment of lumbar side bending with this technique (e.g., rocking the pelvis) is useful for patients with hip pathology (the hip needs to be protected). |

## Lumbar Translatoric Joint Play Segmental Stability Test

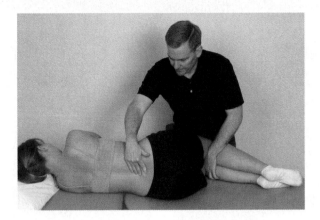

| | |
|---|---|
| **PURPOSE** | The purpose of this test is to evaluate the mobility and stability of the lumbar spinal segments. |
| **PATIENT POSITION** | The patient lies in a side-lying position with the hips and knees flexed. The hips are flexed 60 to 70 degrees to allow the femurs to align with the angle of the vertebral bodies while the lumbar spine is maintained in a neutral position. |
| **THERAPIST POSITION** | The therapist stands with a diagonal stance in front of the patient, and the anterior aspect of the hip of the caudal leg rests firmly against the patient's knees. |
| **HAND PLACEMENT** | **Cranial hand:** The palpating index finger pad is placed at the interspinous space of the segment to be tested with the rest of the hand and fingers stabilizing the spine cranially to the tested segment. |
| | **Caudal hand:** The hand is placed across the posterior aspect of both knees to press the patient's knees firmly into the therapist's hip. |
| **PROCEDURE** | The therapist uses the caudal hand and hip to push and pull the patient's femurs anterior and posterior to create anterior and posterior lumbar spinal forces. The palpating cranial hand assesses for excessive joint play as a sign of instability. |
| **NOTES** | Positive results for instability may be coupled with the presence of a lumbar step, which is often associated with spondylolisthesis. The passive mobility findings should be correlated with other PIVM and active range of motion (AROM) findings. |

## Lumbar Rotation Passive Intervertebral Motion Test: Prone Lying with Rolling the Legs

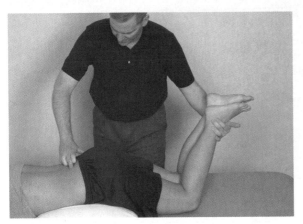

Lumbar right rotation PIVM, prone lying with rolling the legs

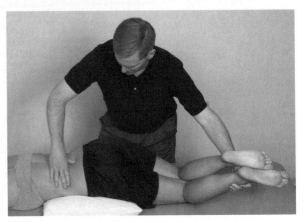

Lumbar left rotation PIVM, prone lying with rolling the legs

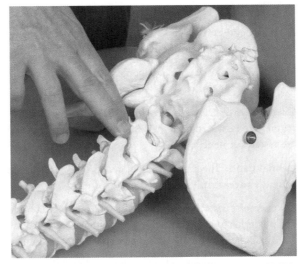

Finger placement for palpation for lumbar rotation PIVM

| | |
|---|---|
| **PURPOSE** | This test evaluates the passive rotation of lumbar segments L5-S1 through T12-L1. |
| **PATIENT POSITION** | The patient is prone with a pillow under the abdomen and pelvis. |
| **THERAPIST POSITION** | The therapist stands next to the patient. |
| **HAND PLACEMENT** | **Caudal hand:** The caudal hand supports both of the patient's legs at the ankles. |
| | **Cranial hand:** The pad of the long finger is used to palpate the lateral aspect of the interspinous space of the lumbar segment. |
| **PROCEDURE** | Both of the patient's knees are flexed to approximately 45 to 60 degrees, and the legs are supported at the ankles with the caudal hand and forearm. Right rotation of the lumbar spine is induced with rolling the legs toward the patient's right side. The pad of the long finger on the cranial hand is used to palpate the right lateral aspect of the interspinous space of the specified segment. The therapist palpates for the spinous process of the lower member of the segment to rotate or press into the palpating finger in relation to the superior member of the segment's spinous process. The amount of right rotation available at |

## Lumbar Rotation Passive Intervertebral Motion Test: Prone Lying with Rolling the Legs—cont'd

each segment is noted and compared. Left rotation is induced with rolling the legs toward the patient's left side. The pad of the thumb can be used to palpate the left lateral aspect of the interspinous space of the specified segment. The therapist palpates for the spinous process of the lower member of the segment to rotate or press into the palpating finger. The amount of left rotation available at each segment is noted and compared. The amount of rotation available in each direction is compared.

NOTES  Assessment of PIVM begins at L5-S1 and proceeds cranially. As the assessment progresses cranially, the amount of rotation of the legs is increased, but the amount of rotation back towards the midline with each successive segment is decreased. This technique follows the rule of the leg, which states that the direction of the movement of the legs is the same as the direction of the rotation of the lumbar spine (i.e., rolling the legs to the right induces right rotation of the lumbar spine). The direction of rotation is based on the direction of rotation of the vertebral body of the superior member of the spinal segment in relation to the inferior member of the segment.

## Lumbar Rotation Passive Intervertebral Motion Test: Prone Lying with Raising the Pelvis

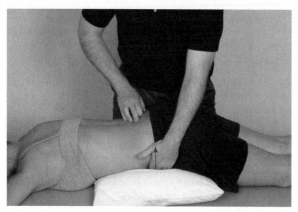

Lumbar right rotation, prone lying with raising the pelvis

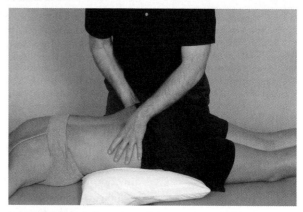

Lumbar left rotation, prone lying with raising the pelvis

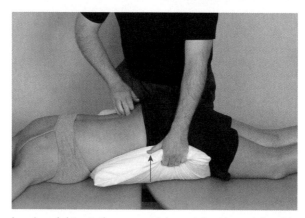

Lumbar right rotation, prone lying raising the pelvis with assist of pillow

|  |  |
|---|---|
| **PURPOSE** | This test is used to evaluate the passive rotation of lumbar segments L5-S1 through T12-L1. |
| **PATIENT POSITION** | The patient is prone with a pillow under the abdomen and pelvis. |
| **THERAPIST POSITION** | The therapist stands next to the patient. |
| **HAND PLACEMENT** | **Caudal hand:** The fingers grasp the patient's pelvis under the ASIS.<br><br>**Cranial hand:** The pad of the long finger palpates the lateral aspect of the interspinous space. |
| **PROCEDURE** | With the therapist standing on the patient's right side, the fingers of the caudal hand are used to grasp the patient's pelvis under the left ASIS. Right lumbar rotation is induced with gentle lifting of the pelvis in a rotary manner. The pad of the long finger on the cranial hand palpates the right lateral aspect of the interspinous space of the specified lumbar segment. The therapist palpates for the spinous process of the lower member of the segment to rotate or press into the palpating finger. The amount of passive rotation available at each segment is noted and compared. Left lumbar rotation is induced with grasping the patient's pelvis under the right ASIS (with the fingers of the caudal hand) and gently lifting the pelvis in a rotary manner. The pad of the long finger or thumb on the cranial hand is used to |

## Lumbar Rotation Passive Intervertebral Motion Test: Prone Lying with Raising the Pelvis—cont'd

palpate the left lateral aspect of the interspinous space of the specified lumbar segment. The therapist palpates for the spinous process of the lower member of the segment to rotate or press into the palpating finger. The amount of passive rotation available at each segment is noted and compared. The amount of rotation available in each direction is compared.

NOTES        Assessment begins at L5-S1 and proceeds cranially. The amount of lifting of the pelvis is increased with assessment of each successive cranial segment. This technique can be performed with the therapist standing on the same side of the patient to assess both right and left rotation (as described), or the therapist can switch sides to assess the rotation available in each direction. When this technique is performed, the therapist should be aware that just placing the hand under the patient's pelvis can induce enough movement to rotate L5-S1. To prevent this occurrence, the therapist should push the hand into the pillow/table to allow the patient's pelvis to remain in a neutral position. This technique can also be performed with the pillow used to lift the pelvis. Assessment of lumbar rotation with this technique (e.g., lifting the pelvis) is useful for patients with hip pathology (the hip needs to be protected).

## Lumbar Rotation Passive Accessory Intervertebral Motion Test: Spring Testing Through the Transverse Processes

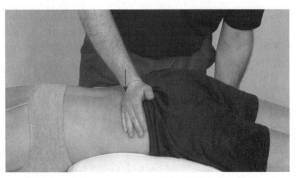

Lumbar rotation, spring testing through left transverse process

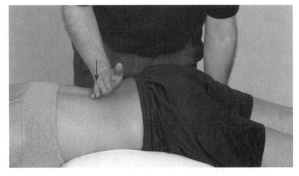

Lumbar rotation, spring testing through right transverse process

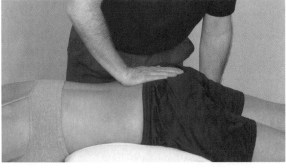

Lumbar rotation, spring testing through right sacral base

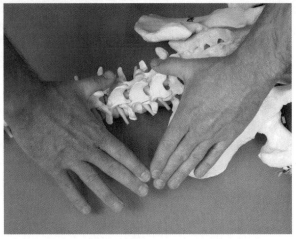

Lumbar rotation, spring testing through transverse processes V to identify L2-L4 transverse processes

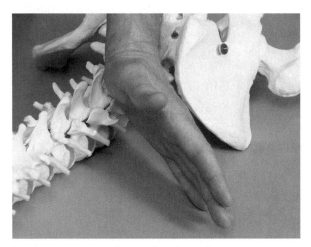

Lumbar rotation, spring testing through transverse process: hand placement

| | |
|---|---|
| **PURPOSE** | This test evaluates the passive rotation of lumbar segments L5-S1 through L2-L3 and assesses the level of reactivity of lumbar segments L5-S1 through L2-L3 (pain provocation test). |
| **PATIENT POSITION** | The patient is prone with a pillow under the abdomen and pelvis. |
| **THERAPIST POSITION** | The therapist stands next to the patient. |
| **HAND PLACEMENT** | **Caudal hand:** This hand supports the therapist's body weight on the edge of the treatment table. |

## Lumbar Rotation Passive Accessory Intervertebral Motion Test: Spring Testing Through the Transverse Processes—cont'd

**Cranial hand:** The proximal ulnar aspect of the fifth metacarpal contacts the transverse process.

**PROCEDURE**

With the therapist standing on the patient's right side, the ulnar aspect of the fifth metacarpal on the caudal hand locates the iliac crest on the patient's left side. The ulnar aspect of the fifth metacarpal locates the 12th rib on the patient's left side. The hands make a V shape. The transverse process of L3 is located at the point of the V. The ulnar aspect of the fifth metacarpal of the cranial hand is used to "sink into" the middle of the V at the location of the L3 transverse process. The therapist should take up the slack and spring (i.e. midrange thrust) the transverse process of L3. The amount of passive right rotation available at the segment is noted (spring testing the transverse process of L3 assesses the mobility of the L3-L4 segment). Also noted is any pain provocation. The procedure is repeated with the transverse processes of L2 (located just inferior to the 12th rib, segment L2-L3) and L4 (located just superior to the iliac crest, segment L4-L5). L5-S1 is tested with placement of the middle crease of the cranial hand on the patient's right PSIS with the thenar eminence on the sacral sulcus. The therapist takes up the slack and springs the L5-S1 segment by giving a posterior to anterior force. The amount of passive right rotation available at the segment is noted. Also noted is pain provocation. The procedure is repeated with assessment of the opposite side spinal segments. The amount of rotation available and the level of reactivity in each direction at each segment are compared.

**NOTES**

The therapist is recommended to spring with the cranial hand to remain specific and consistent with this technique. Spring testing of segments L2-L3 through L4-L5 on the left induces *right* rotation, and spring testing segment L5-S1 (through the PSIS and sacral base) on the left induces *left* rotation. The forearm of the arm that gives the impulse should be near to parallel to the direction of the force applied. Assessment of rotation tests the ability of the facet joint on the ipsilateral side to gap (i.e., right rotation tests the ability of the right facet joint to gap). Pain provocation with spring testing the L5-S1 segment could indicate dysfunction at that segment or the sacroiliac joint.

## Central Posterior-to-Anterior Passive Accessory Intervertebral Motion Test   (DVD)

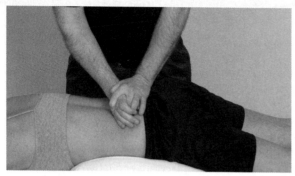

Central posterior-to-anterior PAIVM test, two-handed technique

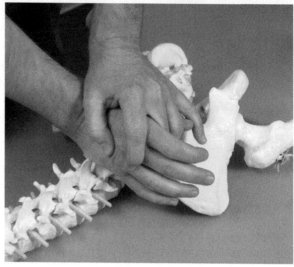

Hand positioning for central posterior-to-anterior PAIVM test, two-handed technique

| | |
|---|---|
| **PURPOSE** | This test is used for passive accessory motion or pain provocation of the lumbar spinal segments. For intervention, the appropriate grade of mobilization (I to IV) to treat pain or hypomobility is used. |
| **PATIENT POSITION** | The patient lies prone over a pillow with the arms by the body or hanging off the edge of the table. A pillow can be placed under the lower legs for comfort. |
| **THERAPIST POSITION** | The therapist stands at the side of patient. |
| **HAND PLACEMENT** | **Right hand:** The right hand is placed on the patient's back so that the ulnar border of the hand just distal to the pisiform is in contact with the spinous process of the vertebrae to be mobilized. The shoulders are directly over the patient. The right wrist is fully extended, with the forearm midway between supination and pronation. |
| | **Left hand:** The right hand is reinforced with the left hand so that the second and third digits of the left hand envelop the second metacarpal phalangeal joint of the right hand. The elbows are allowed to slightly flex. |
| **PROCEDURE** | The therapist applies a posterior-to-anterior force on each spinous process examined and performs a total of three slow repetitions. First pressures should be applied gently; amplitude and depth of the movement are increased if no pain response occurs. The therapist assesses the quality of movement through the range and the end feel and compares it with the levels above and below. |
| **NOTES** | A mid range of passive movement thrust (spring test) could also be used with this technique to assess tissue resistance and pain provocation. |
| | A positive response is movement that reproduces the comparable sign (pain or resistance or muscle guarding). |

## Central Posterior-to-Anterior Passive Accessory Intervertebral Motion Test—cont'd

**ALTERNATIVE ONE-HANDED TECHNIQUE**

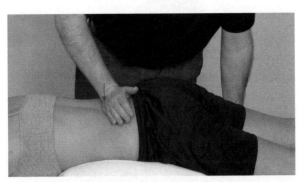

Central posterior-to-anterior PAIVM test, one-handed technique commonly used for spring testing

This technique could also be done as a one-handed technique with the cranial hand contacting the spinous process just distal to the pisiform, the elbow flexed, and the forearm perpendicular with the angle of the contour of the surface of the spine. The caudal hand rests at the edge of the table to support the therapist's upper body weight with leaning over the patient.

The two-handed posterior-anterior PAIVM test was used in development of CPRs for both stabilization and manipulation and has been included as one of the primary findings in clinical decision making for identification of patients who will respond to stabilization if hypermobility is noted and to manipulation if hypomobility is noted with this PAIVM procedure.[30,31] Fritz, Piva, and Childs[114] reported intertester reliability (n = 49 patients with LBP) for findings of hypomobility of 77% agreement with a Kappa value of 0.38 (0.22, 0.54), for findings of hypermobility of 77% agreement with a Kappa value of 0.48 (0.35, 0.61), and for findings of pain provocation of 85% agreement with a Kappa value of 0.57 (0.43, 0.71). The finding of lack of hypomobility with central posterior-anterior PAIVM testing combined with lumbar flexion of more than 53 degrees showed a +LR of 12.8 for correlation with radiographic evidence of lumbar instability.[114]

# MANIPULATION TECHNIQUES FOR LUMBAR SPINE, PELVIS, AND HIPS

## Lumbopelvic (Sacroiliac Region) Manipulation

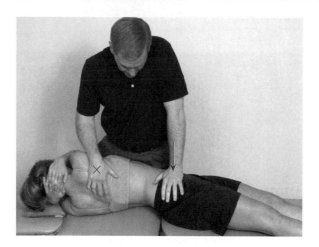

| | |
|---|---|
| **PURPOSE** | This technique restores lumbopelvic mobility and reduces lumbopelvic pain. |
| **PATIENT POSITION** | The patient is supine on the treatment table. |
| **THERAPIST POSITION** | The therapist stands on the side opposite the side to be manipulated. |
| **PROCEDURE** | |

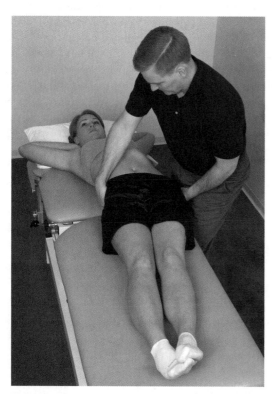

Therapist translates pelvis toward therapist side of table

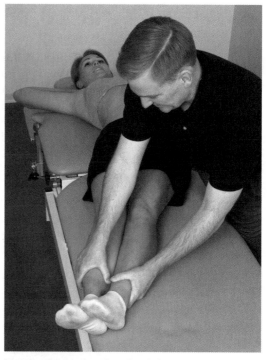

Maximally side bend patient's lower extremities and trunk to the right

## Lumbopelvic (Sacroiliac Region) Manipulation—cont'd

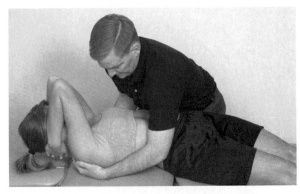

Lift and rotation of patient's upper body

The pelvis is translated toward the therapist's side of the table. The therapist maximally side bends the patient's lower extremities and trunk to the right. Without losing the right side bending, the therapist lifts and left rotates the trunk so that the patient rests on her left shoulder. The patient's right ASIS and ilium is contacted in a broad comfortable manner with the therapist's left hand. The top shoulder and scapula are grasped with the therapist's right hand, and the trunk is rotated to the left with the right side bending maintained. Once the right ASIS starts to elevate, a counter anterior-to-posterior force is applied through the ASIS to further take up the tissue slack, and once a firm barrier to motion is reached, a high-velocity, low-amplitude thrust is performed through the pelvis in an anterior-to-posterior direction.

**ALTERNATIVE TECHNIQUE**   An alternative method is use of the cranial forearm and hand across the scapula, thoracic, and lumbar spine to maintain the locked spinal position.

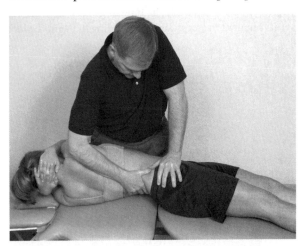

**NOTES**   Flynn and colleagues[30] used this technique to develop the CPR for manipulation for treatment of acute low back pain. This clinical prediction rule was validated by Childs et al,[28] who also used this technique with a different sample of patients and clinicians. This technique could be used to treat hypomobility impairments of the lower lumbar spine, lumbosacral junction, and sacroiliac joint on the targeted side.

## Lumbar Rotation Manipulation in Side Lying

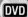

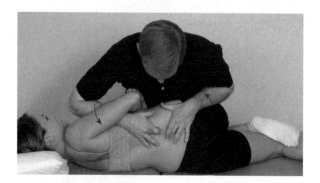

| | |
|---|---|
| **PURPOSE** | This technique manipulates a specific lumbar segment (L1-L2 through L5-S1) into rotation. |
| **PATIENT POSITION** | The patient is positioned side lying facing the therapist with the bottom leg in approximately 30 degrees of hip and knee flexion. |
| **THERAPIST POSITION** | The therapist stands in front of the patient with feet parallel with the table, weight on the balls of the feet, and hips and knees slightly flexed in an athletic stance position. The patient's top knee is positioned in the "hip hollow" at the anterior hip shelf of the therapist created by slight flexing of the hips and knees, and the therapist presses the front of the hip into the patient's knee to support the top leg. |
| **HAND PLACEMENT** | **Caudal hand:** The technique begins with grasping of the patient's top leg just proximal to the ankle to induce hip flexion and lumbar forward bending. |
| | **Cranial hand:** The pad of the long finger contacts the interspinous space of the targeted spinal segment to assess forward bending to begin the technique setup. |
| **PROCEDURE** | |

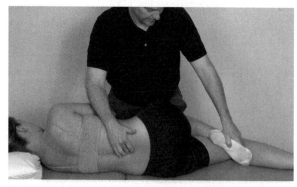

Hook top leg on bottom leg once forward-bending position has been reached for lumbar rotation technique

## Lumbar Rotation Manipulation in Side Lying—*cont'd*

The single leg forward bending PIVM technique is used to forward bend the lumbar spine up to the segment to be manipulated and then the hip and spine are slightly extended to maintain the spinal segment inferior to the targeted segment in a forward bent position and to maintain the targeted segment in neutral. Once this point is reached, the top leg is "hooked" onto the bottom leg (i.e., the foot of the top leg rests behind the knee of the bottom leg).

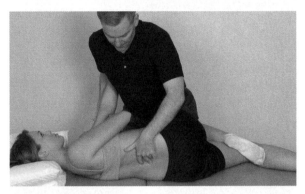

Rotation of spine to include segment above the level to be manipulated

The position of the hands are now switched so that the pad of the third digit of the caudal hand now palpates the interspinous space of the targeted segment and the second digit palpates one segment above. The spine is rotated to include the segment superior to the segment to be manipulated, but the segment to be manipulated is maintained in neutral. This is accomplished by pulling the patient's bottom arm (from proximal to the elbow) in a forward and upward rotary motion with the cranial hand. Next, fold the patient's arms loosely across the patient's chest.

The cranial hand slides underneath the patient's top arm, and the pad of the long finger contacts the top right lateral side of the spinous process of the cranial member of the segment.

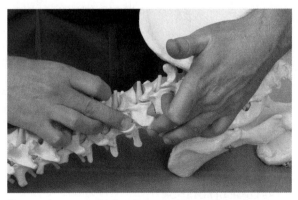

Finger placement for lumbar rotation manipulation

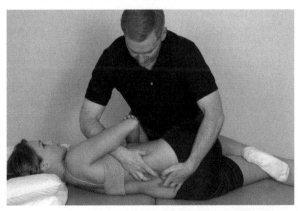

Hand and arm positioning to set up lumbar rotation technique

## Lumbar Rotation Manipulation in Side Lying—cont'd    (DVD)

The pad of the long finger of the caudal hand is used to contact the left lateral (bottom) side of the spinous process of the caudal member of the segment.

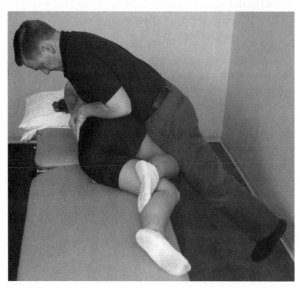

Lumbar rotation manipulation caudal view to illustrate therapist body position

The cranial leg is used to step into the edge of the table toward the patient so that the caudal leg leaves the ground and the knee on the patient's upper leg slides down the thigh of the therapist's caudal leg. Equal and opposite forces through the forearms (with contact with the patient's right anterior shoulder and chest and the right posterior hip and pelvis) are used to take up the slack and induce right rotation of the specified segment. The manipulation is coordinated with the patient's breathing, with progressive oscillation into more rotation each time. The manipulation is repeated through approximately three breathing cycles. Once an end-range barrier is established, a short-amplitude, high-velocity thrust may be imparted. After completion of the manipulation, the spine is derotated to a neutral position and PIVM of the specified segment can be retested. For manipulation of a lumbar segment into left rotation, the procedure is repeated with the patient positioned in right side lying.

**AN ALTERNATIVE CAUDAL HAND/ARM POSITION FOR THE LUMBAR ROTATION MANIPULATION TECHNIQUE**

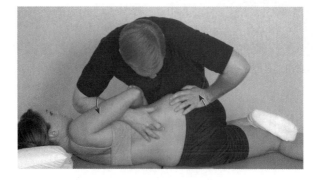

## Lumbar Rotation Manipulation in Side Lying—cont'd

An alternative caudal hand/arm position can assist in creation of greater leverage and can further lock the spine for production of an effective thrust manipulation, especially at the L5-S1 segment.

**NOTES**   Impairment-based indications for use of the right rotation manipulation technique are decreased right rotation PIVM or PAIVM testing and limited AROM of the lumbar spine. Indications for use of the left rotation manipulation technique are decreased left rotation PIVM or PAIVM testing and limited AROM of the lumbar spine. This technique is best performed as a progressive oscillation and is best combined with deep breathing for mechanical effects. Acute disc involvement, spondylolysis, or spondylolisthesis are considered precautions for performance of this technique.

This technique can be modified into an isometric manipulation and further adjustments can be made in the technique to enhance the success of high-velocity thrust manipulation. The technique set up is the same for the thrust, but emphasis is placed on use of the therapist forearms as the points of contact. Once the spinal segment is isolated with locking out the segments above and below as previously described, log-rolling the patient toward the therapist is helpful to create a 45-degree angle of the patient's pelvis in relation to the table and allow better use of gravity. The therapist's caudal forearm and body weight rotate the pelvis and lumbar spine toward the floor, and a counterforce is applied through the thorax with the cranial forearm.

If the patient has difficulty relaxing during a direct manipulation, use of an isometric manipulation technique can be effective. Once the segment is isolated and the spine is locked superior and inferior to the targeted segment as previously described, the patient is instructed to actively press the pelvis back into the therapist's forearm. After this force output (about 50% of maximum) is resisted for 10 seconds, the patient is asked to relax as the therapist takes up the tissue slack to apply a greater stretch and hold for 10 seconds. At this new barrier point, the isometric rotation is repeated and immediately followed by further stretching. After this sequence is repeated three to four times, the therapist applies further end range oscillations, or a sustained stretch, or a thrust manipulation.

After application of the manipulation, the patient is gently repositioned in a neutral side-lying position and muscle tone and passive lumbar mobility are reassessed to determine the effectiveness of the manipulation. If objective or subjective improvements are noted, the patient is progressed to active lumbar range of motion exercises, spinal stabilization exercises, or functional activities, such as walking on a treadmill. In general, it is advisable to have the patient functionally use the new mobility gained with the manipulation after the procedure. The follow-up activities also allow the therapist further opportunity to assess the effectiveness of the manual therapy interventions.

## Modification: Lumbar Rotation Manipulation Initiated Caudally

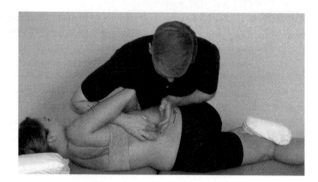

**PROCEDURE**    The setup and hand placement are the same as in the side-lying lumbar rotation manipulation, but instead of equal and opposite forces used with both arms, the cranial arm stabilizes as the caudal forearm provides the manipulative force. This variation should be used when spinal segments cranial to the targeted segment are either highly reactive or unstable.

## Modification: Lumbar Rotation Manipulation Initiated Cranially

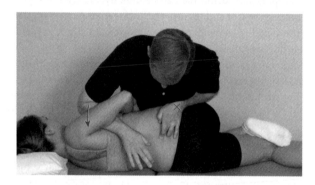

**PROCEDURE**    The setup and hand placement are the same as in the side-lying lumbar rotation manipulation, but instead of equal and opposite forces used with both arms, the caudal arm stabilizes the pelvis and lower spinal segments as the cranial forearm provides the manipulative force. This variation should be used when spinal segments caudal to the targeted segment are either highly reactive or unstable.

## Modification: Lumbar Rotation Manipulation with Lateral Flexion  (DVD)

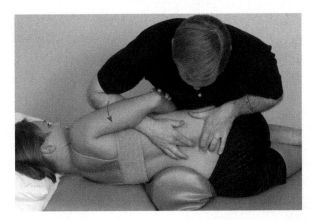

---

**PROCEDURE**   The setup and hand placement are the same as in the side-lying lumbar rotation manipulation, but the patient starts the procedure by lying over a bolster to induce lateral flexion to the opposite direction of the rotation. The caudal forearm can also rock the lateral (top) aspect of the pelvis inferiorly and downward to induce further lateral flexion. Lateral flexion could be used as either the primary or secondary lever with the technique. If lateral flexion is used as the primary lever, the manipulative force is with the caudal arm. If lateral flexion is used as the secondary lever to assist in taking up tissue slack, the manipulative force is with equal and opposite forces from both arms or either the caudal or cranial forces are emphasized. Care must be taken to maintain the lumbar spine in neutral or slight backward bending at the targeted segment when lateral flexion is used as a primary or secondary lever.

## Lumbosacral Lift Manipulation

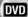

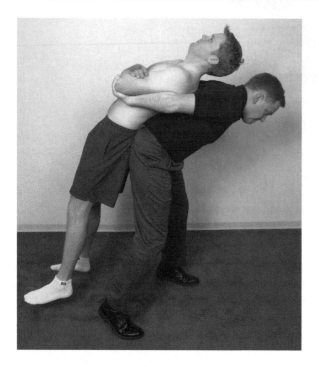

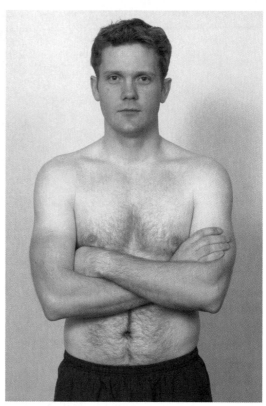

Patient arm position for lumbosacral lift manipulation

|  |  |
|---|---|
| **PURPOSE** | This technique is used to manipulate the lumbosacral junction (L5-S1) with a distractive force. |
| **PATIENT POSITION** | The patient stands with the arms folded firmly across the chest. |
| **THERAPIST POSITION** | The therapist stands with a diagonal stance with the back to the patient. |
| **HAND PLACEMENT** | Each hand is cupped across the inferior aspect of the patient's elbows. |
| **PROCEDURE** | The therapist leans forward, hinging at the hips, with the lumbar spine stabilized in a neutral position, to backward bend the patient to the lumbosacral junction and lift the patient's feet off the floor. The therapist's buttock should contact the patient's lumbosacral junction. The therapist can apply the thrust by rising up on the toes and dropping the heels abruptly to the ground or by jumping off the ground and landing with the legs and trunk held rigidly. In this way, the ground reaction forces cause the manipulative thrust. |
| **NOTES** | If the patient is taller than the therapist, the patient may need to spread the legs to assure the correct alignment of the therapist's buttock to the patient's lumbosacral junction. If the patient is much shorter than the therapist, the therapist needs to flex a greater degree at the hips and knees to create the proper patient-to-therapist alignment. Joint distraction at the lumbosacral junction occurs with the initial lift position and may be all the force that is needed for an effective technique. The therapist is advised to first lift the patient without applying the thrust and to reassess the patient's tolerance to the positioning before resetting the technique and applying the thrust. In addition to restoring mobility at the lumbosacral junction, this technique can be used to correct sacroiliac dysfunctions. |

## Lumbar Rotation Manipulation: Oscillation Through the Transverse Process ▸ DVD

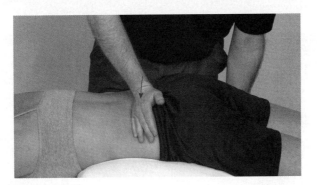

**PURPOSE**

This technique manipulates a specific lumbar segment (L1-L2 though L5-S1) into rotation.

**PATIENT POSITION**

The patient is prone with a pillow under the abdomen and pelvis.

**THERAPIST POSITION**

The therapist stands next to the patient.

**HAND PLACEMENT**

**Caudal hand:** The caudal hand is used to support the therapist's body weight on the edge of the treatment table.

**Cranial hand:** The ulnar proximal aspect of the fifth metacarpal is used to contact and apply force through the transverse process.

**PROCEDURE**

With the therapist standing on the patient's right side, the ulnar aspect of the fifth metacarpal on the caudal hand is used to locate the iliac crest on the patient's left side. The ulnar aspect of the fifth metacarpal locates the 12th rib on the patient's left side. The two hands make a V shape on the patient's back. The transverse process of L3 is located at the point of the V. The ulnar proximal aspect of the fifth metacarpal of the cranial hand is used to "sink into" the middle of the V at the location of the L3 transverse process. For manipulation into right rotation, the therapist takes up the slack and oscillates the left transverse process of L3. On completion of the manipulation, right rotation is retested. The procedure can be repeated with the transverse processes of L2 (located just inferior to the twelfth rib, segment L2-L3) and L4 (located just superior to the iliac crest, segment L4-L5). The therapist manipulates L5-S1 by placing the middle crease of the cranial hand on the patient's right PSIS with the thenar eminence on the sacral sulcus. The therapist takes up the slack and oscillates the L5-S1 segment by giving a posterior-to-anterior force.

For manipulation of the lumbar segments into left rotation, the procedure is repeated by oscillating through the right transverse processes of L2-L4 and through the left PSIS.

**NOTES**

This technique is commonly used to induce grade I and II oscillations for the purpose of pain inhibition. Therefore a painful reactive facet joint or surrounding soft tissues are indications for this technique.

## Lumbar Spine Side-Bending (Lateral Flexion) Manipulation: Prone Abducting the Leg with a Thumb or Finger Block

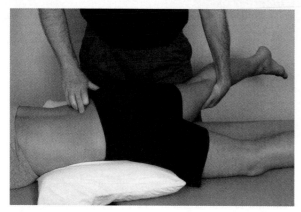

Lumbar spine lateral flexion manipulation, prone abducting the leg with finger block

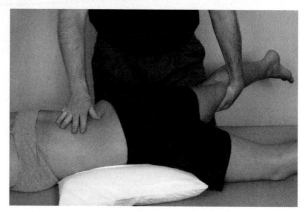

Lumbar spine lateral flexion manipulation, prone abducting the leg with thumb block

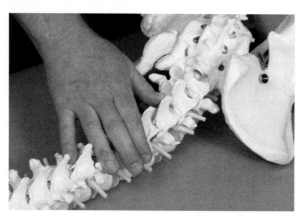

Thumb placement to create fulcrum for lumbar spine lateral flexion manipulation, prone abducting the leg with thumb block

| | |
|---|---|
| **PURPOSE** | This technique is used to manipulate a specific lumbar segment (L1-L2 through L5-S1) into side bending. |
| **PATIENT POSITION** | The patient is prone with a pillow under the abdomen and pelvis. |
| **THERAPIST POSITION** | The therapist stands next to the patient. |
| **HAND PLACEMENT** | **Caudal hand:** The caudal hand supports the patient's right leg at the knee but avoids patella compression. |
| | **Cranial hand:** The pad of the thumb or long finger is used to block the lateral aspect of the spinous process of the cranial member of the segment. |
| **PROCEDURE** | The therapist stands on the patient's right side and uses the pad of the thumb or long finger of the cranial hand to block the right lateral aspect of the spinous process of the cranial member of the specified segment. Lumbar side bending to the right is induced by abducting the patient's right hip with the caudal hand and keeping the leg even with the top of the table to avoid excessive hip extension/lumbar lordosis. The therapist takes up the slack and oscillates. On completion of the manipulation, lumbar side bending is retested. |

## Lumbar Spine Side-Bending (Lateral Flexion) Manipulation: Prone Abducting the Leg with a Thumb or Finger Block—cont'd

The spinal segment is manipulated into side bending to the left with the therapist standing on the patient's left side and repeating the procedure abducting the left hip.

NOTES    Impairment-based indications for use of the right side-bending manipulation technique are decreased lumbar AROM and right side-bending PIVM testing of a specific lumbar segment (L1-L2 through L5-S1). Indications for use of the left side-bending manipulation technique are decreased lumbar AROM and left side bending of a specific lumbar segment (L1-L2 through L5-S1). With proper handling of the patient's leg, excessive hip extension and compression of the patella are avoided. This technique can also be performed with the patient's knee slightly flexed. However, excessive knee flexion with tightness of the rectus femoris muscle should be avoided. This technique is most commonly used as a grade III (nonthrust) manipulation for mechanical effects. Hip pathology is a precaution with this technique.

## Lumbar Spine Side-Bending (Lateral Flexion) Manipulation with a Mobilization Table and a Thumb Block

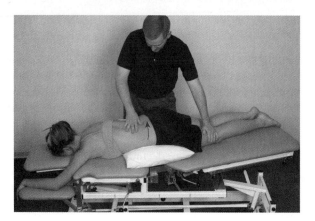

The prone lumbar spine side-bending manipulation is even more effective with use of a mobilization table. The cranial hand function remains the same; but instead of abduction of the hip to induce lateral flexion, the lateral flexion function of the table is used to swing both legs and the lumbar spine into a lateral flexion passive motion.

## Side-Bending Myofascial Stretch

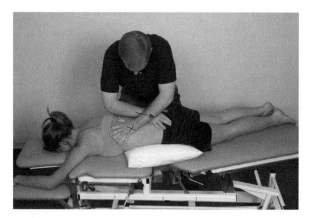

A side-bending myofascial stretch can also be applied with the use of the mobilization table with placement of the hands on the upper and lower lumbar spine as the stretch is applied. The stretch should be sustained for at least 30 seconds and repeated three to four times.

## Prone Lumbar Isometric Manipulation  (DVD)

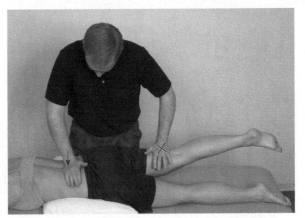

Lumbar isometric manipulation combined with direct mobilization of targeted segment with posterior-to-anterior pressure through transverse process

---

| | |
|---|---|
| **PURPOSE** | The purpose of this technique is to manipulate a lumbar segment (L1-L2 though L5-S1) with a painful facet joint entrapment. |
| **PATIENT POSITION** | The patient is prone with a pillow under the abdomen and pelvis. |
| **THERAPIST POSITION** | The therapist stands next to the patient. |
| **HAND PLACEMENT** | **Caudal hand:** The caudal hand is placed across the posterior aspect of the patient's upper leg. |
| | **Cranial hand:** The ulnar proximal aspect of the fifth metacarpal is used to contact the transverse process of the superior member of the targeted segment. |
| **PROCEDURE** | After the reactive or stiff facet joint is identified with a posterior-to-anterior force at the transverse process with the cranial hand, the posterior-anterior force is held with the cranial hand at the targeted transverse process and the patient is asked to extend the opposite hip. Isometric resistance is applied to the hip extension for a 10-second hold. After the patient rests the leg back on the table, posterior-anterior oscillations are applied to the targeted segment for 10 seconds and then the isometric hip extension is repeated. This sequence is repeated three to four times until improved mobility and reduced joint reactivity is noted with the posterior-anterior force at the transverse process. |
| **NOTES** | Opposite hip extension is used to facilitate an isometric contraction of the multifidus muscle on the side of the targeted facet joint. The patient may have difficulty actively extending the hip for the first one or two isometric contractions. Commonly, the patient is able to generate greater force with each subsequent contraction. The segment can be further isolated by side bending the lumbar spine to the targeted segment. |

## Lumbar Spine Side-Bending Manipulation: Side Lying Raising and Lowering the Legs

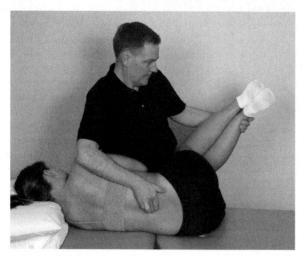

Lumbar spine side-bending manipulation side lying raising the legs

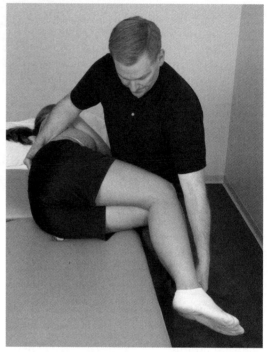

Lumbar spine side-bending manipulation lowering the legs

| | |
|---|---|
| **PURPOSE** | This manipulation is used to move a specific lumbar segment (L1-L2 through L5-S1) into side bending. |
| **PATIENT POSITION** | The patient is positioned side lying facing the therapist with the hips and knees flexed to 90 degrees. |
| **THERAPIST POSITION** | The therapist stands with a diagonal stance in front of the patient facing the patient's thighs with the caudal leg forward, flexed, and supporting the patient's bottom thigh. |
| **HAND PLACEMENT** | **Caudal hand:** This hand holds the patient's bottom leg just proximal to the ankle. |
| | **Cranial hand:** The pad of the long finger is used to block the lateral aspect of the spinous process of the cranial member of the segment. |
| **PROCEDURE** | With the patient in a left side-lying position, both legs are positioned in 90 degrees of hip and knee flexion. For manipulation of the segment into right side bending, the pad of the long finger on the cranial hand is used to block the right lateral aspect of the spinous process of the cranial member of the segment. The patient's legs are lifted until side bending is induced at the targeted segment. The therapist takes up the slack and oscillates through the leg. On completion of the manipulation, side bending to the right is retested. The pad of the long finger of the cranial hand is used to block the left lateral aspect of the spinous process of the cranial member of the segment. The legs are lowered until side bending is induced at the targeted segment. The therapist takes up the slack and oscillates through the leg. On completion of the manipulation, side bending is retested to the left. |

## Lumbar Spine Side-Bending Manipulation: Side Lying Raising and Lowering the Legs—cont'd

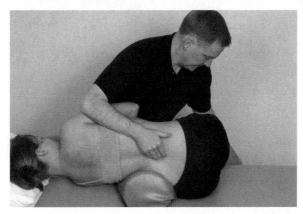

Further stretch can be induced with lowering the legs manipulation technique by having patient lie over a bolster

The leg-lowering manipulation technique can be further facilitated by placing the patient over the top of the bolster, with the apex of the bolster positioned to induce lateral flexion at the targeted segment.

**NOTES** Impairment-based indications for use of the right side-bending manipulation technique are decreased lumbar AROM and right side bending PIVM of a specific lumbar segment (L1-L2 through L5-S1). Indications for use of the left side-bending manipulation technique are decreased lumbar AROM and left side bending PIVM of a specific lumbar segment (L1-L2 through L5-S1).

## Isometric Lumbar Manipulation with the Side-Bending Leg Lowering Technique

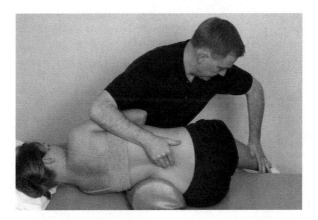

An isometric manipulation can be used with the side-bending leg lowering manipulation by applying resistance in the leg-raising direction followed by further stretching into the leg-lowering direction. The isometric contraction is held for 10 seconds and followed by a 10-second stretch. This sequence is repeated for three to four bouts.

## Lumbar Spine Side-Bending Manipulation: Side Lying Rocking the Pelvis   (DVD)

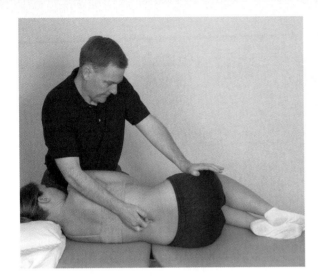

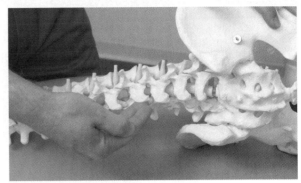

Finger placement for blocking spinous process for lumbar spine side bending, side lying rocking the pelvis

| | |
|---|---|
| **PURPOSE** | The purpose of this technique is to manipulate a specific lumbar segment (L1-L2 through L5-S1) into side bending. |
| **PATIENT POSITION** | The patient is in a side-lying position facing the therapist. |
| **THERAPIST POSITION** | The therapist stands next to the patient. |
| **HAND PLACEMENT** | **Caudal hand:** The palm of the hand is placed on the patient's greater trochanter. |
| | **Cranial hand:** The pad of the long finger is used to block the lateral aspect of the spinous process of the cranial member of the segment. |
| **PROCEDURE** | With the patient in a left side-lying position, both legs are positioned in 90 degrees of hip and knee flexion. The pad of the long finger of the cranial hand is used to block the left lateral aspect of the spinous process of the cranial member of the segment. The superior aspect of the greater trochanter is contacted with the heel of the caudal hand, with the elbow straight and the arm in line with the direction of the force. Lumbar side bending is induced to the left with the caudal hand pushing the patient's greater trochanter caudally. The therapist takes up the slack and oscillates. On completion of the manipulation, side bending to the left is retested. |

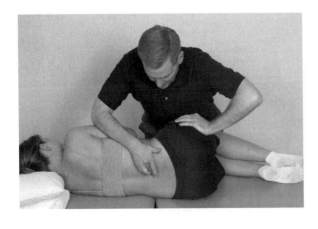

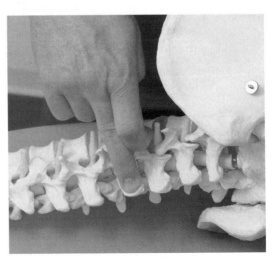

## Lumbar Spine Side-Bending Manipulation: Side Lying Rocking the Pelvis—cont'd

For manipulation of the segment into right side bending, the pad of the long finger on the cranial hand is used to block the right lateral aspect of the spinous process of the cranial member of the segment. The caudal hand pushes the patient's greater trochanter cranially, with the forearm lined up in frontal plane parallel to the direction of the force. The therapist takes up the slack and oscillates. On completion of the manipulation, side bending to the right is retested.

NOTES | Because of the small lever arm, use of grade I and II oscillations is most appropriate for this technique. The forearm should be positioned parallel to the direction of the force applied through the greater trochanter. The procedure can be performed with the patient in a right side-lying position, with caudal movement of the pelvis inducing right side bending and cranial movement of the pelvis inducing left side bending. Manipulation of lumbar side bending with this technique (e.g., rocking the pelvis) is useful for patients with hip pathology (the hip joint is not stressed).

## Posterior Ilial Rotation Sacroiliac Joint Manipulation    (DVD)

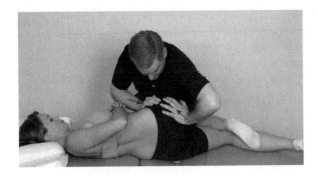

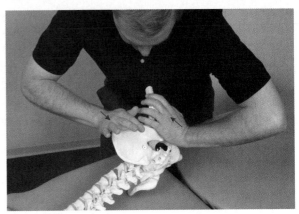

Posterior rotation SIJ manipulation hand placement

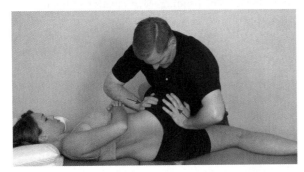

Posterior rotation SIJ manipulation with leg positioned
from isometric manipulation

| | |
|---|---|
| **PURPOSE** | This technique is used to manipulate an anterior ilial rotation displacement sacroiliac joint dysfunction and to restore posterior rotation of the ilium. |
| **PATIENT POSITION** | The patient is positioned side lying facing the therapist. |
| **THERAPIST POSITION** | The therapist stands with a diagonal athletic stance in front of the patient. |
| **HAND PLACEMENT** | **Caudal hand:** The palm is used to contact the patient's ischial tuberosity. |
| | **Cranial hand:** The palm is used to contact the patient's ASIS. |
| **PROCEDURE (PROVOCATION TEST)** | The patient's bottom leg is flexed to approximately 30 degrees of hip and knee flexion. The top hip is flexed to approximately 90 degrees, and the foot of the top leg is hooked at the knee of the bottom leg. The spine is rotated to include the L5-S1 segment with pulling the patient's bottom arm (from proximal to the elbow) in a forward and upward rotary motion with the cranial hand. The patient's arms are loosely folded across the chest. The palm of the cranial hand is used to contact the patient's top ASIS, and the palm of the caudal hand is used to contact the patient's top ischial tuberosity. A force couple is created with pushing the ASIS posteriorly and pushing the ischial tuberosity anteriorly. The force is gradually increased over 10 to 30 seconds. End range oscillations or a thrust can be used. |

For further mechanical advantage and for an isometric manipulation, the therapist should follow the procedure as described previously; but before application of the force couple, the therapist should step inside the patient's top leg and alternate a direct manipulation, using the force couple, with an isometric manipulation by using isometric hip extension of the top leg (patient instructed to push the thigh into the front hip of the therapist). The therapist takes up the slack and holds for 10 seconds and then instructs the patient to isometrically extend the hip for 10 seconds. The force couple of the direct manipulation is

## Posterior Ilial Rotation Sacroiliac Joint Manipulation—cont'd

maintained as the isometric manipulation is performed. The procedure is repeated for a total of three to four repetitions. Once the slack is fully taken up, a small-amplitude, high-velocity thrust manipulation can also be used.

NOTES     Patients who tend to redisplace into anterior rotation of the sacroiliac joint can turn this technique into a self-isometric manipulation: In supine position, the ipsilateral hip is flexed and both hands are used to hold the thigh in a flexed position. The hip is isometrically extended into the hands and held for 10 seconds; repeat three to four times.

## Lumbosacral Manual Traction with a Mobilization Table     DVD

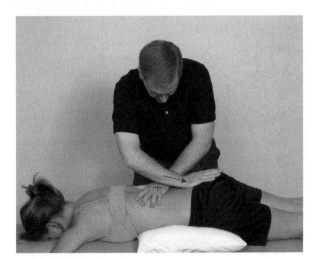

The direct sacral mobilization technique can be modified to apply traction at the lower lumbar spine with use of a mobilization table. The table can be released to allow the lower section to separate as the manual traction force is sustained at the sacrum and counter-force is applied at the upper lumbar spine.

## Anterior Ilial Rotation Sacroiliac Joint Manipulation   **DVD**

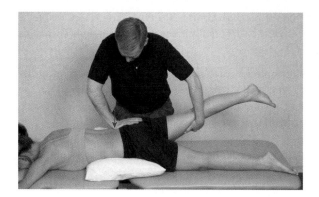

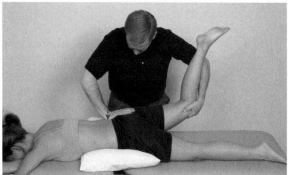

Anterior rotation SIJ manipulation with knee flexed

Anterior rotation SIJ manipulation hand placement

| | |
|---|---|
| **PURPOSE** | The purpose is to manipulate a posterior ilial rotation displacement sacroiliac joint dysfunction and restore anterior rotation of the ilium. |
| **PATIENT POSITION** | The patient is prone with a pillow under the pelvis. |
| **THERAPIST POSITION** | The therapist stands with a diagonal athletic stance next to the patient. |
| **HAND PLACEMENT** | **Caudal hand:** The caudal hand grasps the anterior thigh just proximal to the knee. |
| | **Cranial hand:** The hypothenar eminence is used to contact the PSIS, with the fingers pointing toward the patient's thigh (to keep the hands off the lumbar spine). |
| **PROCEDURE** | The hypothenar eminence of the cranial hand is used to contact the PSIS, and the caudal hand is used to extend the hip just enough to take up the slack in the hip. The cranial hand forces the PSIS towards the table and approximately 10 to 20 degrees laterally. An isometric manipulation can be added by following the procedure as described previously; but before the application of the direct manipulation force, the patient is instructed to isometrically flex the hip into the therapist's hand and hold for 10 seconds. After the isometric hip flexion hold, the therapist further extends the patient's hip and progressively oscillates with the caudal hand to take up the slack and repeats three to four times. At the end range of the available motion, a thrust can be applied with the cranial hand directed to the pelvis. |
| **NOTES** | The fingers of the cranial hand should point toward the patient's feet and should not contact the patient's lumbar spine. The patient's knee can be flexed during the performance of this technique. |

## Anterior Ilial Rotation Sacroiliac Joint Manipulation—cont'd

This technique can be turned into a self-isometric manipulation: In the prone position with a pillow under the pelvis, the unaffected leg is placed off the lateral edge of the bed with the foot on the floor. The hip is isometrically flexed on the affected side by pushing the knee into the bed and holding for 10 seconds. The procedure is repeated three to four times. Patients who tend to stiffen or redisplace between therapy sessions are instructed to perform this self-manipulation as part of a home program.

## Coccyx Direct Internal Manipulation

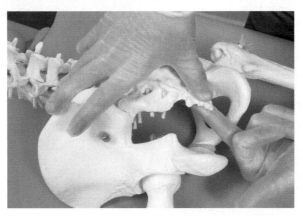

Coccyx direct internal manipulation hand placement

| | |
|---|---|
| **PURPOSE** | This manipulation is used to mobilize the coccyx to correct a coccygeal displacement and to inhibit pelvic floor muscle tone. |
| **PATIENT POSITION** | The patient is prone over two or three pillows with the hips abducted and internally rotated. |
| **THERAPIST POSITION** | The therapist stands at the side of the patient. |
| **HAND PLACEMENT** | **Caudal hand:** With a latex glove with lubricating gel worn on the long finger, the finger is eased through the anus into the rectum, with the volar pad of the finger facing dorsally to palpate the anterior surface of the coccyx. |
| | **Cranial hand:** The thumb is placed on the external dorsal surface of the coccyx. |
| **PROCEDURE** | Once the proper finger placement is obtained, a distraction force is applied along the long axis of the coccyx. If a lateral flexed or rotation deviation is noted, correction can be attempted during application of the distraction force. The distraction force is sustained for 30 seconds for three to four repetitions. |
| **NOTES** | The primary finding for indication of coccyx manipulation is coccyx pain with sitting, pain with contraction of the gluteus maximus muscle, and pain provocation with direct pressure at the coccyx. Pelvic floor muscle dysfunctions can contribute to coccyx pain and should be addressed as part of the treatment plan of care. Stress reduction strategies, such as use of a coccyx pillow with a square cut out of the posterior edge of the cushion, should be used on a consistent basis to unload the coccyx when seated. Modalities such as ionotophoresis may assist in reduction of pain in this region as well. |

## Sacral Mobilization and Myofascial Stretch    DVD

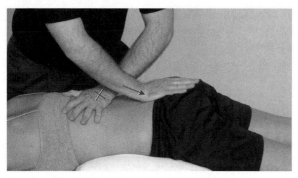

Myofascial stretch and sacral mobilization

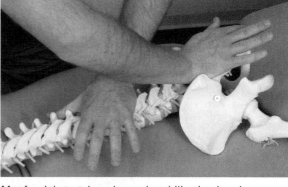

Myofascial stretch and sacral mobilization hand placement

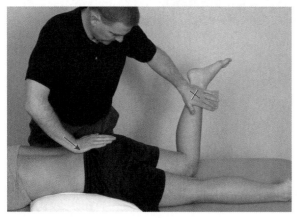

Isometric manipulation of sacrum with hip lateral rotators

| | |
|---|---|
| **PURPOSE** | This manipulation inhibits muscle tone at the lumbosacral junction and, in theory, corrects suspected sacral torsional displacements. |
| **PATIENT POSITION** | The patient is in a prone position with a pillow supporting the pelvis. |
| **THERAPIST POSITION** | The therapist stands with a diagonal athletic stance against the edge of treatment table. |
| **HAND PLACEMENT** | **Cranial hand:** The heel of the hand is placed at the base of the patient's sacrum. |
| | **Caudal hand:** The palm of hand is placed across the upper lumbar spine and erector spinae muscles. |
| **PROCEDURE** | The cranial hand gradually sinks into the myofascial tissues over the base of the sacrum and applies a caudally directed anterior force as the tissue tone relaxes. The caudal hand applies a gradual counterforce directed anteriorly and superiorly. The forces start gentle and gradually are increased as the muscle tone relaxes. For further mobilization of the sacrum, the caudal hand can move the hip into medial rotation and isometrically resist lateral rotation as the cranial hand sustains pressure at the base of the sacrum. In theory, the isometric contraction of the lateral rotators of the hip pulls one side of the base of the sacrum anteriorly to mobilize the SIJ and inhibit muscle tone in the region. The isometric force should be sustained for 10 seconds and repeated three to four times with a 10-second rest between contractions. The sacral force is sustained throughout and between the isometric contractions. |

## Coccyx Isometric Manipulation

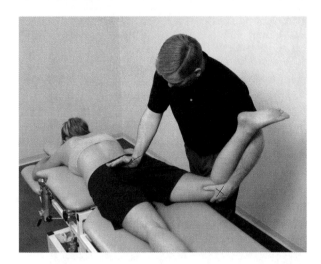

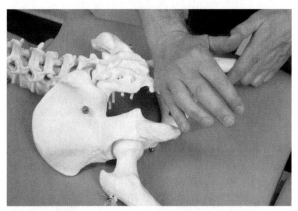

Coccyx isometric manipulation hand placement

| | |
|---|---|
| **PURPOSE** | This technique is used to manipulate the sacrococcygeal joint. |
| **PATIENT POSITION** | The patient is in a prone position lying over a pillow with the knee flexed on the side to be manipulated. |
| **THERAPIST POSITION** | The therapist stands at the side of the patient. |
| **HAND PLACEMENT** | **Cranial hand:** The hypothenar eminence is placed at the lateral edge of the base of the coccyx just distal to the sacrococcygeal joint on the side of the therapist. |
| | **Caudal hand:** The caudal hand cups the medial and anterior aspect of the patient's knee on the leg closest to the therapist. |
| **PROCEDURE** | A medially directed force is applied at the sacrococcygeal joint with the cranial hand as the caudal hand abducts the patient's hip. Once full hip abduction is obtained, hip adduction is resisted isometrically and held for 10 seconds. The patient rests for 10 seconds and then repeats the isometric hold after the tissue slack is taken up with further hip abduction and direct force. The procedure is repeated three to four times, and the direct force is maintained with the cranial hand throughout the hold/relax sequence with the hip. |
| **NOTES** | In theory, gliding the sacrococcygeal joint toward the midline from the right to the left moves the coccyx into right lateral flexion because the proximal coccyx is a convex joint surface moving a concave distal sacrum. Pelvic floor muscle dysfunctions can contribute to coccyx pain and should be addressed as part of the treatment plan of care. Stress reduction strategies, such as regular use of a coccyx pillow with a square cut out of the posterior edge of the cushion, should be used on a consistent basis to unload the coccyx when seated. Modalities such as ionotophoresis may assist in reduction of pain in this region as well. |

## Hip Abduction/Adduction Isometric Manipulation

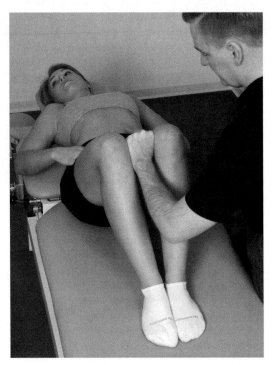

Hip adduction isometric manipulation

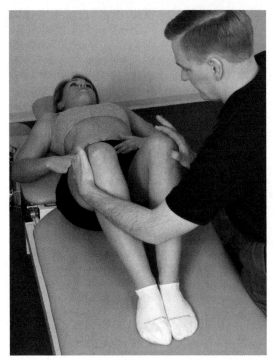

Hip abduction isometric manipulation

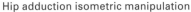

| | |
|---|---|
| **PURPOSE** | General isometric manipulation of the pelvis is used to relax muscle tone and balance alignment of the pelvis and to inhibit pain. |
| **PATIENT POSITION** | The patient is supine in the hook-lying position. |
| **THERAPIST POSITION** | The therapist stands at the edge of the table. |
| **PROCEDURE** | For the hip adduction isometric technique, the therapist places a closed fist between the patient's knees and asks the patient to squeeze the fist between the knees. The isometric contraction is held for 10 seconds and repeated three to four times, with a 10-second rest between contractions. |
| | For the hip abduction isometric technique, the therapist places the hands along the lateral aspect of both of the patient's knees and asks the patient to pull the knees apart. The contraction is held for 10 seconds and repeated three to four times, with a 10-second rest between contractions. |
| **NOTES** | A useful method is to finish a manual therapy session with these isometric techniques to relax muscle tone of the pelvic region before the therapy session is completed. Theoretically, the symphysis pubis and sacroiliac joints are both mobilized with these isometric techniques. Alternating between the abduction and adduction isometric techniques is often helpful. |

## Hip Joint Anterior Glide Manipulation

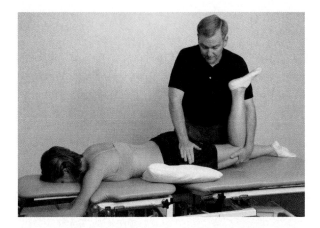

| | |
|---|---|
| **PURPOSE** | This manipulation is used to stretch the anterior hip joint capsule to improve hip extension range of motion. |
| **PATIENT POSITION** | The patient is prone lying over a pillow. |
| **THERAPIST POSITION** | The therapist stands on the side of the table opposite the hip to be manipulated. |
| **PROCEDURE** | The therapist lifts and holds the patient's hip in extension with the caudal hand and applies an anterior lateral force parallel to the angle of the acetabulum at the posterior aspect of the proximal femur near the greater trochanter. |
| **NOTES** | Typically, a progressive oscillation or a grade III mobilization force is used with this technique to attempt to improve hip extension. If the leg is too heavy for the therapist to hold, the femur could be supported in an extended position with a pillow or towel roll. Patients with chronic low back pain conditions such as spinal stenosis commonly have limited hip extension and may benefit from use of an anterior glide manipulation to attempt to improve hip mobility. |

**ALTERNATE TECHNIQUE FOR HIP JOINT ANTERIOR GLIDE MANIPULATION**

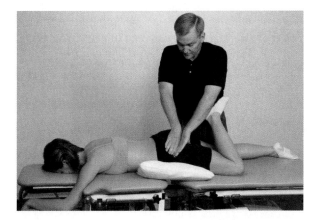

The anterior glide manipulation can be performed with the targeted hip placed in an end range external rotation position with the patient's tibia resting on the opposite leg in a frog leg position. This position allows the therapist to use the web space of both hands to apply an anterior lateral force at the posterior aspect of the proximal femur. Theoretically, this manipulation technique should assist in restoring both hip extension and external rotation.

## Hip Joint Manipulation with a Mobilization Belt   (DVD)

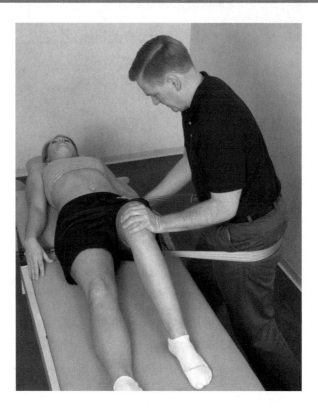

| | |
|---:|:---|
| **PURPOSE** | The purpose of this manipulation is to stretch the hip joint capsule and restore full hip mobility. |
| **PATIENT POSITION** | The patient is supine, lying close to the edge of the table on the side of the hip to be manipulated. |
| **THERAPIST POSITION** | The therapist stands, in a diagonal stance with the caudal foot back, at the edge of the table on the side of the hip to be manipulated. |
| **PROCEDURE** | The mobilization belt is positioned at the proximal thigh near the crease formed by flexing the patient's hip to 30 degrees of flexion and looped around the therapist's buttock. The therapist stabilizes the patient's pelvis and distal femur while leaning in an inferior and posterior direction in line with the 120-degree angle at the neck of the patient's femur. |

## Hip Joint Manipulation with a Mobilization Belt—cont'd

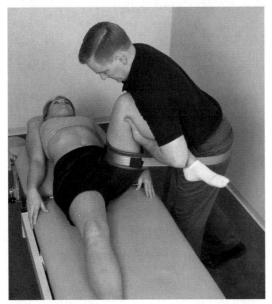

Lateral distraction hip joint manipulation with belt combined with passive hip internal rotation

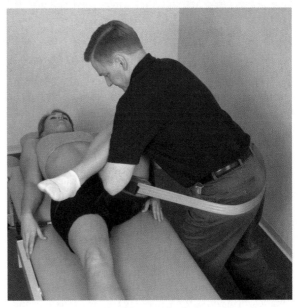

Lateral distraction hip joint manipulation with belt combined with passive hip external rotation

**Mobilization with Movement:** The distraction technique can be modified by flexing the hip to 90 degrees. The therapist uses the chest to stabilize the distal femur, the cranial hand to stabilize the pelvis, and the caudal hand/arm to rotate the hip either into internal or external rotation. The distraction is sustained as the hip is stretched repeatedly into an end range of motion position.

**NOTES**    The therapist should follow the hip mobilization techniques with active range of motion exercises, such as the bent knee fall out exercise, to have the patient move into the new range of motion obtained with the manipulation procedure. Many patients with low back pain have limitations in hip capsular mobility and can benefit from this technique.

# Case Studies and Problem Solving

The following case studies are provided as a way for physical therapy students to practice problem solving with an impairment-based evidence-based approach. Basic objective and subjective information is provided, and students are asked to develop a physical therapy diagnosis, problem list, and treatment plan.

## Mr. Acute Back

### History

A 30-year-old factory worker bent over to put down his dog's dish and strained his lower back 2 weeks before the initial evaluation. The pain is focused in the right lumbosacral (LS) junction and radiates into the right buttock and posterior thigh. Pain is made worse with sitting, bending forward, twisting, and walking and is relieved with lying supine in a 90/90 position. The patient is a heavy smoker and has had LBP episodes in the past but never this intense or prolonged. An MRI scan 2 years previous showed a degenerative disc at L5-S1. FABQ work subscale score is l6.

### Tests and Measures

- Structural examination reveals 1/2 leg length discrepancy, with the left leg shorter, and the patient is shifted to the left in standing, avoiding full weight on the right lower extremity (LE)
- Active motion testing: 50% forward bending with provocation of pain, 25% left sidebending, 50% right sidebending, 25% right rotation, 50% left rotation, and 15% backward bending with provocation of pain
- Quadrant test results are positive right for LBP
- Neurologic testing results are negative
- Palpation: Guarded/tight/tender right L5-S1 area
- PIVM: Significant restriction L5-S1 FB, LSB, and right rotation (RRot)
- PAIVM (spring) test: Positive pain provocation right L5-S1 facet and limited mobility with posterior-anterior testing
- Strength: 4/5 Multifidus, abdominal, and hip muscles
- Muscle length: Moderately tight right psoas and both hamstrings
- Hip AROM: 65 degrees external rotation, 38 degrees internal rotation bilaterally

### Evaluation

Diagnosis
Problem list
Goals
Treatment plan/intervention

## Mr. Chronic Back

### History

A 55-year-old man with a 14-month history of LBP and sciatica received 2 months of physical therapy with good relief of sciatica but still has LBP. The patient works as a machine operator and has to stand on concrete all day and wants to work 6 more years. LBP is constant and focused centrally across the lower lumbar region. Pain is worse with prolonged sitting, standing, or bending. The patient was injured at work by falling on a wet spot left by a leaky air conditioner. The patient works on light duty with a 25-pound lifting restriction. Pain is worse (7/10) at the end of the day.

### Tests and Measures

- Structural examination: Good symmetry, but step noted at L3-L4 with increased lumbar lordosis and rotund abdomen
- AROM: All planes 75% with limited lower lumbar motion and fulcrum at L3-L4
- PIVM: Limited L5-S1 and L4-L5 in all motions; hypermobile L3-L4 all motions with positive pain provocation spring testing results L3-L4
- Palpation: Myofascial tightness with minimal tenderness lumbar paraspinals
- Muscle length: Moderately tight bilateral hamstrings and iliopsoas
- Muscle strength: Abdominals and multifidus 3+/5
- Endurance: Poor

### Evaluation

Diagnosis
Problem list
Goals
Treatment plan/intervention

## Ms. Lucy Goosey

### History

A 25-year-old woman who works at a department store as a cashier has right upper lumbar pain and left upper thoracic area pain that is provoked with prolonged standing and work activities. The patient admits to being fairly sedentary when not at work. The patient describes pain as achiness that intensifies with sustained postures and is relieved with lying down.

### Tests and Measures

- Posture: Moderate forward head posture with protracted scapulas and flat lumbar spine
- Cervical AROM: At 75% in all planes with stiffness noted in upper thoracic spine and pain reported with end range left rotation
- Lumbar AROM: Nearly 100% in all planes with poor muscle control noted with FB and stiffness noted in lower thoracic spine
- Straight Leg Raise: 95 degrees bilaterally
- Prone Instability Test: Positive
- PIVM: Hypermobile in midcervical segments; moderately restricted upper thoracic right rotation and FB; hypermobile upper lumbar; moderately restricted T9-T10 and T10-T11 right rotation
- Palpation: Mildly tender and moderately guarded left upper thoracic tissues and right lower thoracic; moderately tender left lower cervical facet joint tissues and right upper lumbar tissues
- Strength: Poor+ scapular stabilizers, lumbar, and cervical multifidus
- Other observations: System hypermobility noted in fingers, elbows, and knees

### Evaluation

Diagnosis
Problem list
Goals
Treatment plan/intervention

## REFERENCES

1. Burton A, Tollotson K, Main C, et al: Psychosocial predictors of outcome in acute and subchronic low back trouble, *Spine* 20:722-728, 1995.
2. Truchon M: Determinants of chronic disability related to low back pain: towards an integrated biopsychosocial model, *Disabil Rehabil* 23:758-767, 2001.
3. Fenuele J, Birkmeyer N, Abdu W, et al: The impact of spinal problems on the health status of patients: have we underestimated the effect? *Spine* 25:1509-1514, 2000.
4. Deyo R, Gray D, Dreuter W, et al: United States trends in lumbar fusion surgery for degenerative conditions, *Spine* 30:1441-1445, 2005.
5. Cibulka M, Delitto A, Koldehoff R: Changes in innominate tilt after manipulation of the sacroiliac joint in patients with low back pain: an experimental study, *Phys Ther* 68:1359-1363, 1988.
6. Waddell G, Feder G, McIntosh A: *Low back pain evidence review*, London, 1999, Royal College of General Practitioners. Available at http://www.rcgp.org.uk/rcgp/clinspec/guidelines/backpain/backpain5.asp#Guideline.
7. American Medial Association: *Guides to the evaluation of permanent impairment*, ed 3, Chicago, 1988, AMA.
8. Troke M, Moore AP, Maillardet FJ, et al: A normative database of lumbar spine ranges of motion, *Manual Ther* 10:198-206, 2005.
9. Norris CM: Spinal stabilization 2: limiting factors to end-range motion in the lumbar spine, *Physiotherapy* 81(2):64-72, 1995.
10. Inufusa A, An HS, Lim T, et al: Anatomic changes of the spinal canal and intervertebral foramen associated with flexion-extension movement, *Spine* 21(21):2412-2420, 1996.
11. Nachemson A: The load on lumbar disks in different positions of the body, *Clin Orthop* 45:107-122, 1966.
12. Paris SV: Anatomy as related to function and pain, *Orthop Clin North Am* 14(3):475-489, 1983.
13. Pearcy MJ, Tibrewal SB: Axial rotation and lateral bending in the normal lumbar spine measured by three-dimensional radiography, *Spine* 9:582-587, 1984.
14. Panjabi MM, Oxland TR, Yamamoto I, et al: Mechanical behavior of the lumbar and lumbosacral spine as shown by three-dimensional load-displacement curves, *J Bone Joint Surg (Am)* 76:413-424, 1994.
15. Lund T, Nydegger T, Schlenzka D, et al: Three-dimensional motion patterns during active bending in patients with chronic low back pain, *Spine* 27(17):1865-1874, 2002.
16. Legaspi O, Edmond S: Does the evidence support the existence of lumbar spine coupled motion? A critical review of the literature, *JOSPT* 27(4):169-178, 2007.
17. Bergmark A: Stability of the lumbar spine: a study in mechanical engineering, *Acta Orthop Scand Suppl* 230(60):2-54, 1989.
18. Taylor JR, O'Sullivan P: Lumbar segmental instability: pathology, diagnosis, and conservative management. In Twomey LT, Taylor JR, editors: *Physical therapy of the low back*, London, 2000, Churchill Livingstone.
19. Macintosh JE, Bogduk N: The biomechanics of the lumbar multifidus, *Clin Biomech* 1:205-213, 1986.
20. Strruresson B, Selvik G, Uden A: Movements of the sacroiliac joints: a roentgen stereophotogrammetric analysis, *Spine* 14(2):162-165, 1989.
21. Neumann DA: *Kinesiology of the musculoskeletal system*, St Louis, 2002, Mosby.
22. Adams MA, Bogduk N, Burton K, et al: *The biomechanics of back pain*, ed 2, Edinburgh, 2006, Churchill Livingstone.
23. Vleeming A, Snijders CJ, Stoeckart R, et al: The role of the sacroiliac joints in coupling between spine, pelvis, legs and arms. In Vleeming A, et al, editors: *Movement, stability and low back pain*, Edinburgh, 1997, Churchill Livingstone.
24. Richardson CA, Snijders CJ, Hides JA, et al: The relation between the transversus abdominis muscles, sacroiliac joint mechanics, and low back pain, *Spine* 27(4):399-405, 2002.
25. Koes BW, van Tulder MW, Oselo R, et al: Clinical guidelines for the management of low back pain in primary care: an international comparison, *Spine* 26(22):2504-2514, 2001.
26. Airaksinen O, Brox JI, Cedrashi C, et al, on behalf of the COST B13 working group on guidelines for chronic low back pain: European guidelines for the management of chronic nonspecific low back pain, *Eur Spine J* 15:192-300, 2006.
27. Brennan GP, Fritz JM, Hunter SJ, et al: Identifying subgroups of patients with acute/subacute "nonspecific" low back pain: results of a randomized clinical trial, *Spine* 31(6):623-631, 2006.
28. Childs J, Fritz J, Flynn T, et al: A clinical prediction rule to identify patients with low back pain most likely to respond to spinal manipulation: a validation study, *Ann Intern Med* 141(12):922-928, 2004.
29. Delitto A, Erhard RE, Bowling RW: A treatment-based classification approach to low back syndrome: identifying and staging patients for conservative treatment, *Phys Ther* 75(6):470-485, 1995.
30. Flynn T, Fritz J, Whitman J, et al: A clinical prediction rule for classifying patients with low back pain who demonstrate short-term improvement with spinal manipulation, *Spine* 27:2835-2843, 2002.
31. Hicks GE, Fritz JM, Delitto A, et al: Preliminary development of a clinical prediction rule for determining which patients with low back pain will respond to a stabilization exercise program, *Arch Phys Med Rehabil* 86:1753-1762, 2005.
32. Fritz JM, Delitto A, Vignovic M, et al: Interrater reliability of judgments of the centralization phenomenon and status change during movement testing in patients with low back pain, *Arch Phys Med Rehabil* 81:57-61, 2000.
33. McKenzie R: *The lumbar spine: mechanical diagnosis and therapy*, Waikanae, New Zealand, 1981, Spinal Publication Ltd.
34. Werneke M, Hart DL: Centralization phenomenon as a prognostic factor for chronic low back pain and disability, *Spine* 26:758-765, 2001.
35. Werneke M, Hart DL: Categorizing patients with occupational low back pain by use of the Quebec Task Force classification system versus pain pattern classification procedures: discriminant and predictive validity, *Phys Ther* 84:243-254, 2004.
36. Long A, Donelson R: Does it matter which exercise? A randomized trial of exercise for low back pain, *Spine* 29:2593-2602, 2004.
37. Waddell G: Clinical assessment of lumbar impairment, *Clin Orthop Related Res* 221:110-120, 1987.

38. Whitman JM, Flynn TW, Childs JD, et al: A comparison between two physical therapy treatment programs for patients with lumbar spinal stenosis, *Spine* 31(22):2541-2549, 2006.

39. Fritz JM, Delitto A, Erhard RE: Comparison of a classification-based approach to physical therapy and therapy based on clinical practice guidelines for patients with acute low back pain: a randomized clinical trial, *Spine* 28:1363-1372, 2003.

40. Bigos S, et al: *Acute low back problems in adults*, Rockville, MD, 1994, Agency for Health Care Policy and Research, Public Health Service, US Department of Health and Human Services.

41. DoD/VA: *Low back pain guidelines*, Falls Church, VA, 1999, DoD/VA. Available at http://www.qmo.amedd.army.mil/lbpfr.htm.

42. ACC and National Health Committee: *New Zealand acute low back pain guide*, Wellington, NZ, 1997, ACC and National Health Committee. Available at http://www.nzgg.org.nz/library/gl_complete/backpain1/index.cfm#contents.

43. Fritz JM, Whitman JM, Flynn TW, et al: Factors related to the inability of individuals with low back pain to improve with a spinal manipulation, *Phys Ther* 84:173-190, 2004.

44. Cleland J, Fritz JM, Whitman JM, et al: The use of a lumbar spine manipulation technique by physical therapists in patients who satisfy a clinical prediction rule: a case series, *JOSPT* 36(4):209-214, 2006.

45. Panjabi MM: The stabilizing system of spine: part II: neutral zone and instability hypothesis, *J Spinal Disorders* 5:390-397, 1992.

46. Panjabi MM, Lydon C, Vasavada A, et al: On the understanding of clinical instability, *Spine* 23:2642-2650, 1994.

47. Oxland TR, Panjabi MM: The onset and progression of spinal injury: a demonstration of neutral zone sensitivity, *J Biomechanics* 25:1165-1172, 1992.

48. Panjabi MM: The stabilizing system of the spine: part I: function, dysfunction, adaptation, and enhancement, *J Spinal Disorders* 5:383-389, 1992.

49. Hohl M: Normal motions in the upper portion of the cervical spine, *J Bone Joint Surg* 46-A(8):1777-1779, 1978.

50. Panjabi MM, Krag MH, Chung TQ: Effects of disc injury on mechanical behavior of the human spine, *Spine* 9:707-713, 1984.

51. White AA III, Johnson RM, Panjabi MM, et al: Biomechanical analysis of clinical instability in the cervical spine, *Clin Orthop Related Res* 109:85-96, 1975.

52. Frymoyer JW, Selby DK: Segmental instability: rationale for treatment, *Spine* 10:280-286, 1985.

53. Ogon M, Bender BR, Hooper DM, et al: A dynamic approach to spinal instability, part I: sensitization of intersegmental motion profiles to motion direction and load condition by instability, *Spine* 22:2841-2858, 1997.

54. Paris SV: *Introduction to spinal evaluation and manipulation*, Atlanta, 1986, Institute Press.

55. Olson KA, Paris SV, Spohr C, et al: Radiographic assessment and reliability study of the craniovertebral sidebending test, *J Manual Manipulative Ther* 6:87-96, 1998.

56. Fritz JM, Erhard RE, Hagen BF: Segmental instability of the lumbar spine, *Phys Ther* 78: 889-896, 1998.

57. Shippel AH, Robinson GK: Radiological and magnetic resonance imaging of cervical spine instability: a case report, *J Manipulative Physiol Ther* 10:317-322, 1987.

58. Twomey LT: A rationale for the treatment of back pain and joint pain by manual therapy, *Phys Ther* 72:885-892, 1992.

59. Olson KA, Joder D: Cervical spine clinical instability: a resident's case report, *J Orthop Sports Phys Ther* 31(4):194-206, 2001.

60. Gonnella C, Paris SV, Kutner M: Reliability in evaluating passive intervertebral motion, *Phys Ther* 62:436-444, 1982.

61. Richardson CA, Jull GA: Muscle control-pain control: what exercises would you prescribe? *Manual Ther* 1:2-10, 1995.

62. Tippets RH, Apfelbaum RI: Anterior fusion with the caspar instrumentation system, *Neurosurgery* 22:1008-1013, 1988.

63. Jull G, Bogduk N, Marsland A: The accuracy of manual diagnosis for cervical zygapophysial joint pain syndromes, *Med J Aust* 148:233-236, 1988.

64. Pope MH, Frymoyer JW, Krag MH: Diagnosing instability, *Clin Orthop Related Res* 279:60-67, 1992.

65. Teyhan DS, Flynn FW, Childs JD, et al: Arthrokinematics in a subgroup of patients likely to benefit from lumbar stabilization exercise program, *Phys Ther* 87(3):313-325, 2007.

66. Herkowitz HN, Rothman RH: Subacute instability of the cervical spine, *Spine* 9:348-357, 1984.

67. Hodges PW, Richardson CA: Inefficient muscular stabilization of the lumbar spine associated with low back pain: a motor control evaluation of transversus abdominis, *Spine* 21:2640-2650, 1996.

68. Moseley GL, Hodges PW, Gandevia SC: Deep and superficial fibers of the lumbar multifidus muscle are differentially active during voluntary arm movements, *Spine* 27(2):E29-E36, 2002.

69. Kjaer P, Bendix T, Sorensen JS, et al: Are MRI-defined fat infiltrations in the mulfidus muscles associated with low back pain? *BMC Med* 5:1-10, 2007.

70. Hides JA, Jull GA, Richardson CA: Long-term effects of specific stabilizing exercises for first-episode low back pain, *Spine* 26(11):E243-E248, 2001.

71. Hodges PW, Richardson CA: Contraction of the abdominal muscles associated with movement of the lower limb, *Phys Ther* 77:132-142, 1997.

72. Hides J, Wilson S, Stanton W, et al: An MRI investigation into the function of the transversus abdominis muscle during "drawing-in" of the abdominal wall, *Spine* 31(6):E175-E178, 2006.

73. O'Sullivan PB, Twomey LT, Allison GT: Evaluation of specific stabilizing exercise in the treatment of chronic low back pain with radiographic diagnosis of spondylolysis or spondylolisthesis, *Spine* 22(24):2959-2967, 1997.

74. Schmidt RA: *Motor control and learning*, ed 2, Champaign, IL, 1988, Human Kinetics Publishers, Inc.

75. Urquhart DM, Hodges PW, Allen TJ, et al: Abdominal muscle recruitment during a range of voluntary exercises, *Manual Ther* 10:144-153, 2005.

76. Donelson R, April C, Medcalf R, et al: A prospective study of centralization of lumbar and referred pain: a predictor of symptomatic discs and annular competence, *Spine* 22(10):1115-1122, 1997.

77. Aina A, May S, Clare H: Systematic review: the centralization phenomenon of spinal symptoms: a systematic review, *Manual Ther* 9:134-143, 2004.

78. Clare HA, Adams R, Maher CG: A systematic review of efficacy of McKenzie therapy for spinal pain, *Aust J Physiother* 50:209-216, 2004.

79. Miller ER, Schenk RJ, Karnes JL, et al: A comparison of the McKenzie approach to a specific spine stabilization program for chronic low back pain, *JMMT* 13(2):103-112, 2005.

80. Riddle DL, Rothstein JM: Intertester reliability of McKenzie's classifications of the syndrome types present in patients with low back pain, *Spine* 18:1333-1344, 1993.

81. Fritz JM, Erhard RE, Delitto A, et al: Preliminary results of the use of a two-stage treadmill test as a clinical diagnostic tool in the differential diagnosis of lumbar spinal stenosis, *J Spinal Disord* 10(5):410-416, 1997.

82. Fritz JM, Erhard RE, Vignovic M: A nonsurgical treatment approach for patients with lumbar spinal stenosis, *Phys Ther* 77(9):962-972, 1997.

83. Saal JA, Saal JS: Nonoperative treatment of herniated lumbar intervertebral disc with radiculopathy an outcome study, *Spine* 14(4):431-436, 1989.

84. Weber H: Lumbar disc herniation: a controlled prospective study with ten years of observation, *Spine* 8:131-140, 1983.

85. Thomas KC, Fisher CG, Boyd M, et al: Outcome evaluation of surgical and nonsurgical management of lumbar disc protrusion causing radiculopathy, *Spine* 12(13):1414-1422, 2007.

86. Saunders HD, Saunders R: *Evaluation, treatment, and prevention of musculoskeletal disorders*, vol 1, Chaska, Minn, 1993, Saunders.

87. Fritz JM, Lindsay W, Matheson JW, et al: Is there a subgroup of patients with low back pain likely to benefit from mechanical traction? Results of a randomized clinical trial and subgrouping analysis, *Spine* 32(26):E793-800, 2007.

88. Van der Heijden GJMG, Beurskens AJHM, Koes BW, et al: The efficacy of traction for back and neck pain: a systematic, blinded review of randomized clinical trail methods, *Phys Ther* 75(2):93-104, 1995.

89. Paris SV: Physical therapy approach to facet, disc, and sacroiliac syndrome of the lumbar spine. In White AH, editor: *Conservative care of low back pain*, Baltimore, 1990, Williams and Wilkins.

90. Creighton DS: Positional distraction: a radiological confirmation, *JMMT* 1(3):83-86, 1993.

91. Ostelo RWJG, deVet CW, Waddell G, et al: *Rehabilitation after lumbar disc surgery*, Oxford, 2002, The Cochrane Library, 4, Update software.

92. Laslett M, Young SB, April CN, et al: Diagnosing painful sacroiliac joints: a validity study of a McKenzie evaluation and sacroiliac provocation tests, *Aust J Physiother* 49:89-97, 2003.

93. Laslett M, Williams M: The reliability of selected pain provocation tests for sacroiliac joint pathology, *Spine* 19:1243-1249, 1994.

94. Lee D: *The pelvic girdle: an approach to the examination and treatment of the lumbopelvic-hip region*, Edinburgh, 2004, Churchill Livingstone.

95. Mens JMA, Vleeming A, Snijders CJ, et al: Reliability and validity of the active straight leg raise test in posterior pelvic pain since pregnancy, *Spine* 26(10):1167-1171, 2001.

96. Potter NA, Rothstein JM: Intertester reliability for selected tests of the sacroiliac joint, *Phys Ther* 65:1671-1975, 1985.

97. Cibulka M, Koldehoff R: Clinical usefulness of a cluster of sacroiliac joint tests in patients with and without low back pain, *J Orthop Sports Phys Ther* 29(2):83-92, 1999.

98. Riddle DL, Freburger JK, NAORRN: Evaluation of the presence of sacroiliac joint region dysfunction using a combination of tests: a multicenter intertester reliability study, *Phys Ther* 82:772-781, 2002.

99. Stuge B, Lacrum E, Kirkesola G, et al: The efficacy of a treatment program focusing on specific stabilizing exercises for pelvic girdle pain after pregnancy: a randomized controlled trial, *Spine* 29(4):351-359, 2004.

100. Hayne CR: Manual transport of loads by women, *Physiotherapy* 67(8):226-231, 1981.

101. O'Sullivan PB, Beales DJ: Diagnosis and classification of pelvic girdle pain disorders: part I: a mechanism based approach within a biopsychosocial framework, *Manual Ther* 12:86-97, 2007.

102. Mens JM, Damen L, Snijders CJ, et al: The mechanical effect of a pelvic belt in patients with pregnancy-related pelvic pain, *Clin Biomech* 21(2):122-127, 2006.

103. Ostgaard HC, Zetherstrom G, Rooos-Hansen E, et al: Reduction of back and posterior pelvic pain in pregnancy, *Spine* 19(8):894-900, 1994.

104. Waddell G: *The back pain revolution*, Edinburgh, 2004, Churchill Livingstone.

105. O'Sullivan P: Classification of lumbopelvic pain disorders: why is it essential for management, *Manual Ther* 11:169-170, 2006.

106. Janda V: *Postural and phasic muscles in the pathogenesis of low back pain*, Dublin, 1968, Proceedings of the XIth Congress ISRD.

107. Goldby LJ, Moore AP, Doust J, et al: A randomized controlled trial investigating the efficiency of musculoskeletal physiotherapy on chronic low back disorder, *Spine* 11(10):1083-1093, 2006.

108. Fritz JM, George SZ, Delitto A: The role of fear-avoidance beliefs in acute low back pain: relationships with current and future disability and work status, *Pain* 94:7-15, 2001.

109. Sieben JM, Vlaeyen JWS, Portegijs PJM, et al: A longitudinal study on the predictive validity of the fear-avoidance model in low back pain, *Pain* 117:162-170, 2005.

110. Fritz JM, George SZ: Identifying specific psychosocial factors in patients with acute, work-related low back pain: the importance of fear-avoidance beliefs, *Phys Ther* 82:973-983, 2002.

111. Waddell G, Newton M, Handerson I, et al: A fear-avoidance beliefs questionnaire (FABQ) and the role of fear-avoidance beliefs in chronic low back pain and disability, *Pain* 52:157-168, 1993.

112. George SZ, Bialosky JE, Fritz JM: Physical therapist management of a patient with acute low back pain and elevated fear-avoidance beliefs, *Phys Ther* 84(6):538-549, 2004.

113. Hicks GE, Fritz JM, Delitto A, et al: Interrater reliability of clinical examination measures for identification of lumbar segmental instability, *Arch Phys Med Rehabil* 84:1858-1864, 2003.

114. Fritz JM, Piva SR, Childs JD: Accuracy of the clinical examination to predict radiographic instability of lumbar spine, *Eur Spine J* 14:743-750, 2005.

115. Reese N, Bandy W: Use of an inclinometer to measure flexibility of the iliotibial band using the Ober test and the Modified Ober test: difference in magnitude and reliability of measurements, *JOSPT* 33:326-330, 2003.

116. Maitland G, Hengeveld E, Banks K, et al: *Maitland's vertebral manipulation*, ed 7, Edinburgh, 2005, Elsevier Butterworth Heinemann.

117. Urban LM: The straight leg raise test: a review, *JOSPT* 2(3):117-133, 1981.

118. Deville W, van der Windt D, Dzaferagic A, et al: The test of Laseque: systematic review of the accuracy in diagnosing herniated discs, *Spine* 25:1140-1147, 2000.

119. Bandy WD, Irion JM, Briggler M: The effect of time and frequency of static stretching on flexibility of the hamstring muscles, *Phys Ther* 77:1090-1096, 1997.

120. Richardson C, Jull G, Hodges P, et al: *Therapeutic exercise for spinal segmental stabilization in low back pain: scientific basis and clinical approach*, Edinburgh, 1999, Churchill Livingstone.

121. Janda V: *Rational therapeutic approach of chronic back pain syndromes*, Turku, Finland, 1985, Proceedings of the Symposium "Chronic Back Pain, Rehabilitation and Self Help."

122. Oh JS, Cynn HS, Won JH, et al: Effects of performing an abdominal drawing-in maneuver during prone hip extension exercises on hip and back extensor muscle activity and amount of anterior pelvic tilt, *JOSPT* 37(6):320-324, 2007.

123. Dreyfuss P, Michaelson M, Pauza M, et al: The value of medical history and physical examination in diagnosing sacroiliac joint pain, *Spine* 21:2594-2602, 1996.

124. Russell A, Maksymowych W, LeClercq S: Clinical examination of the sacroiliac joints: a prospective study, *Arthritis Rheum* 24:1575-1577, 1981.

125. Wang SS, Whitney SL, Burdett RG, et al: Lower extremity muscular flexibility in long distance runners, *JOSPT* 17:102-107, 1993.

126. Bullock-Saxton J, Bullock M: Repeatability of muscle length measures around the hip, *Physiother Can* 46:105-109, 1994.

## CHAPTER 5

# Examination and Treatment of Thoracic Spine Disorders

## CHAPTER OVERVIEW

This chapter covers the kinematics of the thoracic spine and rib cage, describes common thoracic spine disorders, and provides a detailed description of special tests, manual examinations, manipulations, and exercise procedures for the thoracic spine and ribcage.

## OBJECTIVES

- Describe the significance and impact of thoracic spine disorders
- Describe thoracic spine and rib cage biomechanics
- Classify thoracic spine disorders based on signs and symptoms
- Describe interventions for thoracic spine and rib cage disorders
- Demonstrate and interpret thoracic spine examination procedures
- Demonstrate manipulation techniques of the thoracic spine and rib cage
- Instruct exercises for thoracic spine disorders

## SIGNIFICANCE OF THORACIC SPINE DISORDERS

The impact of thoracic spine disorders is not fully appreciated because little research has been completed on these disorders in comparison with cervical and lumbar disorders. Some data do concern chronic conditions that affect the thoracic spine, such as scoliosis and osteoporosis,[1] but little has been published on the impact of acute thoracic spine disorders.

## THORACIC SPINE AND RIB CAGE KINEMATICS: FUNCTIONAL ANATOMY AND MECHANICS

The thorax consists of the thoracic spine, the rib cage, and the sternum. The thorax is a fairly rigid structure whose function is to provide a stable base for muscles to control the craniocervical region and shoulder girdle, to protect internal organs, and to create a mechanical bellows for breathing.[3] The structure consists of 12 thoracic vertebrae and 12 corresponding ribs on each side. A natural thoracic kyphosis is created by a bony slope of 3.8 degrees from posterior to anterior at each vertebral body,

which creates a 45-degree kyphotic angle for the entire thoracic spine.[4]

Anatomically and functionally, the thoracic spine is commonly divided into the upper thoracic (T1-T4), the middle thoracic (T5-T9), and the lower thoracic (T10-T12), with the upper thoracic functioning as a transition zone from the cervical spine to the thoracic spine and the lower thoracic functioning as a transition zone from thoracic spine to lumbar spine.[4] The middle thoracic region is the most rigid because of the rib articulations, with the T11 and T12 vertebraes being more mobile because of the lack of complete anterior rib attachment with the "floating ribs" at T11 and T12.[4] The upper thoracic region moves with the cervical spine and with similar mechanics to the cervical spine.

The facet joints of the thoracic vertebrae are generally in the frontal plane with a mild slope that varies between 0 and 30 degrees from the vertical.[3] The spinous processes of the thoracic vertebrae tend to angle downward and extend to the level of the caudal vertebrae's transverse processes. In identification of the vertebral level through palpation, the transverse processes can be found lateral to the most prominent aspect of the spinous process of the vertebra one level above.[5] This trend is consistent throughout the upper and middle thoracic spine but is less consistent at lower thoracic levels (especially T11 and T12).[5]

The costotransverse and costovertebral joints allow movement of the ribs in relation to the spine and function during ventilation. The costovertebral joints connect the heads of each of the 12 ribs to the corresponding sides of the bodies of the thoracic vertebrae. The costotransverse joints connect the articular tubercles of the ribs 1 to 10 to the transverse processes of the corresponding thoracic vertebrae. Ribs 11 and 12 usually lack costotransverse joints.[3] The sternocostal joints provide a functional link of the ribs from the sternum to the thoracic spine (Figure 5-1).

The costovertebral joints connect the head of the rib with a pair of costal facets at adjacent vertebral bodies and the adjacent margin of the intervertebral disc. The articular surfaces of the costovertebral joints are slightly ovoid and held together by capsular and radiate ligaments.[3] Costotransverse joints connect the articular tubercle of a rib to the costal facet on the transverse process of a corresponding thoracic vertebra. An articular capsule surrounds this synovial joint, and the costotransverse ligament firmly anchors the neck of the rib to the entire length of a corresponding transverse process.[3]

Approximately 30 to 40 degrees of forward bending and 20 to 25 degrees of backward bending are available throughout the thoracic region.[3] The magnitude of forward and backward bending tends to increase in a cranial to caudal direction.[3] The kinematics of forward bending occur with a superior and slightly anterior sliding (i.e., upglide) of the inferior facet surfaces of the superior member of the vertebral segment moving on the superior facet surfaces of the lower member of the vertebral segment (Figure 5-2). Backward bending occurs with just the opposite movements: inferior and slightly posterior sliding (i.e., downglide) of the inferior facet surfaces of the superior member of the vertebral segment moving on the superior facet surfaces of the lower member of the vertebral segment (Figure 5-3).

Approximately 30 degrees of axial rotation occur to each side throughout the thoracic region.[3] Rotation occurs in the mid-thoracic spine as the frontal plane–aligned inferior articular facets of the superior member of the spinal segment slide a short distance in relation to the superior facets of the inferior member of the vertebral segment.[3] The amount of axial rotation tends to decrease from the upper to lower thoracic spine because the greater vertically oriented facet joints tend to block the horizontal plane movement (Figure 5-4).[3]

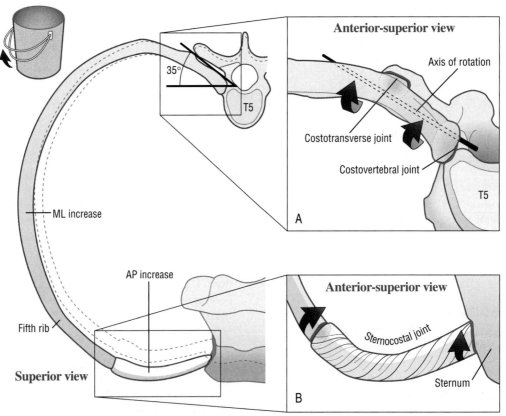

**FIGURE 5-1** Top view of fifth rib shows "bucket-handle" mechanism of elevation of the ribs during inspiration. *Ghosted* outline of the rib indicates its position before inspiration. Elevation of the rib increases both anterior-posterior (AP) and medial-lateral (ML) diameters of thorax. Rib connects to vertebral column via costotransverse and costovertebral joints *(A)* and to sternum via the sternocostal joint *(B)*. During elevation, neck of the rib moves about an axis of rotation that courses between each costotransverse and costovertebral joint. Elevating rib creates torsion in the cartilage associated with sternocostal joint. From Neumann DA: *Kinesiology of the musculoskeletal system*, St Louis, 2002, Mosby.

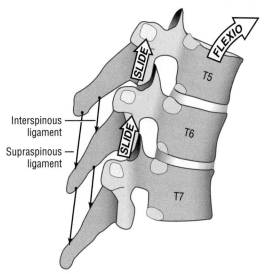

**FIGURE 5-2** Kinematics at thoracic region. Kinematics of thoracolumbar flexion are shown through 85-degree arc: sum of 35 degrees of thoracic flexion and 50 degrees of lumbar flexion. From Neumann DA: *Kinesiology of the musculoskeletal system*, St Louis, 2002, Mosby.

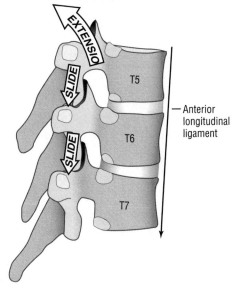

**FIGURE 5-3** Kinematics at thoracic region. Kinematics of thoracolumbar extension are shown through arc of 35 to 40 degrees: 20 to 25 degrees of thoracic extension and 15 degrees of lumbar extension. From Neumann DA: *Kinesiology of the musculoskeletal system*, St Louis, 2002, Mosby.

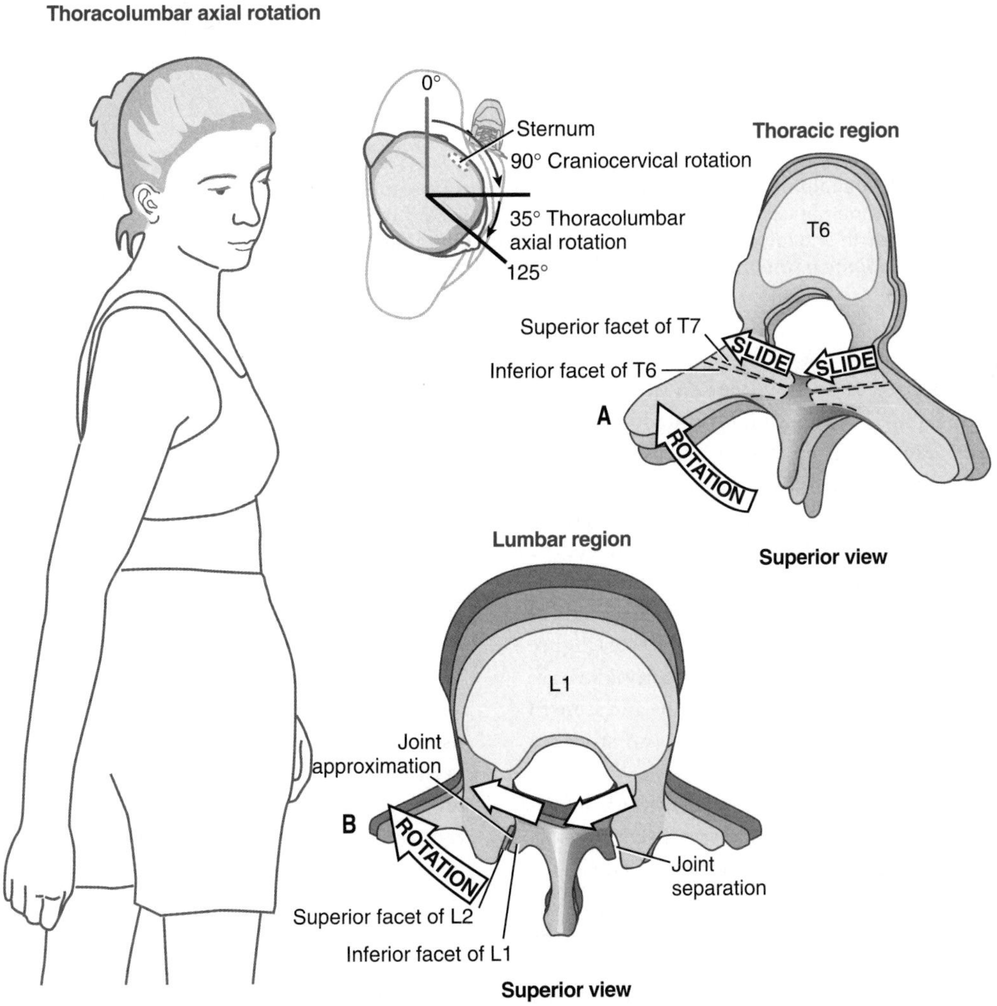

**FIGURE 5-4** Kinematics of thoracolumbar axial rotation are depicted as the subject rotates her face 125 degrees to the right. The thoracolumbar axial rotation is shown through a 35-degree arc: the sum of 30 degrees of thoracic rotation and 5 degrees of lumbar rotation. **A**, Kinematics at the thoracic region. **B**, Kinematics at the lumbar region. From Neumann DA: *Kinesiology of the musculoskeletal system*, St Louis, 2002, Mosby.

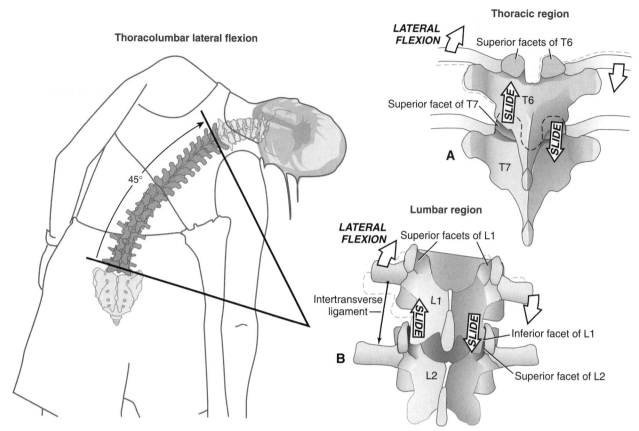

**Thoracolumbar lateral flexion**

**Thoracic region**

**FIGURE 5-5** Kinematics of thoracolumbar lateral flexion are shown through approximate 45-degree arc: sum of 25 degrees of thoracic lateral flexion. **A,** Kinematics at thoracic region. **B,** Kinematics at lumbar region. Note slight contralateral coupling pattern between axial rotation and lateral flexion in lumbar region. Elongated and taut tissue is indicated by *thin black arrow.* From Neumann DA: *Kinesiology of the musculoskeletal system,* St Louis, 2002, Mosby.

Approximately 25 degrees of lateral flexion occur to each side in the thoracic region.[3] The motion is limited by the ribs and remains fairly constant from one segment to another throughout the thorax. Lateral flexion occurs as the inferior facet surface of the superior member of the spinal segment slides superiorly (i.e., upglide) on the opposite direction of the lateral flexion and inferiorly (i.e., downglide) on the same side of the lateral flexion. The ribs drop slightly on the same side of the lateral flexion and rise slightly on the opposite side (Figure 5-5). Coupling patterns for lateral flexion and rotation are inconsistent in the middle and lower thoracic spine and seem to vary from individual to individual and from one study to another.[3,6]

The thorax changes shape during ventilation with movement at five articulations: the manubriosternal, sternocostal, interchondral, costotransverse, and costovertebral joints. During inspiration, the shaft of the ribs elevate in a path perpendicular to the axis of the rotation that courses between the costotransverse and costovertebral joints. The downward-sloped shaft of the ribs rotates upward and outward, increasing the intrathoracic volume in both anterior posterior and medial lateral diameters.[3] During expiration, the muscles of inspiration relax to allow the ribs and sternum to return to their pre-

inspiration positions. The lowering of the body of the ribs combined with the inferior and posterior movements of the sternum decreases the anterior-posterior and medial-lateral diameters of the thorax.[3]

## DIAGNOSIS, CLASSIFICATION, AND MANAGEMENT OF DISORDERS

Thoracic spine pain conditions are commonly caused by mechanical musculoskeletal impairments of the joints and soft tissues. An impairment-based classification system has not been fully developed and validated, and in general, little research is found on the effectiveness of commonly used interventions for thoracic spine pain.[7] The potential causes of thoracic spine pain include referral from other structures, such as the cervical spine; visceral issues; fractures from osteoporosis; and mechanical musculoskeletal issues. Table 5-1 outlines a classification for potential causes of acute thoracic pain.

A number of serious medical conditions can be the source of acute thoracic pain. Table 5-2 provides an outline of the conditions that must be screened before initiation of treatment of the thoracic spine. Appropriate referrals for further medical

| TABLE 5-1 | Classification of Causes of Acute Thoracic Pain |
|---|---|
| **PAINFUL CONDITIONS OF THORACIC SPINE** | |
| Serious conditions | Infection, fracture, neoplastic disorders, inflammatory disorders, disc protrusion |
| Mechanical conditions | Discogenic pain; zygapophyseal joint pain; rib dysfunctions: costotransverse and costovertebral joint pain, muscle imbalances and myofascial pain, postural deviations |
| **CONDITIONS REFERRING PAIN TO THORACIC SPINE** | |
| Somatic conditions | Disorders of cervical facet joints, muscles, and intervertebral discs |
| Visceral conditions | Myocardial ischemia, dissecting thoracic aortic aneurysm, peptic ulcer; acute cholecystitis; pancreatitis; renal colic; acute pyelonephritis |

Adapted from National Health and Medical Research Council: Acute thoracic spinal pain. In *Australian acute musculoskeletal pain guidelines: evidence-based management of acute musculoskeletal pain*, Brisbane, 2003, Australian Academic Press.

| TABLE 5-2 | Alerting Features (Red Flags) of Serious Conditions Associated with Acute Thoracic Spinal Pain | |
|---|---|---|
| **FEATURE OR RISK FACTOR** | | **CONDITION** |
| Minor trauma (if >50 y of age, history of osteoporosis and corticosteroid use) | | Fracture |
| Major trauma in younger population | | Fracture |
| Fever<br>Night sweats<br>Risk factors of infection (e.g., underlying disease process, penetrating wound, tuberculosis) | | Infection |
| History of malignant disease<br>Age >50 y<br>No improvement with treatment<br>Unexplained weight loss<br>Pain at multiple sites<br>Pain at rest<br>Night pain | | Tumor |
| Chest pain or heaviness<br>No effect on pain with movement/change in posture<br>Abdominal pain<br>Shortness of breath, cough | | Other serious conditions |

Adapted from National Health and Medical Research Council: Acute thoracic spinal pain. In *Australian acute musculoskeletal pain guidelines: evidence-based management of acute musculoskeletal pain*, Brisbane, 2003, Australian Academic Press.

diagnostic testing should be made if these features or risk factors are identified in patients with acute thoracic spinal pain. After a screening for red flags associated with these serious conditions, an impairment-based approach is used to address impairments noted in the examination (Table 5-3).

The cervical spine must be screened as a possible source of referral pain to the thoracic spine. Experimental studies in healthy volunteers and in patients have shown that pain from structures in the cervical spine can be referred into the upper thoracic spinal region. Referred pain into the upper thoracic spine region can arise from the lower cervical facet joints,[8-10] the cervical muscles,[11] or the cervical intervertebral discs.[12] Cervical screening examination testing should include active range-of-motion (AROM) testing, Spurling's test, cervical distraction test, palpation, and passive intervertebral joint motion (PIVM) testing.[13] If upper extremity symptoms are reported, upper limb neurodynamic (ULND) testing should also be carried out.[13] Chapter 6 provides a detailed description of these examination procedures.

## Osteoporosis

Osteoporosis is a condition associated with loss of bone density that is most common in women after menopause and that can result in vertebral fractures and excessive thoracic kyphotic deformity. The prevalence rate of vertebral fractures associated with osteoporosis dramatically increases in women aged 65 years and older,[14] with a 6.5% prevalence rate in those 50 to 59 years of age and a 77.8% prevalence rate in those older than 90 years of age.[15] The most common sites of vertebral fractures are at the T7, T8, T11, and L1 vertebra.[15] A triggering event for an osteoporotic fracture is often not present. In a hospital-based case series of 30 patients with acute thoracolumbar vertebral compression fractures, 46% of cases were classified as spontaneous, 36% were associated with a trivial strain, and 18% were

associated with moderate or severe injury.[16] The severity of vertebral deformity has been correlated with more severe back pain and disability. Women with deformities of more than 4 standard deviations (SDs) below the mean had a 1.9 times higher risk of moderate to severe back pain and a 2.6 times higher risk of disability involving the back.[17]

An estimated 30% of postmenopausal white women in the United States have osteoporosis, and 1 in 4 has at least one vertebral deformity; but two thirds of vertebral factures remain undiagnosed.[1] In a group of 3000 American white women aged 65 to 70 years, two thirds reported back pain during the previous 12 months.[2] At least one vertebral deformity was found in 60% of these women, and 24% had deformities 3 SDs or more below the mean.[2] After a clinically diagnosed vertebral fracture, survival rate decreases gradually from the rate expected without fracture.[1] Women with severe vertebral deformities have a consistently higher risk of back pain and height loss.[1] The clinical impact of a single vertebral fracture may be minimal, but the effects of multiple fractures are cumulative and often result in acute and chronic back pain, limitation of physical activity, and progressive kyphosis and height loss. Depression and low self-esteem accompany the loss of functional abilities and the inability to take part in recreational activities. Pain and fear of additional fractures cause decreased physical activity, which in turn exacerbates osteoporosis and increases the risk of fracture.[1]

Osteoporosis is considered a contraindication to thrust manipulation techniques to the thoracic spine and rib cage,

**TABLE 5-3** Impairment-Based Classification for Thoracic Spine Pain Disorders

| CLASSIFICATION | EXAMINATION FINDINGS | PROPOSED INTERVENTIONS |
|---|---|---|
| Thoracic hypomobility | Restricted AROM<br>Restricted PIVM testing in thoracic spine and ribs<br>No UE radicular symptoms<br>Muscle imbalances<br>Postural deviations | Mobility exercises<br>Thoracic<br>spine and rib mobilization/manipulation<br>Self-mobilization techniques<br>Postural exercises |
| Thoracic hypomobility with upper extremity referred pain | Restricted AROM<br>Restricted PIVM testing in upper thoracic spine and ribs<br>UE symptoms<br>Positive ULND test results<br>Muscle imbalances<br>Postural deviations | Mobility exercises<br>Thoracic and rib mobilization/manipulation<br>ULND mobilization/exercise<br>Self-mobilization techniques<br>Postural exercises |
| Thoracic hypomobility with neck pain | Symptoms <30 d<br>No symptoms distal to shoulder<br>No aggravation of symptoms with looking up<br>FABQPA score <12<br>Diminished upper thoracic spine kyphosis (visual estimate)<br>Cervical extension ROM <30 degrees (inclinometer) | Thoracic and rib mobilization/manipulation<br>Mobility exercises<br>Self-mobilization techniques<br>Postural exercises<br>Treatment of cervical impairments |
| Thoracic hypomobility with shoulder impairments | Stiff thoracic spine with shoulder AROM<br>Restricted PIVM testing in upper thoracic spine and ribs<br>Shoulder impingement/rotator cuff signs<br>Muscle imbalances<br>Postural deviations | Mobility exercises<br>Thoracic and rib mobilization/manipulation<br>Self-mobilization techniques<br>Postural exercises<br>Rotator cuff exercises |
| Thoracic hypomobility with low back pain | Stiff thoracic spine with thoracolumbar AROM<br>Restricted PIVM testing<br>Lumbar impairments<br>Muscle imbalances<br>Postural deviations | Mobility exercises<br>Thoracic and rib mobilization/manipulation<br>Lumbar rehabilitation program<br>Self-mobilization techniques<br>Postural exercises |
| Thoracic clinical instability | History of trauma or thoracic surgery<br>Provocation of symptoms with sustained weight-bearing posture<br>Relief of symptoms with non–weight-bearing postures<br>Hypermobility with loose end feel with PIVM testing<br>Poor strength (2/5) of thoracic multifidus, erector spinae, and parascapular muscles<br>Shaking/poorly controlled (aberrant) motion with thoracic active range of motion | Postural education<br>Thoracic stabilization exercise program<br>Parascapular exercises<br>Mobilization/manipulation above and below hypermobilities<br>Ergonomic correction |

*UE,* Upper extremity; *ROM,* range of motion; *ULND,* upper limb neurodynamic test.

especially techniques performed in the prone or supine position. Manual therapy techniques performed to the thoracic spine in the prone position for all patients should be performed with a pillow placed under the thorax as a precaution to cushion the ribs during posterior-to-anterior force application. Gentle nonthrust manual therapy techniques performed to the thorax with the patient in the side-lying position are generally safe for patients with osteoporosis and can be effective in restoring mobility and inhibiting muscle tone and pain in the region. In addition, the sitting thoracic techniques can be performed safely because these techniques involve more lifting distraction forces rather than compressive loading of the vertebra and ribs. Therefore, osteoporosis is a precaution for the nonthrust techniques performed in side-lying and sitting positions, but

osteoporosis is a contraindication for thrust manipulation techniques performed in prone and supine positions.

The physical therapy intervention that can be of greatest assistance for patients with osteoporosis is a program of guided progression of weight-bearing and resistive exercises.[18] Posture, strength, balance, endurance, and bone density can also improve with an exercise program guided by a physical therapist.[18] Results can ultimately prevent falls and fractures, which limits the potential for pain and disability associated with osteoporosis.

## Thoracic Hypomobility

The thoracic spine is by design a fairly rigid structure. With postural stresses and in response to stresses, strains, and injury, regions of the thoracic spine tend to further stiffen and be a source of mechanical pain and stiffness symptoms. No systematic reviews of treatment for thoracic spinal pain are found, and little published research exists on the effectiveness of the most commonly used treatments for thoracic spine pain.[7] Only one randomized controlled trial (RCT) on the effectiveness of manual physical therapy treatment of the thoracic spine could be identified.[19] Schiller[19] compared the use of spinal manipulation with nonfunctional ultrasound placebo in an RCT of 30 patients with mechanical thoracic spinal pain. The group who received manipulation showed significantly better reductions in numeric pain ratings and improvements in lateral flexion at the end of a 2-week to 3-week treatment period.[19] These changes were maintained 1 month later, but results were no longer better than in the placebo group.[19] Oswestry scores and McGill Pain Questionnaire results were the same for both groups throughout the study.[19] Because of the small sample size, it is difficult to draw conclusions from this study. However, some evidence does seem to show that at least short-term pain relief and improvement in mobility can be provided with the use of thoracic spine manipulation.

Once regions of thoracic stiffness are noted with AROM and PIVM testing, further differentiation can be attempted to isolate facet joint versus costotransverse/costovertebral joint hypomobility. Most commonly, both the rib and the thoracic spine PIVM test results show stiffness at the affected spinal segments. Overlying muscle holding is also commonly associated with this condition, as are postural deviations, such as excessive thoracic kyphosis. Muscle imbalances, such as weakness of the parascapular muscles (lower trapezius/middle trapezius) and tightness of the pectoral muscles, are commonly found with an increased thoracic kyphosis and forward head posture.

Pain associated with rib dysfunction is commonly provoked with deep breathing and spring testing the rib as the thoracic vertebra is stabilized. The location of the pain associated with a rib dysfunction is often slightly lateral to the thoracic vertebrae, and symptoms may be referred laterally along the length of the rib angle.

The manual physical therapy approach starts with manipulation to improve thoracic mobility and is followed up with instruction in mobility, self-mobilization, and postural exercises. Once thoracic segmental restrictions are improved, rib techniques can be used to further restore mobility to the region. Case report evidence has shown that nonthrust manipulation to the thoracic spine can decrease tenderness to palpation of the thoracic erector spinae musculature and the associated intercostals spaces of the ribs at the level of the manipulation, increase thoracic side-bending active range of motion, and improve chest expansion that had been limited by pain before the manipulation treatment.[20]

Box 5-1 illustrates self-mobilization and mobility exercises, and Box 5-2 illustrates postural exercises that address common muscle imbalances found with thoracic hypomobility. Thoracic spine PIVM testing for rib and thoracic segmental restrictions and joint manipulation techniques for the ribs and thoracic spine are presented in detail later in this chapter.

## Upper Thoracic Hypomobility with Upper Extremity Referred Pain

Upper thoracic hypomobility with upper extremity referred pain is commonly called T4 syndrome. T4 syndrome is a classification of thoracic spine disorders that involve upper extremity paraesthesia and pain with or without symptoms into the neck or head.[21] This condition is associated with limited upper thoracic mobility, most commonly peak stiffness at T3-T4 or T4-T5 spinal segments and positive upper limb neurodynamic (ULND 1) testing.[22] After manipulation (thrust or nonthrust) of the restricted segment, the upper extremity symptoms subside and an immediate improvement in ULND test results is noted, with improved mobility and reduced upper extremity symptoms.[22] The addition of postural and thoracic mobility exercises can further facilitate recovery (see Boxes 5-1 and 5-2).

The mechanism for the immediate effect of thoracic manipulation on upper extremity symptoms is not completely understood. Speculation exists that upper thoracic manipulation may influence the autonomic nervous system in a therapeutic manner based on the anatomic location of the sympathetic nerve fibers that leave the spinal nerve from levels T1-L2 to join the sympathetic chain via the white rami communicantes. These then travel within the sympathetic chain from up to six segments before synapsing on four to 20 postganglionic neurons.[22] The postganglionic neurons exit via the grey rami communicantes to join a peripheral nerve that is distributed to target tissues.[23] One preganglionic neuron synapses with numerous postganglionic neurons in the sympathetic chain; therefore, it interacts with somatic nerve fibers that supply a variety of target tissues.[22] The head and neck are supplied by levels T1-T4, and the upper trunk and upper limb by T1-T9.[24] Postulation is that dysfunction of the sympathetic nervous system from T4 could result in referred pain in the head, neck, upper thoracic, and upper limbs.

Evans[23] suggests that the joint itself may not be the causative factor but that sustained or extreme postures may lead to relative ischemia in tissues. The sympathetic nerves also form a vasoconstriction network on all arterioles and capillaries that are stimulated in the presence of ischemia. The manipulation techniques are believed to activate descending inhibitory pain pathways,[25] resulting in a hypoalgesic effect. A close relationship is found between pain reduction and sympathetic excitation,[26,27] which supports the role of spinal manipulation as a treatment option for the T4 syndrome. The effectiveness of manipulation for T4 syndrome has only been supported by case report evidence[22,23]; more extensive RCTs are needed to support the use of manipulation and exercise for this condition.

## Thoracic Hypomobility with Neck Pain

Thrust manipulation techniques directed to the thoracic spine have also been shown as an effective means to provide

**BOX 5-1**    Self-Mobilization and Mobility Exercises for the Thoracic Spine

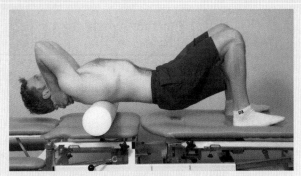

Self soft tissue mobilization of thoracic spine with foam roll. Patient can bridge and glide across foam roll for 1 to 2 minutes as self soft tissue mobilization technique.

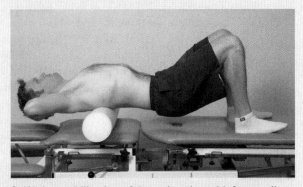

Self joint mobilization of thoracic spine with foam roll. Once patient identifies stiff tender region with initial rolling procedure, sustained pressure can be placed on restricted region and patient can extend with the foam roll focused at targeted stiff region of thorax to attempt to self mobilize the region. Targeted force can be combined with deep breathing. Sustained stretches of 20 to 30 seconds can be applied to two to three targeted areas of stiffness. This technique works best for segments T3-T4 to T7-T8.

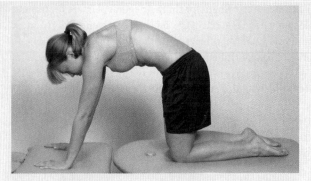

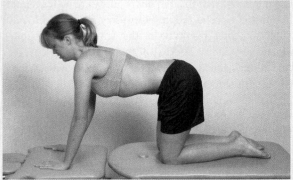

Cat back exercise: arching thoracolumbar spine into flexion/extension positions while in all-fours position can assist in maintaining thoracic spine mobility.

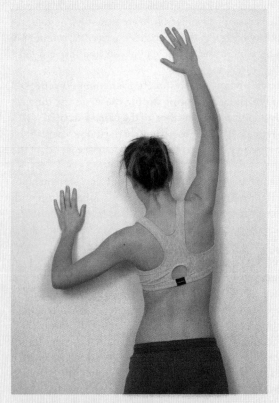

Wall dance exercise. Patient alternately reaches up and across with each arm in attempt to fully elongate and stretch lateral thoracic. This exercise facilitates side bending of thorax.

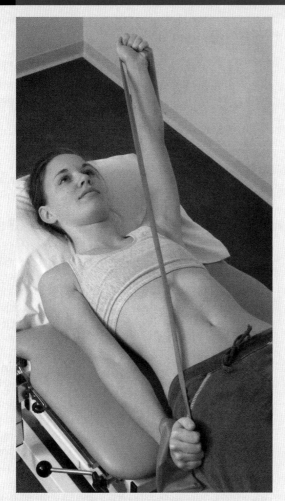

Supine theraband D2 shoulder flexion. This exercise targets lower trapezius muscle.

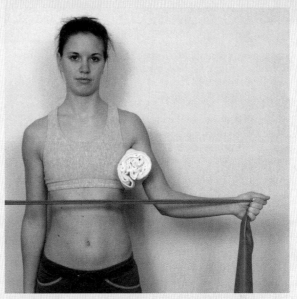

Standing theraband shoulder external rotation. This exercise targets strengthening of the lateral rotators of rotator cuff and scapular stabilizer muscles.

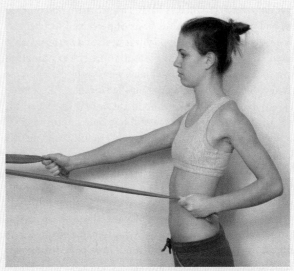

Reciprocal shoulder girdle retraction. Reciprocal motion used with this exercise facilitates thoracic spine rotation motions and at the same time targets strengthening parascapular and thoracic multifidus muscles.

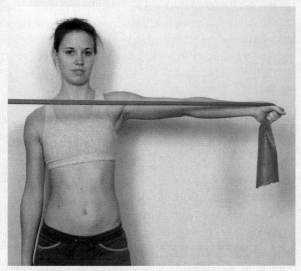

Standing theraband shoulder horizontal abduction. This exercise targets middle trapezius muscle and posterior rotator cuff muscles.

**BOX 5-3**   The Six Variables That Form the Clinical Prediction Rule for Thoracic Manipulation for Treatment of Neck Pain

- Symptoms <30 days
- No symptoms distal to the shoulder
- No aggravation of symptoms with looking up
- FABQPA score <12
- Diminished upper thoracic spine kyphosis (visual estimate)
- Cervical extension range of motion <30 degrees (inclinometer)

Data from Cleland JA, Childs JD, Fritz JM, et al: *Phys Ther* 87(1):9-23, 2007.

immediate relief of neck pain.[28] Cleland[28] developed a clinical prediction rule (CPR) for identification of patients with neck pain who would most likely benefit from thoracic spine thrust manipulation to relieve neck pain. The CPR was developed on a group of 78 patients with neck pain who all received thrust manipulation to the upper and mid thoracic spine. The thoracic spine segments that were regarded as stiff from a clinical examination were targeted for manipulation by the physical therapist. The patients were classified as having a successful outcome on the second or third visit on the basis of perceived recovery. A stepwise logistic regression model was used to determine what common characteristics from the initial patient examination findings predicted a successful outcome with the thoracic manipulation. Six variables were identified for the CPR. If three of six variables (positive likelihood ratio, 5.5) were present (Box 5-3), the chance of a successful outcome improved from 54% to 86%.[28] Further research is ongoing to fully validate this CPR with an RCT.

When a patient with neck pain has signs and symptoms that fit the CPR for thoracic manipulation, thoracic thrust manipulation is indicated at the targeted stiff upper and mid thoracic segments. Additional interventions to treat the neck are dependent on which additional signs and symptoms are identified. A classification system for management of neck pain disorders is outlined in great detail in Chapter 6.

## Thoracic Hypomobility with Shoulder Impairments

Thoracic spine extension and variable amounts of thoracic rotation and lateral flexion are necessary to fully complete unilateral shoulder flexion and abduction movements.[29,30] Crawford and Jull[31] used an inclinometer to measure thoracic motion on 60 women during bilateral shoulder elevation and reported that bilateral shoulder elevation induces 13 to 15 degrees thoracic extension and that a large thoracic kyphosis is associated with reduced arm elevation in older adults.

Loss of upper and mid thoracic mobility is postulated to lead to increased strain and impingement placed on the rotator cuff, especially at the end range of shoulder motions, that may lead to impingement syndrome, tendonitis, and tears of the rotator cuff. Therefore, thoracic mobility should be visually inspected during shoulder AROM testing; if limited mobility is noted with shoulder movements, further examination of the thoracic spine is warranted and should include PIVM testing of the thoracic spinal segments and ribs. If shoulder flexion AROM provokes pain at the end of range, the shoulder girdle should be manually positioned and held into a more retracted position as AROM is retested. If this procedure improves the degree of pain-free AROM, a postural component to the shoulder pain condition is suspected. To improve posture and enhance full shoulder complex flexion/abduction motions, good mobility of the thorax is necessary.

Thoracic hypomobility restrictions should be treated with thoracic manipulation (thrust and nonthrust) techniques. If thoracic and rib restrictions are still evident after the thoracic manipulation, rib manipulation techniques should be used. These techniques can be followed up with postural correction training, thoracic self-mobilization and mobility exercises, and exercises to address muscle imbalances across the shoulder girdle complex (see Boxes 5-1 and 5-2). In addition, a shoulder rehabilitation program designed to address the specific impairments noted at the shoulder, such as rotator cuff muscle strengthening, should be initiated.

## Thoracic Hypomobility with Low Back Pain

Although little has been written on this condition in the low back pain literature, thoracic hypomobility is commonly associated with many low back pain conditions. From a biomechanical impairment-based model, the stiffness in the thoracic spine places increased mechanical loading on the lumbar spine. The stiffness may be caused by muscle holding of the erector spinae muscles that originate in the mid and lower thoracic spine and connect into the thoracolumbar fascia. As these global back muscles guard to protect the painful low back condition or to compensate for weak deep local muscles of the lumbar spine, the thoracic spine tends to stiffen. Therefore, thoracic manipulation can provide reflexive relaxation of these muscles and also reduce mechanical strain on the lumbar spine once the mobility improves.[32] Some hypoalgesic effect may also be seen from manipulation of segments superior to the primary pain symptom.

Therefore, evaluation and treatment of impairments noted in the thoracic spine in patients with lumbar spine conditions is advisable as an adjunct to addressing the primary impairments at the lumbar spine. Further research is needed to further validate this clinical recommendation.

## Thoracic Clinical Instability

Although this condition is thought to be less common than hypomobility disorders of the thoracic spine, clinical instability of the thoracic spine may occur in one or more of the following situations: with systemic hypermobility; with severe postural deviations, such as excessive kyphosis and thoracic scoliosis; after trauma, such as a motor vehicle accident; or after thoracic surgery, such as thoracotomy or thoracic laminectomy. Thoracic laminectomy has been shown on cadavers to increase segmental range of motion by 22% to 30%.[33] Clinical signs and symptoms are similar to instability in other regions of the spine and include achiness with sustained upright postures, relief of pain with recumbent positions, aberrant movements with AROM, and hypermobility noted with PIVM testing. Strength deficits may also be noted with testing the thoracic erector spinae and multifidus and the middle and lower trapezius muscles. Lee[34] describes a mid-thoracic rotation instability syndrome characterized by a "fixation" of the mid-thoracic segment that presents with hypermobility after the fixation is corrected with a manipulation.

Treatment for thoracic clinical instability includes postural education and training, thoracic and parascapular muscle strengthening exercises, mobilization/manipulation techniques for segmental restrictions noted above and below the hypermobile spinal region, and ergonomic corrections at home and work to attempt to reduce the strain associated with a kyphotic thoracic spine posture.

Examination of the thoracic spine starts with structural and postural examination followed by AROM testing of the cervical and thoracolumbar spine as described in Chapter 2. Shoulder screening is also an important component of the thoracic examination for determination of the presence of upper extremity signs/symptoms that could be a contributing or perpetuating factor in the thoracic spine disorder. In addition, primary shoulder impairments may have a thoracic spine hypomobility component that needs to be addressed as part of the plan of care.

## INSPECTION OF THORACIC MOBILITY WITH SHOULDER ELEVATION ACTIVE RANGE-OF-MOTION TESTING

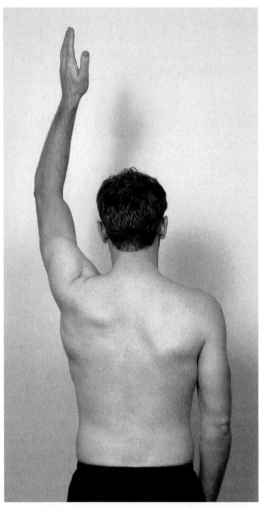

Visual inspection for thoracic extension, lateral flexion, and rotation as patient actively forward flexes shoulder. Compare left versus right to judge for limitations and asymmetries in thoracic motion.

Muscle strength of the parascapular muscles should be tested because weakness of these muscles may be a component of thoracic and shoulder postural deviations (Box 5-4).

Few special tests are described specifically for diagnosis of thoracic spine disorders. The primary objective of the manual portion of the thoracic examination is determination of regions of hypomobility, irritability, tenderness, or instability through the thoracic spine and rib cage. This determination is best done with palpation for tissue condition and PIVM testing.

**BOX 5-4** Parascapular Manual Muscle Tests*

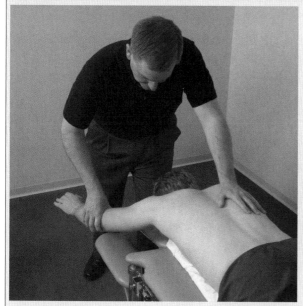

Lower trapezius muscle isometric manual muscle test.

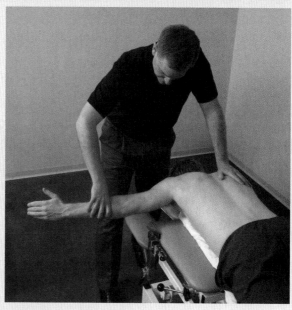

Middle trapezius muscle isometric manual muscle test.

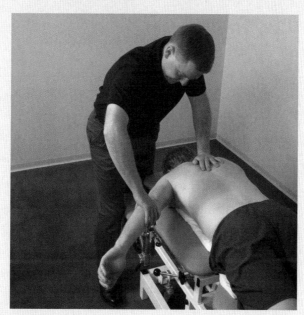

Latissimus dorsi muscle isometric manual muscle test.

*Should be completed as part of the thoracic spine examination.

# THORACIC SPINE PASSIVE INTERVERTEBRAL MOTION TESTING

## Upper Thoracic Forward-Bending Passive Intervertebral Motion Test

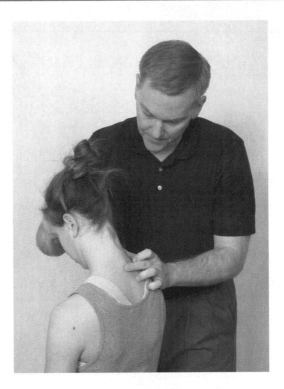

| | |
|---|---|
| **PURPOSE** | This test is used to evaluate the passive forward-bending motion of the thoracic segments C7-T1 through T3-T4. |
| **PATIENT POSITION** | The patient sits with the arms supported on two pillows in the lap. |
| **THERAPIST POSITION** | The therapist stands to the side and slightly behind the patient. |
| **HAND PLACEMENT** | (In reference to the photograph.) |
| | **Right hand:** The right hand supports the patient's forehead. |
| | **Left hand:** The pad of the long finger is used to palpate the interspinous space of the targeted segment. |
| **PROCEDURE** | The pad of the long finger on the left hand is used to palpate the interspinous space of the C7-T1 segment. The right hand is used to passively forward bend the patient's head and neck. The therapist palpates for the C7-T1 interspinous space to expand with forward bending by palpating the relative amount of movement of the superior spinous process of the spinal segment in relation to the inferior member of the segment. The amount of passive forward bending available at the segment is noted. The procedure is repeated one segment at a time with palpation of the interspinous spaces of segments T1-T2 through T3-T4. The amount of passive forward bending available at each segment is compared. |
| **NOTES** | The assessment should begin at C7-T1 and proceed caudally, allowing for easy location of the specified segments with a start at C7, which tends to have a prominent spinous process. The amount of forward bending of the head and neck is increased as the assessment proceeds caudally. However, the head and neck are moved with small oscillations to avoid excessive movement of the patient's neck, which may be painful with large passive movements. Christensen et al[35] reported an intrarater agreement with a Kappa value of 0.60 and an interrater agreement with a Kappa value of 0.22 for a sitting upper thoracic PIVM technique performed by a group of chiropractors. |

## Upper Thoracic Rotation Passive Intervertebral Motion Test (DVD)

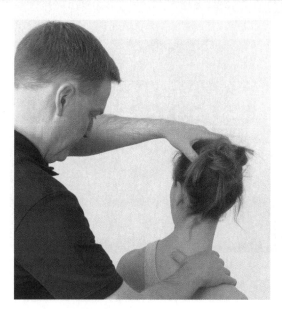

| | |
|---|---|
| **PURPOSE** | The purpose of this test is to evaluate the passive rotation of thoracic segments C7-T1 through T3-T4. |
| **PATIENT POSITION** | The patient sits on a chair or treatment table with the arms resting on two pillows in the lap. |
| **THERAPIST POSITION** | The therapist stands or kneels behind the patient. |
| **HAND PLACEMENT** | (In reference to the picture.) |
| | **Left hand:** The left hand gently grasps the top of the patient's head for left rotation (the right hand is on top of the patient's head for right rotation). |
| | **Right hand:** The pad of the thumb is used to palpate the lateral aspect of the specified segment, and the fingers rest on the patient's shoulder girdle. |
| **PROCEDURE** | The pad of the thumb on the right hand is used to palpate the right lateral aspect of the interspinous space of the C7-T1 segment. Left rotation is induced with the left hand passively rotating the patient's head to the left. The therapist palpates for the spinous process of the superior member of the segment to press into the palpating thumb in relation to the inferior member of the segments spinous process. The amount of passive rotation available at the segment is noted. The procedure is repeated with palpation of the right lateral aspect of interspinous space for segments T1-T2 through T3-T4. The hand placements are reversed, and the procedure is repeated, with rotation of the patient's head to the right. The amount of passive right rotation available at each segment is noted, and the amount of passive rotation available in each direction is compared. |
| **NOTES** | The assessment should begin at C7-T1 and proceed caudally, which allows for easy location of the specified segments with a start at C7. The amount of rotation of the head and neck is increased as the assessment proceeds caudally. However, the therapist should try to move the head and neck as little as possible during the performance of this technique because the patients often have neck pain. During the performance of this technique, the therapist stands directly behind the patient to clearly observe and palpate the motion. If the cervical spine is hypermobile, positioning the cervical spine in a partially forward-bent position can take up tissue slack; then the rotation should occur within the new plane created by the forward-bent position of the neck. |

## Central Posterior-to-Anterior Passive Accessory Intervertebral Motion Test: Backward Bending

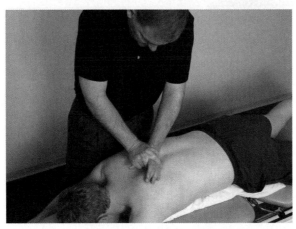

Central PA PAIVM test: two-handed technique.

| | |
|---|---|
| **PURPOSE** | This test is used for passive accessory motion and pain provocation of the thoracic spinal segments. For intervention, one should use the appropriate grade of movement (I to IV) for treatment of pain or hypomobility. |
| **PATIENT POSITION** | The patient lies prone with a pillow under the thorax and with the arms by the body or hanging off the edge of the table. Another pillow can be placed under the lower legs for comfort. |
| **THERAPIST POSITION** | The therapist stands at the side of the patient. |
| **HAND PLACEMENT** | **Left hand:** The left hand is placed on the patient's back so that the ulnar border of the hand just distal to the pisiform is in contact with the spinous process of the vertebrae to be tested. The shoulders are directly over the patient. The wrist is fully extended with the forearm midway between supination/pronation. |
| | **Right hand:** The left hand is reinforced with the right hand so that the second and third digits of the right hand envelop the second metacarpal phalangeal joint of the left hand. The elbows are allowed to slightly flex. |
| **PROCEDURE** | The therapist applies a posterior-to-anterior (PA) force on each spinous process being examined for a total of three slow repetitions. The first pressures should be applied gently; amplitude and depth of the movement is increased if no pain response occurs. The therapist assesses the quality of movement through the range and the end feel and compares it to the levels above and below. |
| **NOTES** | A mid range of movement thrust (spring test) could also be used with this technique for assessment of tissue resistance and pain provocation. A positive response is movement that reproduces the comparable sign (pain or resistance or muscle guarding). The technique assesses for both joint mobility and reactivity. The direction of motion is a direct posterior-to-anterior force that produces a relative backward-bending motion of the targeted vertebra in relation to the vertebra below. Christensen et al[35] reported intrarater reliability with a Kappa value of 0.68 and interrater reliability with a Kappa value of 0.24 for prone passive accessory intervertebral movement (PAIVM) testing; and for agreement in palpation of tenderness over the facet joint, the intrarater reliability was a Kappa value of 0.94 and the interrater reliability was a Kappa value of 0.70. |

## Central Posterior-to-Anterior Passive Accessory Intervertebral Motion Test: Backward Bending—cont'd

**ALTERNATIVE TECHNIQUE**

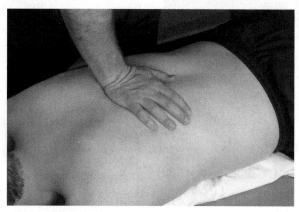

Central PA PAIVM test: one-handed technique commonly used for spring testing.

This technique could also be done as a one-handed technique with the cranial hand contacting the spinous process just distal to the pisiform, the elbow flexed, and the forearm perpendicular with the angle of the contour of the surface of the spine. The caudal hand rests at the edge of the table to support the therapist's upper body weight as the therapist leans over the patient. Application of force could be done as a gradual PA force or a midrange spring test.

## Posterior-Anterior Forward-Bending (Transverse Processes of the Same Vertebra) Passive Accessory Intervertebral Motion Test

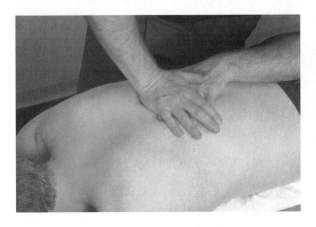

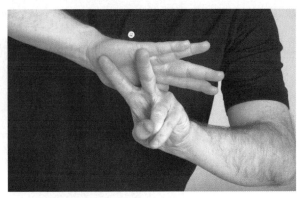

Dummy finger position in relation to manipulative hand for PAIVM test: PA transverse processes of same vertebra.

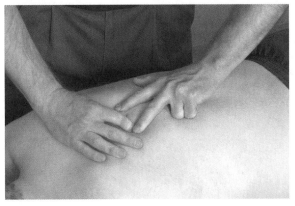

Use of cranial hand to loosely pinch spinous process to find targeted transverse processes for PAIVM test: PA transverse processes of same vertebra.

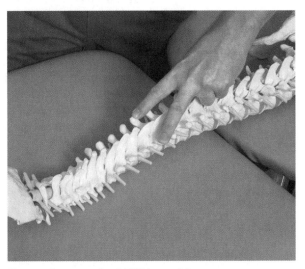

Finger placement for PAIVM test: PA transverse processes of same vertebra.

| | |
|---|---|
| **PURPOSE** | This test assesses passive forward-bending motion and the level of reactivity of thoracic segments T3-T4 through T11-T12. |
| **PATIENT POSITION** | The patient lies prone with a pillow under the chest/trunk. |
| **THERAPIST POSITION** | The therapist stands next to the patient with a diagonal stance. |
| **HAND PLACEMENT** | **Caudal hand:** The second and third digits are used as "dummy" fingers, with the pads of the second and third fingers placed on the transverse processes of the specified vertebra. |
| | **Cranial hand:** The palmar aspect of the fifth metacarpal is placed over the dummy fingers. |
| **PROCEDURE** | The index finger and thumb of the cranial hand gently pinches the lateral edges of the spinous process of T2. The second and third digits of the caudal hand are placed just lateral to the thumb and index finger of the cranial hand, respectively. This position places the dummy fingers over the transverse processes of T3. The volar aspect of the fifth metacarpal |

## Posterior-Anterior Forward-Bending (Transverse Processes of the Same Vertebra) Passive Accessory Intervertebral Motion Test—cont'd

of the cranial hand is placed over the dummy fingers, and the cranial hand takes up the slack (to the joint's mid range) and gives an impulse. The amount of passive forward bending available at the T3-T4 segment and pain provocation are noted. Another variation of this procedure is to gently ease the segment into an end range position to sense the amount of resistance to the passive movement and pain provocation. The procedure is repeated at the transverse processes of T3 through T11 (segments T3-T4 through T11-T12). The amount of passive forward bending available at each segment is compared.

**NOTES**   This technique can be performed by starting at T3 and proceeding caudally, which allows for easy location of the thoracic vertebrae (by counting down from C7). The forearm of the arm that gives the impulse should be perpendicular to the angle of the contour of the spine being examined. One should note that the transverse processes usually are not palpable, but the dummy fingers should feel a firmness when taking up the slack. Also the transverse processes of one thoracic vertebra are located lateral to the spinous process of the superior vertebra.[5] A positive pain provocation test may indicate reactivity of the facet joints and surrounding soft tissues.

**ALTERNATIVE TWO-HANDED TECHNIQUE**

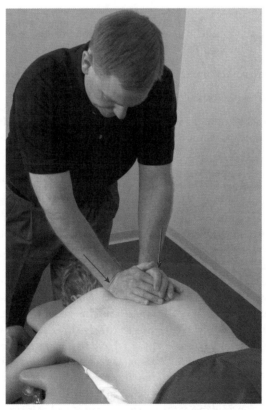

PAIVM test: PA transverse processes of same vertebra.

With the patient lying prone over a pillow, the therapist can stand over the head of the table and position both hypothenar eminences at the transverse processes of the same vertebral. As the therapist keeps both elbows straight, a gradual application of PA pressure can be applied to the targeted thoracic vertebra to assess PAIVM at each thoracic spinal segment.

## Posterior-to-Anterior Rotation (Transverse Processes of Adjacent Vertebrae) Passive Accessory Intervertebral Motion Test

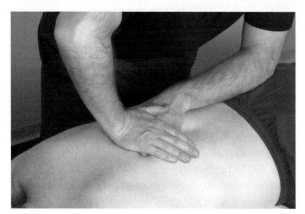

PAIVM test: PA transverse processes of adjacent vertebrae for left rotation.

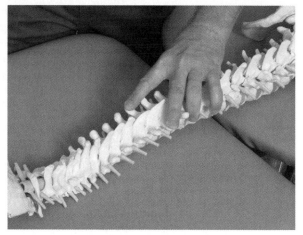

PAIVM test: PA transverse processes of adjacent vertebrae for left rotation finger placement.

| | |
|---|---|
| **PURPOSE** | This test is used to assess the passive rotation and level of reactivity of thoracic segments T3-T4 through T11-T12. |
| **PATIENT POSITION** | The patient is prone with a pillow under the chest/trunk. |
| **THERAPIST POSITION** | The therapist stands with a diagonal stance next to the patient. |
| **HAND PLACEMENT** | **Caudal hand:** The second and third digits are used as dummy fingers, and the pads of the second and third digits are placed on the transverse processes of the specified adjacent vertebrae. |
| | **Cranial hand:** The volar aspect of the fifth metacarpal is placed over the dummy fingers. |
| **PROCEDURE** | The therapist stands on the patient's right side and places the second digit of the caudal hand approximately a finger's width to the right side of the spinous process of T4, which positions the finger over the right transverse process of T5. The third digit of the caudal hand is placed approximately a finger's width to the left side of the spinous process of T5, which positions the third digit over the left transverse process of T6. The therapist places the volar aspect of the fifth metacarpal of the cranial hand over the pads of the dummy fingers and induces left rotation by using the cranial hand to take up the slack (to the joint's mid range) and give an impulse. Another variation is gradual, repeated moving of the segment into an end range position to sense the resistance to movement. The amount of passive rotation available at the targeted segment and pain provocation are noted. Right rotation is tested with placement of the cranial dummy finger on the left transverse process of T5 and the caudal dummy finger on the right transverse process of T6. The cranial hand takes up the slack (to the joint's mid range) and gives an impulse. The amount of passive rotation available at the targeted segment and pain provocation are noted. The procedure is repeated at the appropriate transverse processes of T3-T4 through T11-T12, and the amount of passive rotation available in each direction is compared. |
| **NOTES** | This technique can be performed with starting at T3 and proceeding caudally, which allows for easy location of the thoracic vertebrae (by counting down from C7). The forearm of the arm that gives the impulse should be perpendicular to the angle of the contour of the region of the spine being assessed. This technique follows the *rule of the lower finger:* |

## Posterior-to-Anterior Rotation (Transverse Processes of Adjacent Vertebrae) Passive Accessory Intervertebral Motion Test—cont'd

"the direction of the rotation of the spinal segment is the same as the side of the lower finger" (e.g., if the lower finger is on the right side, right rotation is being induced). The transverse processes usually are not palpable, but the dummy fingers should feel firmness when taking up the slack and the transverse processes of one thoracic vertebra are located lateral to the spinous process of the superior vertebra. Both mobility and pain provocation are tested with this assessment.

**ALTERNATIVE TWO-HANDED TECHNIQUE**

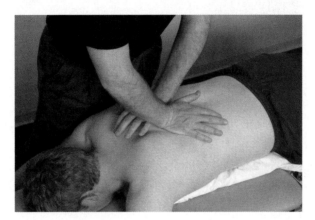

With the patient in a prone-lying position over a pillow, the therapist contacts the adjacent transverse processes of the targeted spinal segment with the hypothenar eminences of each hand. PA force can be applied equally and gradually with both hands or a mid range spring can be applied to assess the PAIVM for thoracic rotation of the targeted segment. It is advisable for students to master the "dummy finger" method before attempting this alternative two-handed technique, because the two-handed technique requires more advanced palpation skills to perform safely and effectively.

# RIB PASSIVE ACCESSORY MOTION TESTS AND MANIPULATION TECHNIQUES

## Rib Posterior-Anterior Accessory Motion Test

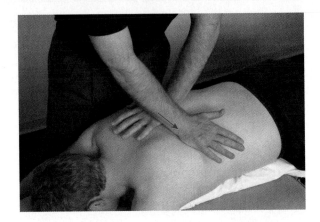

| | |
|---|---|
| **PURPOSE** | This test assesses the mobility and level of reactivity of the costotransverse and costovertebral joints of the targeted rib. If hypomobility is noted, the forces can be modified to convert this technique to a manipulation. |
| **PATIENT POSITION** | The patient is prone with a pillow under the chest/trunk. |
| **THERAPIST POSITION** | The therapist stands with a diagonal stance next to the patient on the opposite side of the targeted rib. |
| **HAND PLACEMENT** | **Caudal hand:** Hypothenar eminence is placed on the opposite transverse process of the corresponding vertebra. |
| | **Cranial hand:** The arm crosses over the top of the caudal hand to place the hypothenar eminence at the posterior rib angle of the targeted rib. |
| **PROCEDURE** | As the therapist sustains a firm stabilizing pressure on the transverse process with the caudal hand, the cranial hand applies a PA force to the rib. Either a mid-range thrust (i.e., spring) force or a gradually intensified PA force can be used. The amount of passive rib mobility available at the targeted segment and pain provocation are noted. The procedure is repeated from the third to the twelfth rib, and left versus right is compared. |
| **NOTES** | If pain is provoked with this procedure, but not with PA PAIVM tests of the thoracic spine, the more irritable joints at the involved segment are likely the rib joints (costotransverse and costovertebral). If pain is provoked with both the thoracic vertebra PAIVM and the rib accessory motion tests, the irritable joints could be either rib or vertebral facet joints or both. This technique can be converted to a mobilization/manipulation technique by varying the depth and frequency of the oscillations. |

## Rib Forward Rotation Passive Motion Test and Manipulation

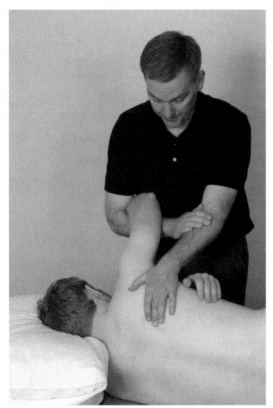

Rib forward rotation passive mobility assessment for middle ribs.

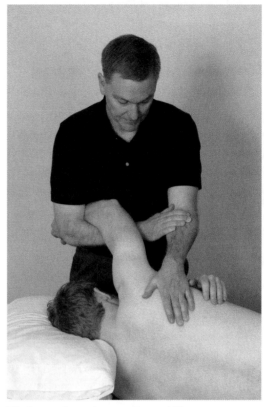

Rib forward rotation passive mobility assessment for lower ribs.

| | |
|---|---|
| **PURPOSE** | This test is used to assess the mobility of the ribs and surrounding soft tissues. If hypomobility is noted, the forces can be modified to convert this technique to a manipulation. |
| **PATIENT POSITION** | The patient is in a side-lying position facing the therapist, with the side to be tested on top. |
| **THERAPIST POSITION** | The therapist stands with a diagonal stance facing the patient. |
| **HAND PLACEMENT** | **Caudal hand:** The pads of the second and third digits contact the posterior angle of the targeted rib. |
| | **Cranial hand:** The therapist hooks the patient's top arm with the forearm and holds the forearm of the caudal arm. |
| **PROCEDURE** | As the targeted rib is contacted, the therapist shifts weight posteriorly to move the patient's top arm/shoulder girdle complex forward and pulls the targeted rib forward to assess the ability of the rib to rotate forward. |
| **NOTES** | This technique can easily be converted to a rib mobilization technique with holding and pulling the targeted stiff rib into an anterior rotation direction. As lower ribs are targeted, the therapist should progressively flex the patient's top arm and shift the body cranially to maintain the therapist's body in the direction of the manipulative force. |

## Rib Bucket-Handle Passive Motion Test and Manipulation

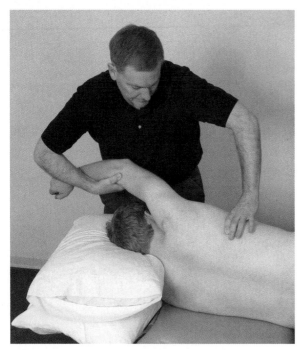

Rib bucket-handle passive motion assessment.

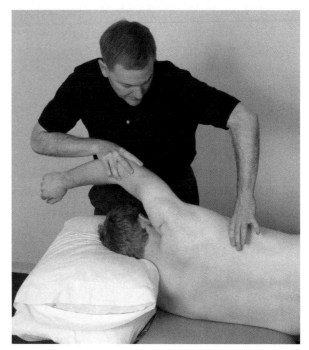

Rib bucket-handle technique converted to isometric manipulation of targeted rib.

| | |
|---|---|
| **PURPOSE** | This test is used to assess the mobility of the ribs and surrounding soft tissues in a bucket-handle motion direction. If hypomobility is noted, the forces can be modified to convert this technique to a manipulation. |
| **PATIENT POSITION** | The patient is in a side-lying position facing the therapist, with the side to be tested on top. |
| **THERAPIST POSITION** | The therapist stands with a diagonal stance facing the patient. |
| **HAND PLACEMENT** | **Caudal hand:** The radial aspect of the index finger is placed between the targeted ribs to be tested.<br><br>**Cranial hand:** This hand holds the patient's top arm above the elbow. |
| **PROCEDURE** | As the therapist palpates the space between the targeted ribs, the patient's shoulder is abducted into end range and overpressure is applied to induce lateral flexion of the thorax to the targeted segment. The therapist attempts to palpate the bucket-handle motion of the superior rib in relation to the adjacent inferior rib. |
| **NOTES** | This technique can be easily converted to a rib mobilization technique with holding the inferior of the rib pairs and applying overpressure either through the rib or through the arm. This technique can be converted to an isometric manipulation (see the figure above right) with resisting the patient's shoulder into adduction as firm pressure is applied to the lower member of the rib pair. The isometric muscle action theoretically pulls the superior rib of the pair superiorly and applies a stretch to the joints and soft tissues of the targeted rib pair. After a 10-second isometric hold, further passive stretch is applied for 10 seconds. This sequence is repeated three to four times. |

## Rib Exhalation Passive Accessory Motion Test and Manipulation    DVD

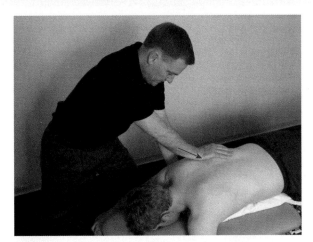

Rib exhalation passive accessory motion test.

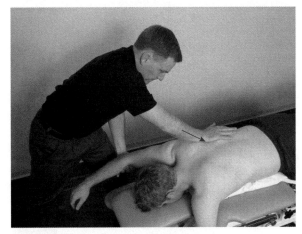

Rib exhalation manipulation with use of upper extremity to provide added leverage.

| | |
|---|---|
| **PURPOSE** | The test assesses the mobility and level of reactivity of the costotransverse and constovertebral joints of the targeted rib. If hypomobility is noted, the forces can be modified to convert this technique to a manipulation. |
| **PATIENT POSITION** | The patient is prone with a pillow under the chest/trunk and the arm off the side of the table or supported by the armrest on a mobilization table. |
| **THERAPIST POSITION** | The therapist stands with a diagonal stance at the side of the head of the patient on the same side of the targeted rib. |
| **HAND PLACEMENT** | **Caudal hand:** This hand supports the therapist's own body weight with positioning of the hand along the side of the treatment table. |
| | **Cranial hand:** The hypothenar eminence is placed at the superior aspect of the posterior rib angle of the targeted rib. |
| **PROCEDURE** | The therapist gradually applies force in an inferior and anterior direction to move the posterior rib angle in an inferior direction. Either a mid-range thrust (i.e., spring) force or a gradually intensified force can be used. The amount of passive rib mobility available at the targeted segment and pain provocation are noted. The procedure is repeated from the third to the twelfth rib and left versus right is compared. |
| **NOTES** | If pain is provoked with this procedure, but not with PA PAIVM tests of the thoracic spine, the more irritable joints at the involved segment are likely rib joints (costotransverse and costovertebral). If pain is provoked with both the thoracic vertebra PAIVM and the rib accessory motion tests, the irritable joints could be either rib or vertebral facet joints or both. This technique can be converted to a mobilization technique by varying the depth and frequency of oscillations. The arm of the side being mobilized can be used to improve the mechanical advantage of the manipulation technique (see the figure above right). The therapist can lift the same side arm into end-range forward flexion to assist in taking up the tissue slack above the rib level to be manipulated. Once this position is attained, an isometric shoulder extension force can be resisted as the exhalation rib force is held at the targeted rib. The isometric force can be held 10 seconds and followed by a 10-second stretch with the hand on the rib. This sequence can be repeated for three to four cycles. Caution should be used in forcing the shoulder to end range of motion if the patient has any signs of shoulder impingement, instability, or pain. |

# SCAPULOTHORACIC SOFT TISSUE TECHNIQUES

## Scapular Passive Mobility Assessment and Mobilization

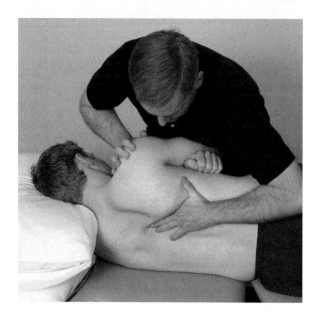

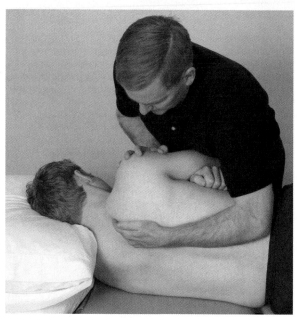

Parascapular soft tissue mobilization, bordering the scapula.

| | |
|---|---|
| **PURPOSE** | The purpose of this test is to assess and treat muscular and connective tissue restrictions of the parascapular tissues. |
| **PATIENT POSITION** | The patient is in a side-lying position facing the therapist, with the targeted scapula on top. |
| **THERAPIST POSITION** | The therapist stands in front of the patient very close to edge of the table. |
| **HAND PLACEMENT** | **Caudal hand:** The web space is positioned at the edge of the inferior angle of the scapula. |
| | **Cranial hand:** The hand is placed across the anterior aspect of the patient's shoulder. |
| **PROCEDURE** | The therapist gradually applies an anterior-to-posterior force of the shoulder girdle complex with the cranial hand as the caudal hand presses anterior and superior to slide the hand under the inferior angle of the scapula. Once the caudle hand is positioned under the inferior angle of the scapula, the pads of the fingers and thumb can be pressed into the thorax to lift the anterior aspect of the scapula away from the thorax with the dorsal aspect of the caudal hand. |
| **NOTES** | If restricted soft tissue mobility or muscle guarding is noted, soft tissue mobilization techniques such as the "bordering the scapula" technique shown in the figure to the right above may be needed before performance of this technique to allow further mobilization of the scapular tissues. The "bordering the scapula" soft tissue mobilization technique is performed by rhythmically gliding the caudal hand along the medial border of the scapula as the cranial hand presses the shoulder girdle into a retracted position. The soft tissue mobilization is repeated multiple times until the muscle tone in the region begins to relax. |

## Pectoralis Minor Muscle Length Test and Stretch

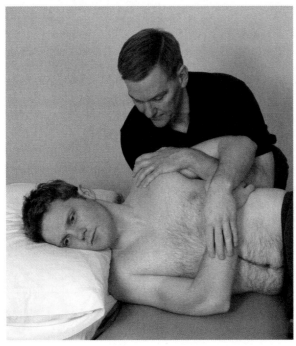

Pectoralis minor muscle length test and stretch.

| | |
|---|---|
| **PURPOSE** | The test assesses and treats muscle length restrictions of the pectoralis minor muscle. |
| **PATIENT POSITION** | The patient is side lying and facing away from the therapist, with the targeted pectoralis minor muscle on top. |
| **THERAPIST POSITION** | The therapist stands behind the patient very close to edge of the table. |
| **HAND PLACEMENT** | **Caudal hand:** The forearm is placed under the patient's top arm, and the hand is positioned at the anterior aspect of the shoulder. |
| | **Cranial hand:** The hand is placed on the posterior aspect of the scapula. |
| **PROCEDURE** | The therapist gradually applies a posterior force with the caudal hand and creates a force couple with the cranial hand to move the scapula into retraction. |
| **NOTES** | Normal muscle length of the pectoralis minor muscle should allow full passive shoulder girdle retraction motion with this passive motion test. If restricted soft tissue mobility or muscle guarding is noted, soft tissue mobilization techniques may be needed to allow further mobilization of the pectoralis tissues with this technique. A hold-relax stretch technique can be used to stretch the pectoralis minor muscle by asking the patient to press the shoulder forward into protraction as the therapist resists for a 10-second hold. This technique is followed by a 10-second stretch into further retraction. The sequence is repeated three to four times. |

# THORACIC SPINE MANIPULATION

## Central Posterior-to-Anterior (Backward-Bending) Manipulation in Prone

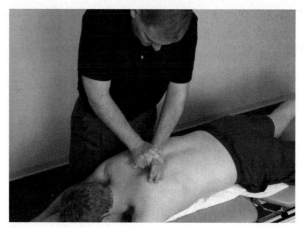

Central PA backward-bending manipulation: two-handed technique.

| | |
|---|---|
| **PURPOSE** | The purpose of this technique is to manipulate a specific thoracic segment (T3-T4 though T12-L1) into backward bending. |
| **PATIENT POSITION** | The patient lies prone with a pillow under the thorax with the arms along the side of the body, hanging off the edge of the table, or supported on the arm rests of the mobilization table. A pillow can be placed under the lower legs for comfort. |
| **THERAPIST POSITION** | The therapist stands at the side of the patient. |
| **HAND PLACEMENT** | **Left hand:** This hand is placed on the patient's back so that the ulnar border of the hand just distal to the pisiform is in contact with the spinous process of the vertebrae to be mobilized. The shoulders are directly over the patient. The left wrist is fully extended with the forearm midway between supination/pronation. |
| | **Right hand:** The left hand is reinforced with the right hand so that the second and third digits of the right hand envelop the second metacarpal phalangeal joint of the left hand. The elbows are allowed to slightly flex. |
| **PROCEDURE** | The therapist takes up the slack and induces posterior to anterior force at the specified segment. The manipulation is coordinated with the patient's breathing, with progressive oscillation into slightly more backward bending with each oscillation. The procedure is repeated through approximately three breathing cycles. On completion of the manipulation, posterior to anterior PAIVM is retested. The depth and frequency of the forces can be modified to perform graded oscillations I to IV or a thrust manipulation with this technique. |
| **NOTES** | Indication for use of this manipulation technique is decreased backward bending (central PA PAIVM motion) at a specific thoracic segment (T3-T4 through T12-L1) or pain provocation with PAIVM motion testing. The force should be perpendicular to the angle of the contour of the region of the spine being manipulated. |

## Central Posterior-to-Anterior (Backward-Bending) Manipulation in Prone—cont'd

**ALTERNATIVE TECHNIQUE**

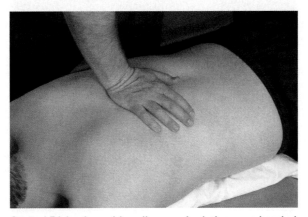

Central PA backward-bending manipulation: one-handed technique.

This technique could also be done as a one-handed technique with the cranial hand contacting the spinous process with the hypothenar eminence, the elbow flexed, and the forearm perpendicular with the angle of the contour of the surface of the spine. The caudal hand rests at the edge of the table to support the therapist's upper body weight as the therapist leans over the patient.

## Thoracic Posterior-Anterior Forward-Bending Manipulation in Prone

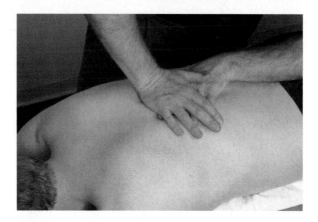

| | |
|---|---|
| **PURPOSE** | This technique is used to manipulate a specific thoracic segment (T3-T4 though T12-L1) into forward bending. |
| **PATIENT POSITION** | The patient is prone with a pillow under the chest/trunk. |
| **THERAPIST POSITION** | The therapist stands with a diagonal stance next to the patient. |
| **HAND PLACEMENT** | **Caudal hand:** The second and third digits are used as dummy fingers, with the pads of the second and third fingers placed on the transverse processes of the specified vertebra. |
| | **Cranial hand:** The palmar aspect of the fifth metacarpal is placed over the dummy fingers. |
| **PROCEDURE** | The manipulation is coordinated with the patient's breathing, with progressive oscillation into slightly more forward bending each repetition. As the patient inhales, the therapist holds against the expansion of the thorax. As the patient exhales, more force is applied to take up the tissue slack and mobilize the spinal segment. The procedure is repeated through approximately three breathing cycles. On completion of the manipulation, forward bending is retested. This manipulation can be used for segments T4-T5 through T11-T12. The depth and frequency of the forces can be modified to perform graded oscillations I to IV or a thrust manipulation with this technique. |
| **NOTES** | Indication for use of this technique is decreased forward bending of a specific thoracic segment (T3-T4 through T12-L1). The forearm of the arm that applies the force should be perpendicular to the surface contour of the region of the spine to be manipulated. The transverse processes usually are not palpable, but the dummy fingers should feel a firmness as the fingers sink into the tissue. Also, the transverse processes of one thoracic vertebra are located lateral to the spinous process of the superior vertebra. |

## Thoracic Posterior-Anterior Forward-Bending Manipulation in Prone—cont'd

**ALTERNATIVE TWO-HANDED TECHNIQUE**

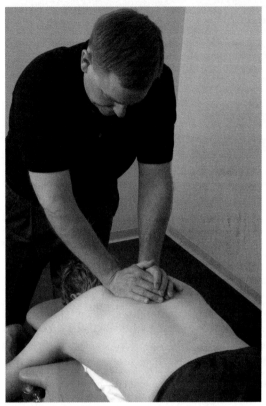

PA forward-bending manipulation: alternative two-handed technique.

With the patient lying prone over a pillow, the therapist can stand at the head of the table and position both hypothenar eminences at the transverse processes of the same vertebra. As the therapist keeps both elbows straight, a gradual application of PA pressure can be applied to the targeted thoracic vertebra with a force that is perpendicular to the contour of the spine being manipulated. The depth and frequency of the forces can be modified to perform graded oscillations I to IV or a thrust manipulation with this technique. This technique can also be used as a PAIVM test.

## Thoracic Rotation Manipulation in Prone

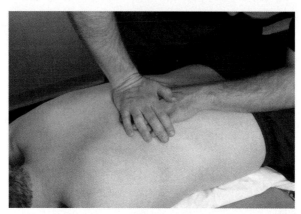

Thoracic rotation manipulation in prone for right rotation.

| | |
|---|---|
| **PURPOSE** | This technique is used to manipulate a specific thoracic segment (T3-T4 though T12-L1) into rotation. |
| **PATIENT POSITION** | The patient is prone with a pillow under the chest/trunk. |
| **THERAPIST POSITION** | The therapist stands with a diagonal stance next to the patient. |
| **HAND PLACEMENT** | **Caudal hand:** The second and third digits are used as dummy fingers, and the pads of the second and third digits are placed on the transverse processes of specified adjacent vertebrae. |
| | **Cranial hand:** The volar aspect of the fifth metacarpal is placed over the dummy fingers. |
| **PROCEDURE** | The cranial hand is used to take up the slack and oscillate the T3-T4 segment. The manipulation is coordinated with the patient's breathing, with progressive oscillation into deeper posterior-anterior pressure and creation of slightly more rotation with each oscillation. As the patient inhales, the therapist holds down the force against the rising thorax; as the patient exhales, the force is deepened further. The procedure is repeated through approximately three breathing cycles. On completion of the manipulation, rotation is retested. A thrust manipulation can also be used at mid range for PIVM testing or end range for treatment effects. Use of a progressive oscillation first is advisable to attain an end range position before application of the thrust manipulation. |
| **NOTES** | The indication for use of this technique is decreased rotation of a specific thoracic segment (T3-T4 through T12-L1). The forearm of the arm that applies the force should be perpendicular to the contour surface of the region of the spine being treated. The transverse processes usually are not palpable, but the dummy fingers should feel a firmness as the fingers sink into the soft tissue. Also, the transverse processes of one thoracic vertebra are located lateral to the spinous process of the superior vertebra. This technique follows the *rule of the lower finger*, which states that the direction of the rotation is the same as the side of the lower finger (e.g., if the lower finger is on the right side, right rotation is being induced). |

## Thoracic Rotation Manipulation in Prone—cont'd

**ALTERNATIVE TWO-HANDED TECHNIQUE**

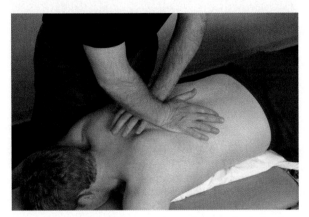

Posterior-anterior two-handed rotation manipulation in prone for left rotation.

With the patient in prone-lying position over a pillow, the therapist contacts the adjacent transverse processes of the targeted spinal segment with the hypothenar eminences of each hand. The therapist is positioned with elbows extended and shoulders placed directly over the targeted segment. PA force can be applied, and the depth and frequency of the forces can be modified to perform a progressive oscillation, graded oscillations II or III, or a thrust manipulation with this technique. Often helpful is combination of the manipulation with the patient's breathing cycle with application of PA force against the chest expansion and further force applied as the breath is released. Osteoporosis is a contraindication for this technique and all manipulation techniques performed in the prone position.

## Thoracic Side-Bending Manipulation in Prone    DVD

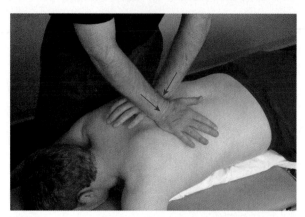

Thoracic posterior-anterior two-handed side-bending manipulation in prone for left side bending.

| | |
|---|---|
| **PURPOSE** | The technique is used to manipulate a specific thoracic segment (T3-T4 though T11-T12) into side-bending (lateral flexion) direction. |
| **PATIENT POSITION** | The patient is prone with a pillow under the patient's chest. |
| **THERAPIST POSITION** | The therapist stands with a diagonal athletic stance next to the patient. |
| **HAND PLACEMENT** | **Caudal hand:** The hand contacts the transverse process of the vertebra with the hypothenar eminence. |
| | **Cranial hand:** This hand contacts the opposite side transverse process of the same vertebrae with the hypothenar eminence and with the arms crossed. |
| **PROCEDURE** | The therapist takes up the tissue slack with a PA force to reach a barrier. Once PA force slack is taken up, the hands are rotated in a clockwise direction to twist the skin for the purpose of taking up more tissue slack to reach a firm barrier. The cranial hand is directed into a caudal direction and the caudal hand is directed into a cranial direction to create a side-bending/gliding force. The body weight of the shoulders/thorax is shifted into a downward direction to add a thrust. The therapist should consider combining the technique with breathing to first create a progressive oscillation before providing the thrust. |
| **NOTES** | Osteoporosis is a contraindication. Most of the force is into an anterior-to-posterior direction at the targeted vertebra. Because of the natural angle of the forearms in this position, frontal plane cranial- and caudal-directed forces create a slight side-bending motion at the targeted spinal segment. |

## Rib Posterior-Anterior Manipulation in Supine

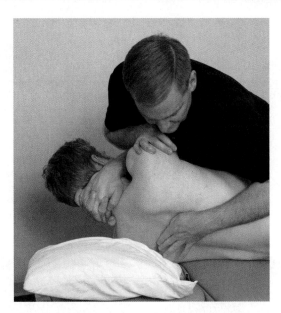

The supine thoracic manipulation technique can be modified to manipulate a rib by placing the thumb on the posterior aspect of the rib just lateral to the transverse process. The force application is combined with breathing as a progressive oscillation or thrust is applied.

## Thoracic Rotation Manipulation in Supine    DVD

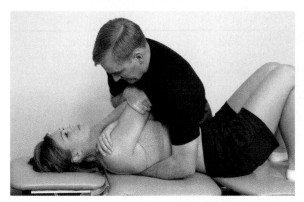

Thoracic supine rotation manipulation in supine with arms folded.

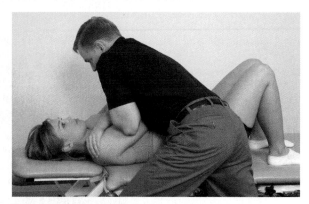

Therapist body position for thoracic supine rotation manipulation.

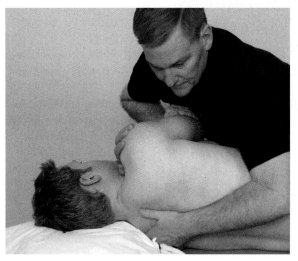

Roll patient to position hand for thoracic supine rotation manipulation.

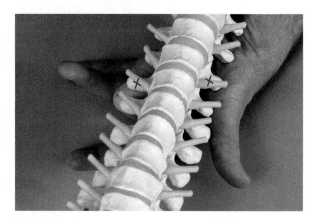

Hand placement on spine model for thoracic supine rotation manipulation.

| | |
|---|---|
| **PURPOSE** | The purpose of this technique is to manipulate a specific thoracic segment (T3-T4 though T11-T12) into rotation. |
| **PATIENT POSITION** | The patient is supine. |
| **THERAPIST POSITION** | The therapist stands next to the patient. |
| **HAND PLACEMENT** | **Caudal hand:** The thenar eminence is placed on the transverse process of the caudal member of the spinal segment, and the dorsal aspect of the middle phalanx of the third digit is placed on the transverse process of the cranial member of the segment. |
| | **Cranial hand:** The hand and forearm are used to maneuver the patient's upper body, head, neck and upper extremities. |
| **PROCEDURE** | The patient's arms are folded across the chest. The arm closest to the therapist should be crossed underneath. The therapist stands on the patient's left side and uses the cranial hand to reach under the patient's shoulders and support the upper body or places the therapist's forearms over the patient's elbows. The cranial hand is used to roll the patient slightly toward the left side, and the index finger of the caudal hand is used to palpate the |

## Thoracic Rotation Manipulation in Supine—cont'd

specified segment. Once the segment is located, both the distal interphalangeal (DIP) and proximal interphalangeal (PIP) joints of the long finger of the caudal hand are flexed. The dorsal aspect of the middle phalanx of the third digit is placed on the left transverse process of the cranial member of the segment. The thenar eminence of the caudal hand is placed on the right transverse process of the caudal member of the segment. The patient is gently rolled back into the supine position onto the caudal hand, and the chest is used to apply force through the patient's forearms to take up the slack and oscillate or thrust the segment.

The manipulation is coordinated with the patient's breathing, with progressive oscillation into slightly more rotation each repetition. The procedure is repeated through approximately three breathing cycles. Once all the tissue slack is taken up, a short-amplitude high-velocity thrust can be imparted. On completion of the manipulation, right rotation is retested.

Additional tissue tension can be created by side bending the patient's thoracic spine superior to the level to be manipulated in the opposite direction of the rotation followed by dropping the same side shoulder girdle (of the direction of rotation) toward the table just prior to application of the manipulation forces. Skin slack can be taken up by pulling the hand contact slightly inferior just before imparting the thrust.

**THORACIC ROTATION MANIPULATION IN SUPINE: HANDS BEHIND THE HEAD VARIATION**

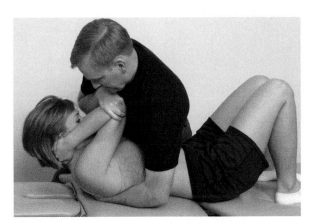

Another variation can be made with this technique to flex the spine superior to the level to be manipulated to add further tissue tension above the level to be manipulated. Changing the patient's hand position to interlock fingers behind the patient's head/neck can facilitate the addition of flexion to this technique.

## Thoracic Rotation Manipulation in Supine—cont'd

**BOX 5-5**  Variations of Hand Positions and Use of Towel to Protect Joints of Hand for the Supine Thoracic Manipulation Techniques

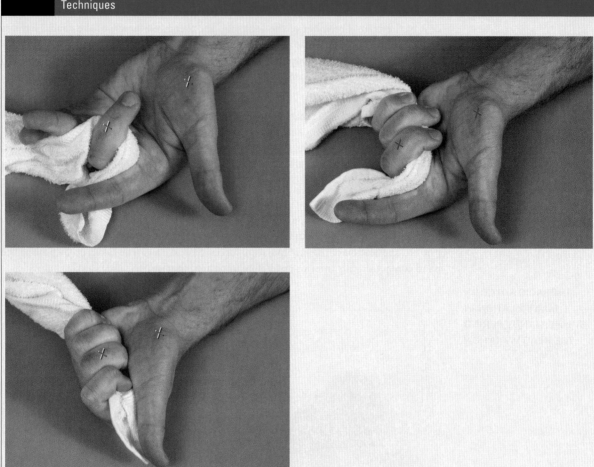

**NOTES**    Indication for use of this technique is decreased rotation of a specific thoracic segment (T3-T4 through T11-T12). The procedure can be performed with the cranial hand used to contact the segment (with the same contact points described previously). This modification prevents the therapist from reaching around the patient to perform the technique. The long finger of the caudal hand (or cranial hand if the modified technique is used) is flexed around a towel or pillowcase to protect the joints from hyperflexion (Box 5-5). The procedure can also be performed with the patient's arms folded across a pillow to create a barrier between the therapist and patient for patient comfort. This technique follows the *rule of the lower finger*, which states that the direction of the rotation is the same as the side of the lower finger (e.g., if the lower finger is on the right side, right rotation is being induced). This technique is commonly used to induce a high-velocity thrust manipulation or as a progressive oscillation.

## Upper Thoracic Rotation Manipulation in Prone

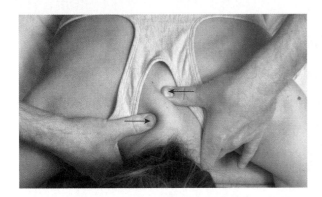

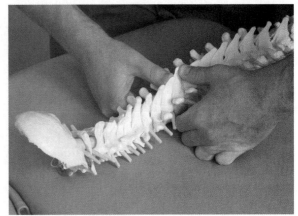

Finger placement for prone upper thoracic rotation manipulation.

| | |
|---|---|
| **PURPOSE** | The purpose is manipulation of a specific thoracic segment (C7-T1 though T3-T4) into rotation. |
| **PATIENT POSITION** | The patient is prone with a pillow under the chest/trunk and the neck in a neutral position. |
| **THERAPIST POSITION** | The therapist stands with a diagonal athletic stance next to the patient. |
| **HAND PLACEMENT** | **Caudal hand:** The pad of the thumb is used to contact the lateral aspect of the spinous process of one member of the segment. |
| | **Cranial hand:** The pad of the thumb is used to contact the lateral aspect of the spinous process of the other member of the segment. |
| **PROCEDURE** | The therapist stands on the patient's side and uses the pad of the thumb of the caudal hand to contact the left lateral aspect of the spinous process of the caudal member of the segment. The pad of the thumb of the cranial hand is used to contact the right lateral aspect of the spinous process of the cranial member of the segment. The therapist manipulates into right rotation by pushing each member of the segment toward the opposite side by using the thumbs to apply an equal and opposite force through the spinous processes. On completion of the manipulation, right rotation is retested. |
| | Manipulation into left rotation is accomplished with repeating the procedure with the caudal thumb contacting the left lateral aspect of the spinous process of the cranial member of the segment and the cranial thumb contacting the right lateral aspect of the spinous process of the caudal member of the segment. On completion of the manipulation, left rotation is retested. |
| **NOTES** | Indication for use of this technique is decreased rotation of a specific thoracic segment (C7-T1 through T3-T4). A flexed index finger can be used to reinforce and support the thumb during the performance of this technique. The therapist should avoid applying the force to the tips of the spinous processes because this is usually uncomfortable to the patient. Grade III oscillations are usually used with this technique. This technique follows the *rule of the upper thumb*, which states that the direction of the rotation is the same as the side of the upper thumb (e.g., if the upper thumb is on the right side, right rotation is being induced). |

## Upper Thoracic Rotation Mobilization with Movement

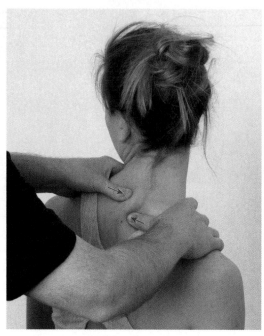

Mobilization with movement for left rotation.

The upper thoracic rotation mobilization technique can be followed up with a mobilization with movement in which the same contact and force are used on an upright patient; as the patient actively rotates the neck into the direction of the manipulation, the therapist applies overpressure through the spinous processes at the targeted segment.

## Upper Thoracic Gap Manipulation with Facet Locking

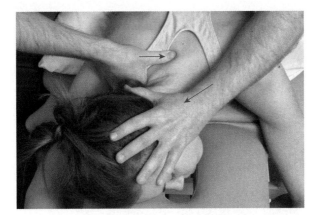

| | |
|---|---|
| **PURPOSE** | This test is used to gap/manipulate the targeted upper thoracic facet joint. |
| **PATIENT POSITION** | The patient is prone with a pillow under the chest. |
| **HAND PLACEMENT** | **Right hand:** The thumb contacts the lateral aspect of the spinous process of the inferior member of the targeted segment on the side opposite the joint to be manipulated. |
| | **Left hand:** The palm is placed across the posterior lateral aspect of the patient's occiput. |
| **PROCEDURE** | The therapist uses the left hand to passively side bend the patient's neck away from the targeted facet joint and then rotates the neck toward the targeted facet joint to take up the slack of the cervical and upper thoracic spine down to, but not including, the targeted segment. The therapist presses superiorly with the left hand along the angle of the neck/head and presses laterally with the right thumb across the spinous process with equal forces. Once the slack is taken up, an oscillatory or a thrust force may be imparted. |
| **NOTES** | This technique is most effective if the positioning allows maximum tension to the targeted facet joint. The therapist should verbally monitor the patient throughout the technique because the prone position hides facial expressions. |

## Variation: Upper Thoracic Gapping Manipulation in Sitting

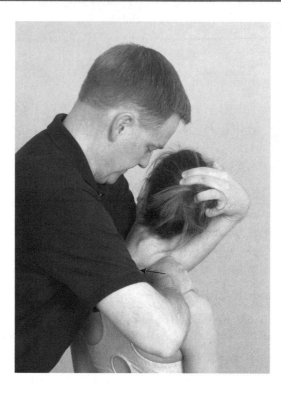

The same facet locking can be used with the patient in the seated position. A cradle hold of the patient's head with the therapist's arm can facilitate the technique. The forces are the same, with lateral force with the thumb across the spinous process combined with a lifting/distraction force imparted with the therapist's other arm/hand on the patient's head.

This advanced technique is most commonly used as a thrust technique.

## Upper Thoracic Press/Kneading Manipulation in Sitting

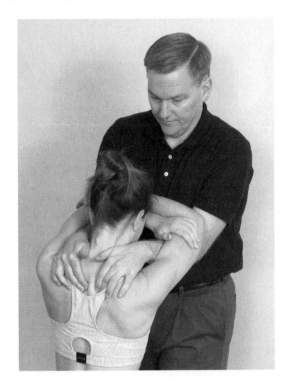

| | |
|---|---|
| **PURPOSE** | The technique is used to manipulate a specific thoracic segment (T1-T2 though T4-T5). |
| **PATIENT POSITION** | The patient sits on a treatment table with the arms folded and the head resting on the forearms. |
| **THERAPIST POSITION** | The therapist stands with a diagonal athletic stance directly in front of the patient. |
| **HAND PLACEMENT** | The therapist's arms are placed under the patient's forearms to support the weight of the patient's head, neck, and shoulders. The pads of digits two and three of both hands are placed at the targeted upper thoracic transverse processes. |
| **PROCEDURE** | The therapist presses the fingers into the targeted thoracic vertebrae while shifting the weight backward to lean away from the patient and lifting the patient's head/neck/upper thorax from flexion into slight extension. |
| **NOTES** | This technique can be used as a general soft tissue technique or made more specific to target a spinal segment. Firm support of the patient's arms/head/neck and convincing the patient to relax into the rhythmic motions of the mobilization are important. The therapist can modify his force application into asymmetrical or diagonal directions to induce lateral flexion and rotation motions at the targeted upper thoracic segments. For instance, the patient's head and neck gliding motion could be angled toward the patient's left as the therapist presses more firmly on the patient's right transverse process to facilitate left rotation at the targeted spinal segment. |

## Upper Thoracic Lift Manipulation    DVD

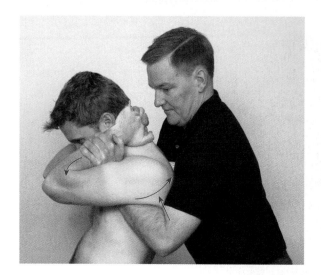
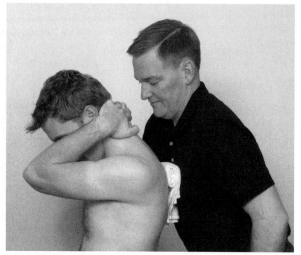

Towel placement for upper thoracic lift manipulation technique.

| | |
|---|---|
| **PURPOSE** | The technique is used to manipulate a specific thoracic segment (T1-T2 though T4-T5). |
| **PATIENT POSITION** | The patient sits on a treatment table with the fingers interlocked behind the neck. |
| **THERAPIST POSITION** | The therapist stands with a diagonal athletic stance behind the patient, and the chest is placed against a rolled hand towel against the targeted spinal segment. |
| **HAND PLACEMENT** | The hands are used to grasp the patient's forearms in each hand. |
| **PROCEDURE** | The patient's neck and upper thoracic spine are fully flexed to the targeted spinal level, and the patient is asked to squeeze the elbows together into a horizontal adduction motion as the therapist lifts the patient in a superior and posterior direction into the counterforce of the rolled towel and the therapist's chest. |
| **NOTES** | This technique is often combined with deep breathing with the manipulative thrust applied as the patient exhales. This technique tends to be safer for patients who may have suspected weakened skeletal structure than the prone techniques because minimal loading forces are used on the thorax and rib cage. |

## Mid Thoracic Lift Manipulation

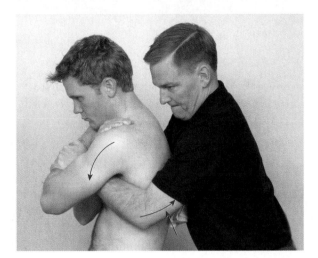

|                        |                                                                                                                                                                                                                                                                                                   |
| ---------------------- | ------------------------------------------------------------------------------------------------------------------------------------------------------------------------------------------------------------------------------------------------------------------------------------------------- |
| **PURPOSE**            | This technique is used to manipulate a specific thoracic segment (T3-T4 through T10-T11).                                                                                                                                                                                                          |
| **PATIENT POSITION**   | The patient sits on a treatment table with the arms folded across the chest and the hands grasping each opposite shoulder.                                                                                                                                                                          |
| **THERAPIST POSITION** | The therapist stands with a diagonal athletic stance behind the patient, and the chest is placed against a rolled hand towel at the targeted spinal segment.                                                                                                                                        |
| **HAND PLACEMENT**     | The patient's forearms are grasped in each hand, with the arms looped inferior and anterior to the patient's arms.                                                                                                                                                                                  |
| **PROCEDURE**          | The patient's upper thoracic spine is flexed to the targeted spinal level as the therapist lifts and squeezes the patient in a superior and posterior direction into the counterforce of the rolled towel and the therapist's chest.                                                                |
| **NOTES**              | This technique is often combined with deep breathing with the manipulative thrust applied as the patient exhales. This technique tends to be safer for patients who may have suspected weakened skeletal structure (such as osteopenia) than the prone techniques because minimal loading forces are used on the thorax. This technique can be modified to have the therapist contact the patient's elbows to apply the superior/posterior directed force to apply the thrust. |

# CASE STUDIES AND PROBLEM SOLVING

The following patient case reports can be used by the student to develop problem-solving skills by considering the information provided in the patient history and tests and measures and developing appropriate evaluations, goals, and plans of care.

## MRS. THORACIC KYPHOSIS

### History

An 83-year-old woman has a 2-year history of progressively increasing intensity lumbar and thoracic pain. The patient needs a walker for ambulation but states that her thoracic area pain is worse with lifting the walker. The patient is very limited functionally and needs assistance for all self-care activities because of pain provocation with all functional mobility, especially attempting to roll over and lie supine.

What diagnostic tests should be done on this patient before beginning treatment?

### Tests and Measures

- Observation: The patient is a frail-looking female with moderately increased thoracic kyphosis and tends to use the upper extremities to support the trunk in sitting
- Gait: Slow and laborious with a grimace each time she lifts the walker
- Functional mobility: The patient is unable to tolerate supine or prone positions because of pain
- Thoracolumbar AROM: Limited in all planes because of pain, with patient demonstrating approximately 20%-25% of expected AROM in all planes of motion
- Palpation: Tender and guarded mid thoracic and lower lumbar paraspinal muscles
- Strength: Grossly fair throughout trunk and extremities; poor strength in lower and middle trapezius
- Balance: Good static, fair + dynamic

### Evaluation
Diagnosis
Problem list
Goals
Treatment plan/intervention

## MRS. C P RULE

### History

A 35-year-old acute care nurse has tightness and discomfort in the mid thoracic spine and mid cervical area that is provoked with prolonged sitting and work activities. Symptoms started 24 days before the initial evaluation after the nurse transferred a heavy patient. The Fear Avoidance Beliefs Questionnaire physical activity (FABQPA) score was 11.

### Tests and Measures

- Structural examination results: Mild forward head posture (FHP) with diminished (flattened) upper thoracic kyphosis
- Cervical AROM in standing: 75% in all planes of motion with mid cervical pain reported at the end range of each motion
- Cervical extension: 25 degrees
- Thoracic AROM: 60% Backward bending, 85% forward bending, 80% bilateral rotation and sidebending with ipsilateral mid thoracic pain reported with bilateral rotation
- PIVM testing: Hypomobility and mild reactivity noted with PA testing T3-T4 and T5-T6 segments with bilateral rotation and forward-bending PAIVM testing; downglide PIVM hypomobility noted C2-C3 and C6-C7 bilaterally
- Shoulder screen: Active shoulder forward flexion and abduction full ROM and pain free
- Muscle length: No limitations noted
- Strength: Lower and middle trapezius are 4−/5; deep neck flexors are 3+/5
- Neurologic screen: Negative
- Palpation: Tender and guarded bilateral mid thoracic and mid cervical paraspinal muscles

### Evaluation
Diagnosis
Problem list
Goals
Treatment plan/intervention

## MR. STIFF THORAX

### History

A 50-year-old college professor has tightness and discomfort in the mid thoracic spine that is provoked with taking a deep breath and with prolonged sitting.

### Tests and Measures

- Structural examination results: Moderate FHP with protracted scapulas
- Cervical AROM in standing: 85% in all planes of motion and pain free
- Thoracic AROM: 25% Backward bending, 85% forward bending, 50% bilateral rotation and side bending with ipsilateral mid thoracic pain reported with bilateral rotation
- PIVM testing: Hypomobility and moderate reactivity noted with PA testing T4-T5 and T5-T6 segments with bilateral rotation and forward-bending PAIVM testing

- Shoulder screen: Active shoulder forward flexion and abduction are 145 degrees bilaterally with a mild symptom of mid thoracic tightness at end range of motion
- Muscle length: Moderately tight right levator scapula and minimally tight bilateral pectoralis major and minor
- Strength: Lower and middle trapezius are 4−/5; deep neck flexors are 3+/5
- Neurologic screen: Negative
- Palpation: Tender and guarded bilateral mid thoracic paraspinal muscles

### Evaluation

Diagnosis
Problem list
Goals
Treatment plan/intervention

## REFERENCES

1. Cooper C: The crippling consequences of fractures and their impact on quality of life, *Am J Med* 103(2A):12S-19S, 1997.

2. Ettinger B, Black DM, Nevitt MC, et al: Contribution of vertebral deformities to chronic back pain and disability, *J Bone Mineral Res* 7:449-456, 1992.

3. Neumann DA: *Kinesiology of the musculoskeletal system*, St Louis, 2002, Mosby.

4. Panjabi MM, Koichiro T, Goel V, et al: Thoracic human vertebrae, quantitative three-dimensional anatomy, *Spine* 16(8):888-901, 1991.

5. Geelhoed MA, McGaugh J, Brewer PA, et al: A new model to facilitate palpation of the level of the transverse processes of the thoracic spine, *JOSPT* 36(11):876-881, 2006.

6. Sizer PS, Brismee JM, Cook C: Coupling behavior of the thoracic spine: a systematic review of the literature, *J Manipulative Physiol Ther* 30(5):390-399, 2007.

7. National Health and Medical Research Council: Acute thoracic spinal pain. In: *Australian acute musculoskeletal pain guidelines: evidence-based management of acute musculoskeletal pain*, Brisbane, 2003, Australian Academic Press.

8. April C, Dwyer A, Bogduk N: Cervical zygapophyseal joint pain patterns II: a clinical evaluation, *Spine* 15:458-461, 1990.

9. Dwyer A, Aprill C, Bogduk N: Cervical zygapophyseal joint pain patterns I: a study in normal volunteers, *Spine* 15:453-457, 1990.

10. Fukui S, Ohseto K, Shiotani M, et al: Referred pain distribution of the cervical zygapophseal joints and cervical dorsal rami, *Pain* 68:79-83, 1996.

11. Hockaday JM, Whitty CWM: Patterns of referred pain in the normal subject, *Brain* 90:481-495, 1967.

12. Schellhas KP, Pollei SR: Thoracic discography: a safe and reliable technique, *Spine* 19:2103-2109, 1994.

13. Wainner RS, Fritz JM, Irrgang JJ, et al: Reliability and diagnostic accuracy of the clinical examination and patient self-report measures for cervical radiculopathy, *Spine* 28(1):52-62, 2003.

14. Santavirta S, Konttinene YT, Heliovaara M, et al: Determinants of osteoporotic thoracic vertebral fracture: screening of 57,000 Finnish women and men, *Acta Orthop Scand* 63:198-202, 1992.

15. Melton LJ, Kan SH, Frye MA, et al: Epidemiology of vertebral fractures in women, *Am J Epidemiol* 129:1000-1011, 1989.

16. Patel U, Skingle S, Campbell GA, et al: Clinical profile of acute vertebral compression fractures in osteoporosis, *Br J Rheumatol* 30:418-421, 1991.

17. Hauag C, Ross PD, Wasnich RW: Vertebral fractures and other predictors of back pain among older women, *J Bone Mineral Res* 11:1026-1032, 1994.

18. Bennell K, Larsen J: Osteoporosis. In Boyling JD, Jull GA, editors: *Grieve's modern manual therapy: the vertebral column*, ed 3, Edinburgh, 2004, Churchill Livingstone.

19. Schiller L: Effectiveness of spinal manipulative therapy in the treatment of mechanical thoracic spine pain: a pilot randomized clinical trial, *J Manipulative Physiol Ther* 24(6):394-401, 2001.

20. Kelly JL, Whitney SL: The use of nonthrust manipulation in an adolescent for the treatment of thoracic and rib dysfunction: a case report, *JOSPT* 36(11):887-892, 2006.

21. Maitland GD: *Vertebral manipulation*, ed 5, Oxford, 1986, Butterworth Heinemann.

22. Conroy JL, Schneiders AG: The T4 syndrome, *Manual Ther* 10:292-296, 2005.

23. Evans P: The T4 syndrome, *J Manipulative Physiol Ther* 18(1):34-37, 1995.

24. Bogduk N: Innervation and pain patterns of the thoracic spine. In Grant R, editor: *Physical therapy of the cervical and thoracic spines*, ed 3, Edinburgh, 2002, Churchill Livingstone.

25. Zusman M: Forebrain-mediated sensitization of central pain pathways: 'non-specific' pain and a new image for MT, *Manual Ther* 7(2):80-88, 2002.

26. Sterling M, Jull G, Wright A: Cervical mobilization: concurrent effects on pain, sympathetic nervous system activity and motor activity, *Manual Ther* 6(2):72-81, 2001.

27. Vincenzino B, Collins D, Benson H, et al: An investigation of the interrelationship between manipulative therapy-induced hypoalgesia and sympathoexcitation, *J Manipulative Physiol Ther* 21(7):448-453, 1998.

28. Cleland JA, Childs JD, Fritz JM, et al: Development of a clinical prediction rule for guiding treatment of a subgroup of patients with neck pain: use of thoracic spine manipulation, exercise, and patient education, *Phys Ther* 87(1):9-23, 2007.

29. Olson KA, Gilette J: Videoflouroscopic evaluation of spine motion during shoulder elevation: a pilot study [abstract], *JMMT* 6(4):206, 1998.

30. Stewart SG, Jull GA, Ng JKF, et al: An initial analysis of thoracic spine movement during unilateral arm elevation, *JMMT* 3(1):15-20, 1995.

31. Crawford HJ, Jull GA: The influence of thoracic posture and movement on range of arm elevation, *Physiother Theory Pract* 9:143-148, 1993.

32. Shambaugh P: Changes in electrical activity in muscles resulting from chiropractic adjustment: a pilot study, *J Manipulative Physiol Ther* 10:300-304, 1987.

33. Oda I, Abumi K, Cunningham BW, et al: An in vitro human cadaveric study investigating the biomechanical properties of the thoracic spine, *Spine* 27(3):E64-E70, 2002.

34. Lee DG: Rotational instability of the mid-thoracic spine: assessment and management, *Manual Ther* 1(5):234-241, 1996.

35. Christensen HW, Vach W, Vach K, et al: Palpation of the upper thoracic spine: an observer reliability study, *J Manipulative Physiol Ther* 25(5):285-292, 2002.

## CHAPTER 6

# Examination and Treatment of Cervical Spine Disorders

### CHAPTER OVERVIEW

This chapter covers the spinal kinematics of the cervical spine, describes common cervical spine disorders with a diagnostic classification system to guide clinical decision making, and provides a detailed description of manual examination, manipulation, and exercise procedures for the cervical spine.

### OBJECTIVES

- Describe the significance and impact of cervical spine disorders
- Describe cervical spine kinematics
- Classify cervical spine disorders based on signs and symptoms
- Describe interventions for cervical spine disorders
- Demonstrate and interpret cervical spine examination procedures
- Describe contraindications and precautions for cervical spine manipulation
- Demonstrate manipulation techniques of the cervical spine
- Instruct exercises for cervical spine disorders

## SIGNIFICANCE OF CERVICAL SPINE DISORDERS

Neck pain is reported to be the second most common musculoskeletal disorder that leads to disability and injury claims.[1] The economic burden of neck pain is second only to low back pain in workers' compensation claims in the United States.[2] Neck pain affects approximately 10% of the North American and Western European populations at any one time, and as much as 45% to 54% each year.[3,4] According the National Center for Health Statistics (NCHS) National Health Interview Survey (NHIS), 28,401,000 persons (13.8% of the population) aged 18 years and older in the United States in 2002 reported having neck pain.[5] As much as 50% to 75% of individuals have neck or shoulder pain at least once in their life.[6] Cervical spine–related musculoskeletal disorders account for approximately 25% of the patients seen in outpatient physical therapy in the United States.[7]

### Cervical Spine Kinematics: Functional Anatomy and Mechanics

The cervical spine is designed for a great deal of mobility and is susceptible to the development of instability impairments.

Among male and female subjects of the same age group, female subjects have greater active range of motion (AROM) than male subjects for all AROM except neck flexion.[8] Table 6-1 shows the mean cervical AROM for 20-year-old to 29-year-old men. Cervical AROM tends to decrease with age.

The intervertebral discs of the cervical spine by middle age develop clefts that appear in the posterolateral aspect of the cervical disc and are thought to occur as a result of the shearing forces associated with cervical spine rotation.[9] The disc's gelatinous nucleus pulposis shows evidence of fibrosis by the mid teens and is replaced with fibrocartilaginous uncovertebral clefts that allow further mobility at the spinal segment.[9] The intervertebral disc is reinforced at the anterolateral aspect by the uncovertebral joints of von Luschka, which allow motion in multiple planes and assist in limiting extreme range of motion.

The zygapophyseal facet joints of the middle and lower cervical spine (C2-C3 to C7-T1) are angled upward and forward at approximately a 45-degree angle.[10] The motions of forward and backward bending occur parallel with the plane of the facet joints as either a bilateral upglide (forward and upward) motion for forward bending or a bilateral downglide (backward and downward) motion for backward bending.[11] At the end range of the upgliding motion, the cervical vertebrae tilts to create

| TABLE 6-1 | AROM as Measured with CROM Device for Men Aged 20 to 29 y[8] | | |
|---|---|---|---|
| MOTION | MEAN | STANDARD DEVIATION | RANGE |
| Flexion | 54.3 | 8.8 | 42-68 |
| Extension | 76.7 | 12.8 | 60-108 |
| Left LF | 41.4 | 7.1 | 30-58 |
| Right LF | 44.9 | 7.2 | 30-58 |
| Left rotation | 69.2 | 7.0 | 52-83 |
| Right rotation | 69.6 | 6.0 | 59-80 |

*LF*, Lateral flexion.
AROM measurements of cervical spine with CROM instrument showed good intratester and intertester reliability with intraclass correlation coefficients greater than 0.80.

| TABLE 6-2 | Cervical Spine Segmental Flexion-Extension | | | |
|---|---|---|---|---|
| SPINAL SEGMENT | PENNING[11] | DVORAK ET AL[12] (SD) | PANJABI ET AL[79] | KOTTKE & MUNDALE[80] |
| Occ-C1 | 30 | | 24 | 22 |
| C1-C2 | 30 | 12 | 24 | 11 |
| C2-C3 | 12 | 10 (3) | | 11 |
| C3-C4 | 18 | 15 (3) | | 16 |
| C4-C5 | 20 | 19 (4) | | 18 |
| C5-C6 | 20 | 20 (20) | | 21 |
| C6-C7 | 15 | 19 (4) | | 18 |

| TABLE 6-3 | Mean Degrees of Rotation in One Direction (Standard Deviation) and Coupled Lateral Flexion (Standard Deviation) as Calculated with Biplanar Radiography in 20 Live Subjects[13] | | | |
|---|---|---|---|---|
| LEVELS | MEAN ROTATION | STANDARD DEVIATION | MEAN COUPLED LATERAL FLEXION | STANDARD DEVIATION |
| Occiput-C2 | 37.5 | 5.9 | −2.4 | 6.0 |
| C2-C3 | 3.7 | 3.2 | −1.6 | 7.7 |
| C3-C4 | 2.9 | 2.5 | 6.2 | 7.1 |
| C4-C5 | 2.1 | 2.9 | 6.2 | 7.1 |
| C5-C6 | 2.7 | 2.2 | 4.0 | 7.9 |
| C6-C7 | 3.2 | 1.3 | 2.7 | 6.5 |

Positive degrees of lateral flexion indicate in same direction as rotation.

| TABLE 6-4 | Segmental Cervical Rotation (Degrees) in One Direction | | |
|---|---|---|---|
| SPINAL SEGMENT | DUMAS ET AL[15] (MEAN [SD]) | PENNING[11] (MEAN [RANGE]) | PANJABI ET AL[79] |
| Occiput-C1 | 1.4 (2.7) | 1.0 (−2-5) | 7.2 |
| C1-C2 | 37.0 (5.8) | 40.5 (29-46) | 38.9 |
| C2-C3 | 0.6 (3.4) | 3.0 (0-10) | |
| C3-C4 | 4.9 (3.7) | 6.5 (3-10) | |
| C4-C5 | 5.2 (4.2) | 6.8 (1-12) | |
| C5-C6 | 5.1 (4.5) | 6.9 (2-12) | |
| C6-C7 | 3.4 (2.7) | 5.4 (2-10) | |
| C7-T1 | 1.5 | 2.1 (−2-7) | |

gapping of the posterior aspect of the facet joint with end range forward bending.[12] The amount of cervical spine segmental motion for sagittal plane motions measured in radiographic and computed tomography (CT) scan studies are described in Table 6-2. The angular plane of the facet joints is important to consider not only in understanding joint mechanics but also in application of passive intervertebral motion (PIVM) testing and joint mobilization/manipulation technique application. The most effective and most comfortable mobilization/manipulation techniques of the cervical spine for the patient commonly require application of forces parallel with the angle formed by the plane of the facet joints.

The facet joints for C1-C2 are oriented more horizontally than the middle and lower cervical spine facet joints to allow greater mobility and pure translation.[12] The occiput-C1 joints are formed by a pair of convex-shaped occipital condyles and the concave-shaped superior articular surfaces of the atlas. Therefore, the occipital condyles glide in the opposite direction of the motion direction, which follows the convex/concave rule (Figures 6-1 and 6-2). For instance, the occipital condyles glide posterior with forward bending and glide anterior with backward bending.

Middle and lower cervical rotation and lateral flexion motions are coupled motions from C2-T1, with lateral flexion and rotation occurring toward the same side. The axis of the motion is perpendicular to the angle of the cervical facet joints, with an upglide on the contralateral facet joint and a downglide on the ipsilateral facet joint (Figures 6-3 and 6-4).[9] Table 6-3 shows the mean range of rotation motion with the mean amount of coupled lateral flexion at each cervical spine segment measured with biplanar radiographs at the end range of rotation of middle-aged men.[13] At several cervical spine levels, the standard deviation is greater than the mean of the motion, which indicates a great deal of variability in healthy subjects. However, the means can provide a general idea of the proportion of motion at each segment and the coupling that occurs. Tables 6-4 and 6-5 show findings from multiple studies of the mean segmental motion for cervical rotation and lateral flexion. Although some variability is noted, the C1-C2 segment allows the greatest amount of rotation (approximately 50%). The studies that have measured cervical segmental motion

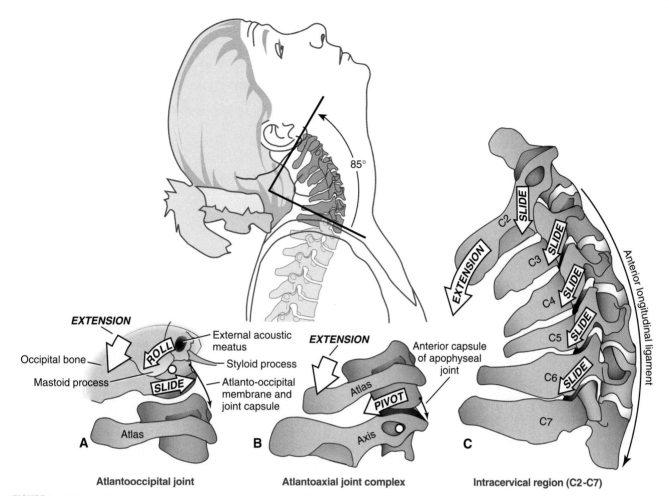

**FIGURE 6-1** Kinematics of craniocervical extension. **A,** Atlantooccipital joint. **B,** Atlantoaxial joint complex. **C,** Intracervical region (C2-C7). Elongated and taut tissues are indicated with *thin black arrows*. From Neumann DA: *Kinesiology of the musculoskeletal system*, St Louis, 2002, Mosby.

| TABLE 6-5 | Cervical Spine Range of Motion: Lateral Flexion in One Direction | | |
|---|---|---|---|
| **SPINAL SEGMENT** | **PENNING**[11] | **WHITE & PANJABI**[81] | **PANJABI ET AL**[79] |
| Occiput-C1 | 6 | 7 | 5.5 |
| C1-C2 | 6 | 0 | 6.7 |
| C2-C3 | 6 | 10 | |
| C3-C4 | 6 | 11 | |
| C4-C5 | 6 | 11 | |
| C5-C6 | 6 | 8 | |
| C6-C7 | 6 | 7 | |
| C7-T1 | 6 | 4 | |

count C6-C7 as the last moving segment with cervical active movements, but clinically, motion is noted in the vertebral segments as caudal as T3-T4 with cervical active motion. The active and passive mobility of the upper thoracic spinal segments should be evaluated and treated with the cervical spine.

The occiput-C1 and C1-C2 spinal segments allow for fine tuning of the head position during neck motion and create a distinction between axial cervical rotation and lateral flexion. A relative lateral flexion of the cranium occurs to the contralateral side of the cervical spine rotation, which functions to keep the eyes level with an axial rotation movement of the head.[13] In the process, the atlas glides in the relative opposite direction of the cervical rotation. During cervical lateral flexion, a relative rotation occurs to the opposite side of the lateral flexion at the C1-C2 and occiput-C1 segments to allow the face to remain facing forward in a frontal plane during the lateral flexion.

In the upper cervical spine (occiput-C1, C1-2), the atlas vertebra may be considered an interposed bearing between the axis vertebra and the occipital condyles that guides and limits

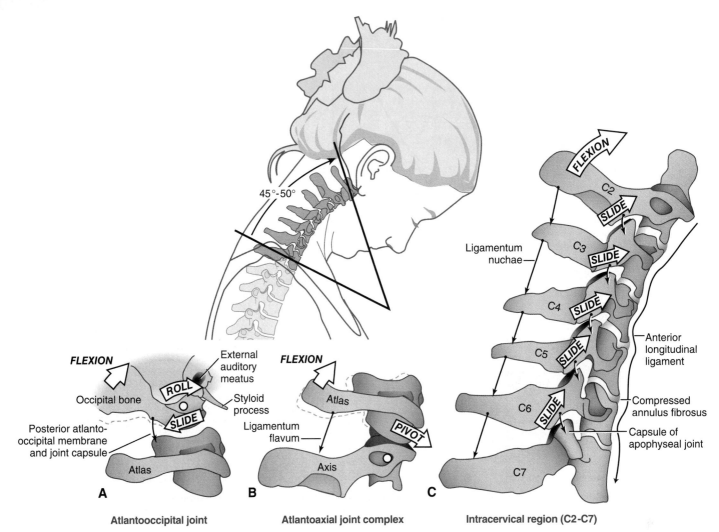

**FIGURE 6-2** Kinematics of craniocervical flexion. **A,** Atlantooccipital joint. **B,** Atlantoaxial joint complex. **C,** Intracervical region (C2-C7). Note in **C** that flexion slackens anterior longitudinal ligament and increases space between adjacent laminae and spinous process. Elongated and taut tissues are indicated with *thin black arrows*; slacked tissue is indicated with *wavy black arrow*. From Neumann DA: *Kinesiology of the musculoskeletal system*, St Louis, 2002, Mosby.

the movement between C2 and the occiput.[11] In flexion-extension, the position of the atlas is relatively independent of the actual relationship between the occiput and C2. In any position of the craniocervical region, the posterior atlantal arch may be found somewhere between the occiput and the spinous process of C2 and not necessarily halfway between.[11]

In lateral bending, the atlas has a more rigidly prescribed position[11] because of the shape of the lateral masses of the atlas as seen in anteroposterior (open-mouth view) radiographic projection. During lateral flexion movement, the odontoid must remain midway between the occipital condyles because of its fixation by the alar ligaments. Thus, lateral flexion in the occipit-C1 segment is always combined with lateral flexion in the atlantoaxial segment and vice versa. Also, a relative lateral glide of the atlas toward the side of the lateral flexion occurs.[14] Craniovertebral lateral flexion is also facilitated by simultaneous contralateral atlantoaxial rotation as a result of the orientation and function of the alar ligament (Figure 6-5).

The C2 vertebra actually rotates toward the side of craniovertebral lateral flexion in relation to C3, which creates a relative contralateral rotation of C1-C2 spinal segment. The cruciate (transverse portion) ligament also assists in stabilization of the craniovertebral complex, especially to prevent excessive anterior shear of C1 in relation to C2 (Figure 6-6). If the cruciate ligament is lax or torn, the dens of C2 is no longer held firmly against the anterior arch of C1.

The coupled movement patterns of the cervical spine have been documented with cadaver studies and CT scan and radiographic studies and can assist in clinical evaluation of movement restrictions.[13-17] For instance, if cervical spine motion is limited with lateral flexion and rotation to the same side, a mid or lower cervical facet joint restriction is suspected (cervical facet capsular pattern). However, if the most significant limitations in cervical active range of motion are noted with lateral flexion and rotation to the opposite direction, upper cervical joint restrictions are suspected (i.e., craniovertebral capsular

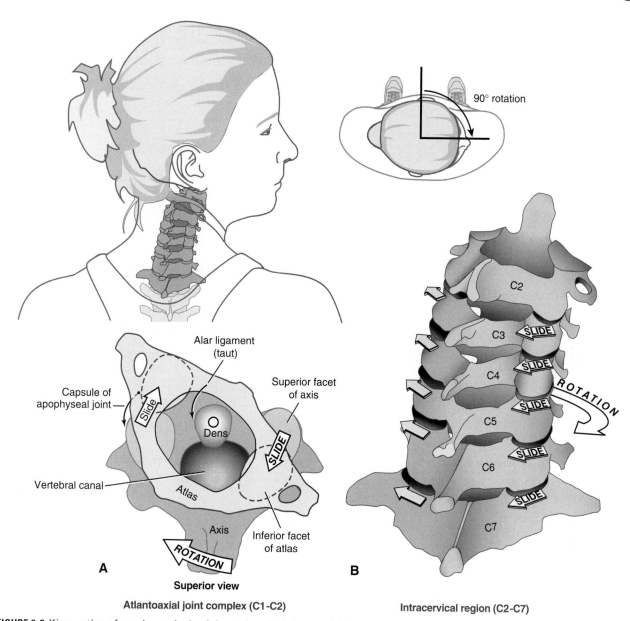

**FIGURE 6-3** Kinematics of craniocervical axial rotation. **A,** Atlantoaxial joint complex. **B,** Intracervical region (C2-C7). From Neumann DA: *Kinesiology of the musculoskeletal system*, St Louis, 2002, Mosby.

pattern). Jarrett, Olson, and Bohannon[18] used this finding as part of the criteria to identify craniovertebral motion restrictions and were able to show good reliability in detection of this type of motion impairment with a cervical range-of-motion (CROM) device.

Neumann[19] attributes the craniovertebral coupling pattern of contralateral lateral flexion with cervical rotation to the motor control exhibited by the upper cervical muscles that create this side-bending motion. Specifically, the rectus capitus lateralis muscle on the left produces left lateral flexion torque to the head via the atlantooccipital joints, and the left obliquus capitis inferior muscle creates left axial rotation of the craniocervical region during right lateral flexion of the cervical spine. The craniovertebral joints must have adequate joint mobility

and motor control to smoothly and fully produce these movements. If these active motions are less than full, passive motion assessment of the craniovertebral motion segments assists in differentiation between a motor control deficit and a joint mobility deficit.

## Diagnosis and Treatment of Cervical Spine Disorders

Cervical spine–related disorders are not a homogeneous group of conditions. Many factors must be considered to arrive at a physical therapy diagnostic classification and to develop a treatment plan of care. Classification systems should adequately define the primary signs and symptoms and guide therapeutic interventions. Once red flags have been screened and the

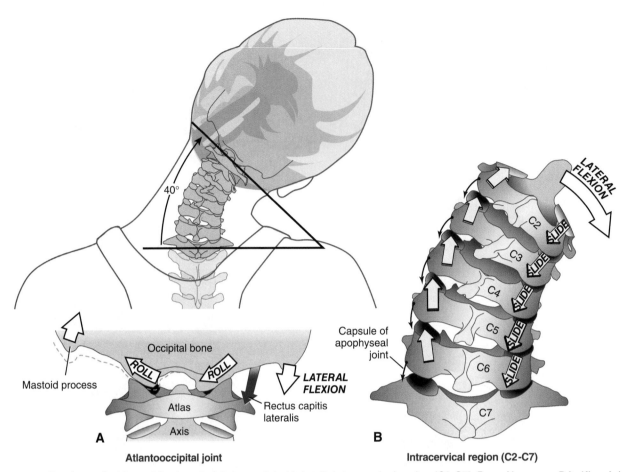

**FIGURE 6-4** Craniocervical lateral flexion. **A,** Atlantooccipital joint. **B,** Intracervical region (C2-C7). From Neumann DA: *Kinesiology of the musculoskeletal system*, St Louis, 2002, Mosby.

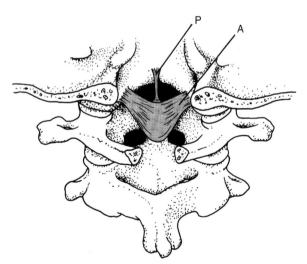

**FIGURE 6-5** Attachments of alar and apical ligaments. *A,* Alar ligament; *P,* apical ligament. From Porterfield JA, DeRosa C: *Mechanical neck pain*, Philadelphia, 1995, Saunders.

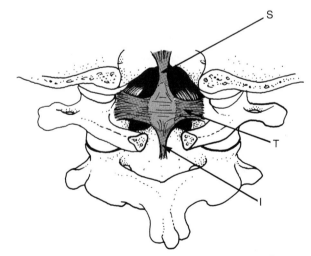

**FIGURE 6-6** Components of the cruciate ligament. *I,* Inferior band of cruciate ligament; *S,* superior longitudinal band of cruciate ligament; *T,* transverse band of cruciate ligament. From Porterfield JA, DeRosa C: *Mechanical neck pain*, Philadelphia, 1995, Saunders.

patient, through medical screening procedures, is determined to be an appropriate candidate for physical therapy, further information should be gathered to arrive at a diagnosis or classification of the condition.

After a traumatic event, such as a whiplash injury from a motor vehicle accident, the patient should be screened for a vertebral fracture with use of the Canadian C-spine rule. The Canadian C-spine rule was developed and validated to enhance clinical decision making for determination of when to obtain cervical spine radiographs for patients who have had trauma.[20] The decision to order conventional radiographs is made on the answers to the following three questions:

1. Do any high-risk factors mandate radiography? Examples include age 65 years or older, a dangerous mechanism of injury, or paresthesias in the extremities. Examples of a dangerous mechanism of injury include: a fall of more than 1 m or five stairs; an axial load to the head; a high-speed motor vehicle accident, rollover, or ejection; a motorized recre-ational vehicle accident; or a bicycle collision. If the answer is yes, then radiographs should be obtained.

2. Do any low-risk factors allow safe assessment of range of motion? Examples include a simple rear-end motor vehicle accident, a normal sitting position in the emergency department, ability of the patient to ambulate, delayed onset of neck pain, and absence of midline cervical spine tenderness. If the answer is yes, then the clinician can move on to question 3. If the answer is no, then radiographs should be obtained.

3. Is the patient able to rotate the neck actively at least 45 degrees to the right and left? If the patient is unable, then radiographs should be obtained. If the patient is able, then no radiographs are necessary.

According to a study by Stiell et al,[20] the Canadian C-spine rule has a sensitivity of 100% and a specificity of 43%.

The following classification system (see Table 6-6) is based on the treatment-based classification system proposed by

| TABLE 6-6 | Classification of Cervical Spine Disorders | |
| --- | --- | --- |
| **CLASSIFICATION** | **EXAMINATION FINDING** | **PROPOSED INTERVENTIONS** |
| Cervical hypomobility | Restricted AROM<br>Restricted PIVM testing cervical or upper thoracic<br>No UE radicular symptoms<br>Sudden or gradual onset | AROM exercises<br>Cervical and thoracic mobilization/manipulation isometric or thrust manipulation techniques<br>Nonthrust manipulation |
| Cervical radiculopathy | Positive Spurling's A test<br>Positive neck distraction test<br>Positive ULNT 1<br><60 degrees ipsilateral neck rotation | Cervical traction (manual/mechanical)<br>ULNT 1 AROM<br>Thoracic spine manipulation<br>Postural exercises |
| Clinical instability | Remote history of trauma<br>Symptoms provoked with sustained weight-bearing posture<br>Symptoms relieved with non–weight-bearing postures<br>Hypermobility with loose end feel of mid cervical segments<br>Poor strength (2/5) of cervical spine multifidus, longus colli, and longus capitus muscles<br>Shaking/poorly controlled (aberrant) motion with cervical active range of motion<br>Greater cervical active range of motion in supine (non–weight-bearing) position than in standing (weight-bearing) position | Postural education<br>Cervical stabilization exercise program<br>Mobilization/manipulation above and below hypermobilities<br>Ergonomic corrections |
| Acute pain (including whiplash)* | High pain and disability scores<br>Recent history of trauma<br>Referred symptoms into upper quarter<br>Poor tolerance to examination and most interventions | Gentle AROM within patient tolerance<br>Activity modification to control pain<br>Relative rest<br>Physical modalities<br>Intermittent use of cervical collar<br>Gentle manual therapy and exercises, but avoidance of pain-inducing manual therapy techniques or exercises |
| Cervicogenic headache | Unilateral headache with onset preceded by neck pain<br>Headache pain triggered by neck movement or positions<br>Headache pain elicited by pressure on posterior neck, especially at 1 of 3 upper cervical joints[55] | Cervical and thoracic mobilization/manipulation<br>Strengthening neck and postural muscles<br>Postural education |

Adapted from Childs JD, Fritz JM, Piva SR, et al: *JOSPT* 34(11):686-700, 2004.
*See Tables 6-7 and 6-8 for further classification of whiplash-associated disorders.
*UE*, Upper extremity.

Childs et al,[21] but the title of each category has been changed to reflect more standard medical and physical therapy terminology to describe each disorder. For instance, Childs et al[21] used the category name of "reduce headache" for what is commonly referred in the literature as a cervicogenic headache. In this text, we use the more common impairment-based terminology. Fritz and Brennan[22] recently presented preliminary data that showed superior treatment outcomes with patients with neck pain disorders who were classified by a physical therapist into a treatment-based classification and received a matched intervention as compared with patients who received unmatched interventions.

## ACUTE PAIN AND WHIPLASH-ASSOCIATED DISORDERS

Most people with whiplash injuries from motor vehicle accidents fully recover within a few weeks, but a significant proportion (14% to 42%) have persistent ongoing pain develop, with 10% reporting constant pain.[23] The Quebec Task Force (QTF) classification of whiplash-associated disorders (WAD) was developed to standardize the terminology associated with diagnosis and management of WAD (Table 6-7).

Based on studies that examined the complex clinical features of patients with WAD and tracked the outcomes of these patients, Sterling[24] came to the conclusion that the Quebec Task Force classification system (see Table 6-7) is too simplified and does not adequately classify patients with WAD to guide clinical decision making. In particular, Sterling[24] found that WAD II is the most common classification and should be subdivided further on the basis of specific clinical findings

within the classification that alter the treatment approach and potentially predict treatment outcomes. The clinical outcomes of patients within the WAD II classification vary greatly from full recovery at 6 months after injury to reports of continued moderate/severe symptoms.[24]

Sterling[24] has proposed three subclassifications for WAD II based on motor, sensory, and psychological impairments (Table 6-8). Patients with chronic WAD with moderate/severe ongoing symptoms have been shown to have higher levels of posttraumatic stress and high levels of persistent fear of movement/reinjury. When these factors are identified in a patient with acute WAD, an early psychological consultation is indicated.[25]

High sensory hyperalgia in the neck is common with most WAD II subclassifications, but the more severe WAD IIC classification also has sensory hyperalgia throughout the body (i.e., generalized). Treatment of this patient population is challenging, and recommendations are to avoid treatments that are noxious and pain provoking for these patients.[24] Only the most gentle manual therapy techniques should be used, combined with active movement within the patient's tolerance. Positioning can be helpful; the neck and shoulder girdle muscles can be supported at rest with use of a folded pillowcase wrapped around the patient's neck and use of pillows to support the arms in sitting when possible. Movement and activity should be encouraged, but overstraining the painful structures of the neck should be avoided. Frequent short doses of exercise and activity are encouraged throughout the patient's day. Activities

| TABLE 6-7 | Quebec Task Force Classification for Whiplash-Associated Disorders[82] |
|---|---|
| **QFT CLASSIFICATION GRADE** | **CLINICAL PRESENTATION** |
| 0 | No symptom of neck pain<br>No physical signs |
| I | Neck symptom of pain, stiffness, or tenderness only<br>No physical signs |
| II | Neck symptom<br>Musculoskeletal signs including:<br>　Decreased range of movement<br>　Point tenderness |
| III | Neck symptom<br>Musculoskeletal signs<br>Neurological signs including:<br>　Decreased or absent deep tendon reflexes<br>　Muscle weakness<br>　Sensory deficits |
| IV | Neck symptoms and fracture or dislocation |

| TABLE 6-8 | Sterling[24] Proposal to Further Subdivide WAD II |
|---|---|
| WAD II A | Neck pain<br>Motor impairment<br>　Decreased range of motion<br>　Altered muscle recruitment patterns (CCFT)<br>Sensory impairment<br>　Local cervical mechanical hyperalgia |
| WAD II B | Neck pain<br>Motor impairment<br>　Decreased ROM<br>　Altered muscle recruitment patterns (CCFT)<br>Sensory impairment<br>　Local cervical mechanical hyperalgia<br>Psychological impairment<br>　Elevated psychological distress |
| WAD II C | Neck pain<br>Motor impairment<br>　Decreased ROM<br>　Altered muscle recruitment patterns (CCFT)<br>　Increased joint positioning errors<br>Sensory impairment<br>　Local cervical mechanical hyperalgia<br>　Generalized sensory hypersensitivity (mechanical, thermal, bilateral upper limb neurodynamic test 1 limitation)<br>　Some may show sympathetic nervous system disturbances<br>Psychological impairment<br>　Elevated psychological distress<br>　Elevated levels of acute posttraumatic stress |

that the patient fears should be gradually introduced as the patient gains range of motion and motor control to assist the patient in overcoming fears of movement and activity. Early active exercise within the patient's tolerance has been shown to result in more favorable patient outcomes.[26,27]

A key feature regarding motor impairments of patients with WAD can be evaluated with the craniocervical flexion test (CCFT) as described by Jull, Kristjansson, and Dall'Alba.[28] The test assesses precision and control to determine whether a patient can use the deep neck muscles and hold a contraction. In motor control problems of the neck, a higher level of use of the superficial neck flexors compensates for inadequate contractile properties of the deep neck flexor muscles.[28] The deep neck flexors include the longus colli, longus capitus, and rectus capitus major and minor; these muscles work with the neck extensor muscles as dynamic stabilizers of the cervical segments. The CCFT has been developed by Jull and colleagues to assess the function of the deep neck flexor muscles (see Box 6-1).

The airbag and biofeedback device can be used as a training tool to recruit deep neck flexor muscles to control for potential cervical instability and also can be used to retrain joint position sense of the cervical spine by attempting to reproduce neck positions as visual feedback is provided by the biofeedback device (Figure 6-7). Jull, Kristjansson, and Dall'Alba[28] also advocate use of the airbag biofeedback device as a strengthening tool; the patient holds the targeted pressure for 10 seconds for up to 10 repetitions.

An equally effective means to strengthen the anterior cervical flexor muscles is to have the patient maintain craniocervical neutral in the supine position as the patient lifts the head off the folded towel (or pillow) and repeat for up to three sets of 12 repetitions (Figure 6-8). Repeated use of this exercise was shown to be just as effective at training neck flexor muscle strength as the Jull protocol.[29] This exercise might be considered a progression from the isolated craniocervical flexion exercise.

Higher levels of pain and disability, older age, cold hyperalgia, impaired vasoconstriction, and moderate posttraumatic stress symptoms have been shown to be associated with poor

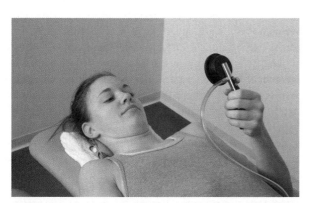

**FIGURE 6-7** Craniocervical flexion test and training program with airbag pressure biofeedback device.

---

**BOX 6-1** The Craniocervical Flexion Test[28]

1. The starting position:
   a. The testing position is in crook lying with the craniocervical and cervical spine in a mid range neutral position. For the neutral neck position, position with a horizontal face line and a horizontal line bisecting the neck longitudinally.
   b. Layers of towel may be placed under the head to achieve the neutral position. Ensure that the towel is aligned with the base of the occiput and the upper cervical region is free to move.
2. Preparation of the stabilizer (pressure biofeedback unit):
   a. Fold the blue airbag of the stabilizer and clip it together.
   b. Place the stabilizer behind the suboccipital region of the neck.
   c. Inflate the stabilizer to 20 mm Hg.
3. The formal test:
   Stage 1: The craniocervical flexion action:
   a. Explain that the test is assessing the precision and control to determine whether the patient can use the deep neck muscles and hold a contraction.
   b. Explain the movement to the patient and describe the craniocervical flexion as "gently nodding your head as though you were saying yes."
   c. Let the patient practice the movement to ensure that the patient is performing a pure nod but not head retraction or lifting of the head.
   d. Instruct the patient to place the front one third of the tongue on the roof of the mouth, with the lips together but the teeth slightly separated to relax the jaw.
   e. The movement should be performed gently and slowly.
   f. Turn the dial to the patient.
   g. Ask the patient to slowly nod to target 22 mm Hg and then 24 mm Hg and in turn 26, 28, and 30 mm Hg. The therapist observes the head movement and watches for a pattern of progressively increasing craniocervical flexion with each stage of the test. The therapist does not watch the dial but observes for proper head movements.
   Stage 2: Testing the holding capacity of the deep neck flexors:
   a. Instruct the patient to gently and slowly nod to target 22 mm Hg and attempt to hold the position steadily for 10 seconds with a good quality craniovertebral nodding movement.
   b. If successful at 22–mm Hg pressure, have the patient relax and repeat at each target pressure separately at 2–mm Hg increments up to a maximum of 30 mm Hg.
   c. Once the maximum pressure that the patient can hold steady with a good quality of movement and with minimal superficial muscle activity is determined, use this pressure level to measure endurance capacity (i.e., 10 repetitions of 10-second holds).
4. Normal performance of deep neck flexors:
   Normal performance is the achievement of pressure of at least 26 mm Hg with the pressure held steady for 10 seconds with 10 repetitions. Ideal performance is to successfully target and hold 28 to 30 mm Hg. The craniocervical flexion action should be able to be performed without dominant activity in the superficial muscles of the neck.

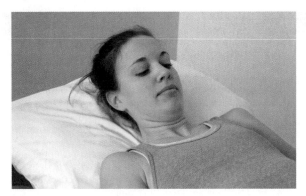

**FIGURE 6-8** Strengthening exercise for anterior neck flexor muscles.

outcomes 6 months after whiplash injury.[25] Patients with ongoing moderate/severe symptoms at 2 to 3 years after the initial injury continue to have decreased range of motion (ROM), increased electromyographic (EMG) activity of the superficial neck muscles during the craniocervical flexion test (an indication of inhibition of the deep neck flexors), sensory hypersensitivity, and elevated levels of psychological distress when compared with individuals with full recovery or milder symptoms.[25] Higher initial neck disability index (NDI) scores (>30), older age, cold hyperalgia, and posttraumatic stress symptoms are significant predictors of poor outcomes.[25] Therefore, motor, sensory, and psychological factors should be assessed during the acute stage after whiplash injury.

Gentle manual therapy techniques, including isometric manipulation, may be helpful to restore limited mobility associated with WAD, but the patient must be monitored closely to ensure pain is not provoked with the treatment approach. Intermittent use of a cervical collar may be beneficial to provide relative rest through the day. Frequent short doses of exercises (10 repetitions, 4 to 5 times per day) with emphasis on training the deep neck flexors and the postural scapular muscles can assist in motor retaining, postural correction, and pain inhibition. More vigorous manipulation techniques can be used to the thoracic spine to inhibit neck pain[30] and restore thoracic mobility. Gradual progression of an aerobic exercise program that is enjoyable for the patient, such as walking or biking within the patient's pain tolerance, can also assist in pain management.

## CERVICAL SPINE INSTABILITY

Clinical instability is defined by Panjabi[31] as the inability of the spine under physiological loads to maintain its pattern of displacement so that no neurological damage or irritation, no development of deformity, and no incapacitating pain occur.

The total range of motion of a spinal segment may be divided into the neutral zone and the elastic zone.[32,33] Motion that occurs in and around the neutral mid position of the spine is produced against minimal passive resistance (i.e., neutral zone), and motion that occurs near the end range of spinal motion is produced against increased passive resistance (i.e.,

elastic zone).[31,34] Clinical instability is believed to be a result of increase in the size of the neutral zone and reduction in the passive resistance to motion created in the elastic zone.

Panjabi[31] conceptualized the components of spinal stability into three functionally integrated subsystems of the spinal stabilizing system. According to Panjabi,[31] the stabilizing system of the spine consists of the passive, active, and neural control subsystems.

The passive subsystem consists of the vertebral bodies, facet joints and joint capsules, spinal ligaments, and passive tension from spinal muscles and tendons. The passive subsystem provides significant stabilization of the elastic zone and limits the size of the neutral zone. Also, the components of the passive subsystem act as transducers and provide the neural control subsystem with information about vertebral position and motion.

The active subsystem, which consists of spinal muscles and tendons, generates the forces needed to stabilize the spine in response to changing loads. The active subsystem is primarily responsible for controlling the motion that occurs within the neutral zone and contributes to maintaining the size of the neutral zone. The spinal muscles also act as transducers that provide the neural control subsystem with information about the forces generated by each muscle.

Through peripheral nerves and the central nervous system, the neural control subsystem receives information from the transducers of the passive and active subsystems about vertebral position, vertebral motion, and forces generated by spinal muscles. With that information, the neural control subsystem determines the requirements for spinal stability and acts on the spinal muscles to produce the required forces.

Clinical spinal instability occurs when the neutral zone increases relative to the total range of motion, the stabilizing subsystems are unable to compensate for this increase, and the quality of motion in the neutral zone becomes poor and uncontrolled.[31-33] Degeneration and mechanical injury of the spinal stabilization components are the primary causes of increases in neutral zone size.[31] Factors that contribute to degeneration or mechanical injury of the stabilizing components are poor posture, repetitive occupational trauma, acute trauma, and weakness of the cervical musculature.[31,35-37]

Because poor quality of motion is a key aspect of clinical instability, the presence of aberrant motions during active movement has been suggested by several authors to be a cardinal sign of clinical instability.[38,39] Aberrant motions are described as either sudden accelerations or decelerations of movement or motions that occur outside the intended plane of movement.[38,40] Other signs and symptoms of cervical clinical instability are general tenderness of the cervical region, referred pain in the shoulder and parascapular area, cervical radiculopathy, cervical myelopathy, occipital and frontal/retroorbital headaches, paraspinal muscle spasm, decreased cervical lordosis, and pain with sustained postures.[33,35,38,41-43] Also, passive intervertebral motion and joint play test results may reveal hypermobility and decreased passive restraints to motion at the end range of passive spinal segmental motion (i.e., a loose end feel).[44] Imaging studies may show alterations of the components of the passive subsystem, such as ligament damage, osteophytes, vertebral fractures, disc degeneration, vertebral displacement, and facet subluxation.[31,32,36,45-47]

Cook et al[48] used a Delphi survey method to establish consensus among orthopaedic manual physical therapy (OMPT) experts on the signs and symptoms of clinical cervical spine instability and reported the following symptoms as reaching the highest consensus: "intolerance to prolonged static postures"; "fatigue and inability to hold head up"; "better with external support, including hands and collar"; "frequent need for self-manipulation"; "feeling of instability, shaking, or lack of control"; "frequent episodes of acute attacks"; and "sharp pain, possibly with sudden movements."[48] The physical examination findings related to cervical instability that reached highest consensus among the clinical OMPT experts were: "poor coordination/neuromuscular control, including poor recruitment and dissociation of cervical segments with movement"; "abnormal joint play"; "motion that is not smooth throughout range of motion, including segmental hinging, pivoting, and fulcruming"; and "aberrant movement."[48]

Objective criteria have been established in the analysis of end-range flexion and extension radiographs for diagnosis of cervical spine instability.[38,42,49,50] However, radiographs do not yield information about the quantity or quality of motion that occurs in the neutral zone (i.e., mid range), which limits the value of radiographs in the diagnosis of cervical spine clinical instabilities.[38,46] Video fluoroscopy shows some promise as a means to analyze the quality of spine motion at mid range, but its use is still experimental for this purpose. Passive intervertebral motion and joint play testing have diagnostic value with assessment of neutral zone size, but the tests have poor interrater reliability and only assess passive motion.[34,51] Because a definitive diagnostic tool for cervical spine clinical instability has not been established, cervical clinical instability continues to be diagnosed on clinical findings, including history, subjective symptoms, visual analysis of active motion quality, and manual examination methods.[44]

When cervical clinical instability does not severely involve or threaten neurological structures, nonsurgical treatment is indicated. The goal of nonsurgical treatment is to enhance the function of the spinal stabilizing subsystems and to decrease the stresses on the involved spinal segments. With proper training, the subsystems are more capable of compensating for an increase in neutral zone size.[31]

Posture education and spinal manipulation may decrease stresses on the passive subsystem.[52] Proper posture reduces the loads placed on spinal segments at end-ranges and returns the spine to a biomechanically efficient position.[52] Spinal manipulation can be performed on hypomobile segments above and below the level of instability.[52] With improved mobility of these segments, spinal movement is thought to be more evenly distributed across several segments and mechanical stresses on the level of clinical instability are thought to be decreased.[52]

Strengthening exercises enhance the function of the active subsystem.[31] The cervical multifidus may provide stability via segmental attachments to cervical vertebrae, and the longus coli and longus capitus may provide anterior stability as a result of the position of the muscle anterior to the cervical vertebral bodies. Strengthening the stabilizing muscles of the cervical spine enables these muscles to improve the quality and control of movement that occurs within the neutral zone.[44] Jull, Kristjansson, and Dall'Alba[28] identified muscle synergy impairments between the superficial and deep anterior cervical spine muscles in patients with both insidious onset and whiplash neck pain disorders. When compared with a healthy population, both groups of patients excessively activated the sternocleidomastoid (SCM) muscles when performing an active craniocervical flexion motion in supine. Previous research by Falla[53] showed that when there is overactivation of the SCM measured with a surface EMG, underactivation of the deep anterior neck muscles tends to occur; the longus capitis in synergy with the longus colli.[53] Falla[53] also showed deficits in the motor control of the deep and superficial cervical flexor muscles in people with chronic neck pain, characterized by a delay in onset of neck muscle contraction associated with movement of the upper limb, cognitive activity, and functional tasks; Falla suggests a rehabilitation program to address retraining to restore the coordination of the deep neck flexor muscles and inhibit the superficial anterior neck muscles. Ylinen et al[54] showed positive outcomes in treatment of patients with chronic neck pain with more gross dynamic neck exercises and less attention to the activation and coordination of the deep neck flexors. Falla[53] suggests starting with a retraining/coordination approach and then progressing into an endurance and strengthening approach.

Jull et al[55] performed a randomized controlled trial to compare the effects of manipulation, manipulation combined with specific postural and deep neck flexor strengthening, specific neck exercises alone and a control group. In all outcome measures, both the specific exercise and the manipulation combined with specific exercise treatment groups showed superior outcomes. This study showed the importance and effectiveness of an approach that uses specific training of the deep neck flexors and postural muscles in the rehabilitation of patients with neck pain.[55]

When cervical spine instability is seen with severe neurological involvement, surgery is the primary treatment intervention. The anterior cervical fusion is the most common surgical intervention.[56] Postsurgical rehabilitation involves a similar approach as treatment of instability with progression of low level strengthening exercises for the anterior cervical and parascapular postural muscles.

## CERVICAL RADICULOPATHY

Cervical radiculopathy (CR) is a disorder of the spinal nerve root commonly caused by cervical disc herniation or other space-occupying lesion, such as spondylitic spurs or cervical osteophytes, resulting in nerve root inflammation, impingement, or both.[57,58] CR is usually present with pain in the neck and one arm, loss of motor function, or reflex changes in the affected nerve root distribution. The most common cause of CR (in 70% to 75% of cases) is foraminal encroachment of the spinal nerve from a combination of factors, including decreased disc height and degenerative changes of the uncovertebral joints anteriorly and zygapophysial joints posteriorly (i.e., cervical spondylosis).[58] Herniation of the intervertebral disc is responsible for only about 25% of the cases.[58] Other space-occupying lesions such as tumors are rarely the cause of CR.[59]

Cervical radiculopathy must be differentiated from other possible causes of upper extremity pain, which might include thoracic outlet syndrome; referral patterns from cervical and upper thoracic anatomical structures; shoulder girdle impairments, such as a rotator cuff impingement; elbow impairments, such as lateral epicondylitis; and wrist/hand impairments, such as carpal tunnel syndrome. Chapter 2 describes upper extremity screening examination procedures. At the very least, active and passive range of motion and palpation should be carried out to screen each region of the upper quarter. Depending on the pain pattern, symptom behavior, and response to these initial screening procedures, additional upper extremity special tests and accessory motion testing should also be carried out. The goal of the examination is differentiation of local pain from referred pain and referred pain from true radicular (i.e., nerve root) pain.

Wainner et al[60] identified a test item cluster of four clinical examination procedures for identification of patients with cervical radiculopathy that was confirmed and correlated with electrodiagnostic testing if all four test items were positive. The four test items include positive Spurling A, neck distraction test, upper limb neurodynamic test 1 (ULNT 1), and limited ipsilateral cervical spine active range of motion of 60 degrees or less.[60]

The single best test in Wainner et al's study[60] for screening for CR was ULNT 1, with a change in probability of the presence of the condition from 23% to 3% when the test results were negative. If the ULNT 1 results are negative, CR can be essentially ruled out. If three of the four test cluster items are positive, the probability of the condition increases to 65%. If all four variables are present, the probability increases to 90%.[60]

Waldrop[61] used the test item cluster developed by Wainner and colleagues and reported on a case series of six patients who met the diagnostic criteria for CR. The six patients were treated for a mean of 10 visits (range, 5 to 18) over an average of 33 days (range, 19 to 56 days). Four of the six patients had a magnetic resonance imaging (MRI) scan performed that confirmed cervical nerve root encroachment or impingement. Reductions in pain and disability were reported with all six patients with a treatment approach that included thoracic thrust manipulation techniques, patient education on proper posture, cervical range of motion and deep neck flexor strengthening exercises, and mechanical cervical traction (Figure 6-9). Cleland et al[57] reported on a similar treatment approach that combined manual physical therapy, cervical traction, and specific neck and parascapular muscle exercises to successfully treat a case series of 10 of 11 patients who met the criteria for cervical radiculopathy.[57] The multimodular intervention approach in this case

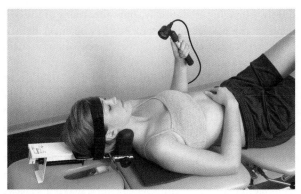

**FIGURE 6-9** Cervical mechanical traction with portable hydraulic traction device.

series was based on available evidence and clinical experience and is a reasonable approach to consider for physical therapy management of this condition. Upper-extremity neurodynamic active and passive motion exercises can also be added to the treatment program. The upper-limb neurodynamic test positions that reproduce upper-extremity symptoms are used to the point of tension (i.e., "neural glide mobilizations") and performed repeatedly as part of the treatment program. Randomized controlled trials (RCTs) need to be performed to determine the best evidence-based approach for CR.

## CERVICAL HYPOMOBILITY

When the primary dysfunction is stiffness of the cervical spine, as noted with active, passive, and passive intervertebral motion testing, and in the absence of arm symptoms, specific spinal manipulation techniques are indicated as the primary intervention. The specific application of technique depends on a number of factors. Skilled manual physical therapists tend to base their clinical judgment of technique selection on multiple factors, including joint mobility and end feel assessment, tissue reactivity, acuity of onset, nature of the symptoms, the patient's emotional state and expectations, and the clinician's manual skill level.

Hoving et al[62] recently showed in a high-quality RCT that physical therapists with advanced training in specific manipulation skills produced significantly better outcomes in treating patients with neck pain compared with both physical therapists with more general training and general medical practitioners. At the 7-week follow-up examination, the results showed a 68% success rate for the patients treated with specific nonthrust manipulation techniques and specific exercises provided by the physical therapists with advanced training in manual therapy compared with a 51% success rate for the patients treated by the physical therapists with more general training and a 36% success rate for patients treated by a general medical practitioner. Korthals-de Bos et al[63] published a cost-analysis study based on the Hoving clinical trial and reported that manual physical therapy required fewer treatment sessions for a more favorable outcome, with the cost of the manual physical therapy about one third the cost of the other two treatment groups. Korthals-de Bos et al[63] concluded that manual physical therapy was more cost effective for treatment of neck pain than general physical therapy or general practitioner care.

A recent Cochrane systematic review of randomized clinical trials concluded that thrust or nonthrust manipulation techniques used with exercise are beneficial for persistent mechanical neck disorders with or without headache.[64] Performed alone, when compared with each other, neither thrust nor nonthrust techniques were superior for treatment of cervical spine disorders.[64] At this time, research data have not been fully developed to identify subgroups of patient who will respond more favorably to various types of manipulation techniques, such as thrust versus nonthrust versus isometric manipulations. These decisions are based more on clinical decision making with clinician experience, the opinions of clinical experts, and the comfort level/skill of the practitioner with various techniques.

Isometric manipulation procedures tend to be most effective when a high level of reactivity has been identified at the hypomobile joint (e.g., when the patient has pain before engaging the barrier to the passive joint motion and reflexive muscle guarding is noted with the passive motion). In this situation, the patient may not tolerate direct sustained force at the joint and the isometric forces likely are tolerated more effectively. This type of situation is often found when the patient has a recent sudden onset of sharp localized neck pain that was brought on by a minor incident, such as suddenly looking up to reach for a cup on a high shelf. The active and passive motion is painful and limited with lateral flexion and rotation toward the painful side. A specific area of tenderness with overlying muscle holding is noted at a particular facet joint. Once the segment is isolated, an isometric manipulation can be used to restore motion and at the same time enhance neuromuscular control of the targeted segment.

Theoretically, the anatomical cause of this type of sudden onset of neck pain is the result of the entrapment of the facet joint meniscus. With a sudden awkward movement, the meniscus becomes entrapped within the edge of the facet joint, which can cause severe pain with attempts to load or move the involved joint. The entrapment can be released with use of the isometric forces directed to the targeted joint or with a thrust manipulation technique that creates joint distraction or gapping. Often, dramatic restoration of joint motion is noted after the first intervention. Subsequent treatments can assist in correcting surrounding joint and muscle impairments as needed for full rehabilitation.

A more gradual onset of joint stiffness is characteristic of osteoarthritic joint changes, adaptive shortening of joint connective tissues, or adhesion formation after recovery from trauma to the spinal segment or surrounding soft tissues. Postural stresses are believed to contribute to these impairments. Various degrees of joint hypomobility can be identified throughout the spine and various levels of joint reactivity are noted at the hypomobile spinal segments. The stronger thrust and nonthrust manipulation techniques tend to be used to target the less reactive joints with hypomobility. The lighter oscillatory nonthrust techniques can be used on joints with higher levels of reactivity and surrounding muscle guarding.

A clinical prediction rule has been developed to identify patients who are likely to report immediate positive response to a cervical thrust manipulation.[65] If four of the six variables are present, an 89% chance exists of an immediate positive response to the manipulation, which was measured in the study as either a 50% reduction in pain scale score, a 4-point change in global perceived effect, or a report of high satisfaction with the treatment.[65] Box 6-2 outlines the six variables that make up the clinical prediction rule. The rule has not yet been validated with a clinical trial, but it provides some preliminary data to predict which patients are likely to have a dramatic immediate response to a thrust manipulation of the cervical spine.

Thrust manipulation techniques directed to the thoracic spine have also been shown as an effective means to provide immediate relief of neck pain.[30] Cleland et al[30] developed a clinical prediction rule (CPR) to identify patients with neck pain who will most likely benefit from thoracic spine thrust manipulation for relief of neck pain. The clinical prediction rule was developed on a group of 78 patients with neck pain who all received thrust manipulation to the upper and mid thoracic spine. The thoracic spine segments that were regarded as hypomobile from a clinical examination were targeted for manipulation by the physical therapist. The patients were classified as having had a successful outcome on the second or third visit based on patient perceived recovery using the global rating of change scale. A stepwise logistic regression model was used to determine what common characteristics from the initial patient examination findings predicted a successful outcome with the thoracic manipulation. Six variables were identified for the CPR. If three of six variables (positive likelihood ratio, 5.5) were present (Box 6-3), the chance of a successful outcome improved from 54% to 86%.[30]

In summary, for patients with neck pain and no symptoms beyond the shoulder, thoracic and cervical spine manipulation techniques can be used to effectively restore spinal mobility, reduce pain, and improve perceptions of disability. Spinal segments that have hypomobility with passive intervertebral motion testing are targeted for manipulation. The manipulation technique can be modified with variations in depth of force, duration of force, speed of application of force, and use of isometric versus direct forces. High levels of fear-avoidance

| **BOX 6-2** | CPR to Identify Patients with Immediate Response to a Cervical High-Velocity Thrust Manipulation[65] |
|---|---|

Initial NDI, <23%
Bilateral involvement pattern
Not performing sedentary work >5 hours per day
Feeling better while moving the neck
Not feeling worse when extending the neck
Diagnosis of spondylosis without radiculopathy

---

**BOX 6-3    Six Variables That Form the Clinical Prediction Rule for Thoracic Manipulation to Treat Neck Pain[30]**

- Symptoms <30 days
- No symptoms distal to the shoulder
- Looking up does not aggravate symptoms
- Fear Avoidance Beliefs Questionnaire Physical Activity (FABQPA) score <12
- Diminished upper thoracic spine kyphosis (visual estimate)
- Cervical extension ROM <30 degrees (inclinometer)

---

beliefs with high levels of anxiety over movement seem to influence the potential effectiveness of manipulation procedures. This influence has come out as a factor in clinical prediction rules for both the cervical spine and the lumbar spine.[21,30,53] Manipulation can still be used with patients with high levels of fear-avoidance beliefs, but other strategies may be needed to effectively deal with the fear of movement, such as a positive reinforcement for active participation in the rehabilitation process, active exercise programs, and perhaps psychological counseling.

The Cochrane systematic review of RCTs on treatment of cervical spine disorders clearly states that mobilization/manipulation is most effective if combined with exercise.[64] Some variability exists in the literature regarding specifically what type of exercise should be used to create the most effective clinical outcomes. Jull and colleagues[28] advocate specific strengthening exercises to target the deep anterior neck flexor muscles combined with stretching muscles that tend to tighten, such as the levator scapulae and the upper trapezuis, and strengthen the scapular adductor and retractor muscles. Cleland et al[30] had the patients in their study follow up the thoracic spine manipulation with more general cervical range-of-motion exercise that combined a nodding motion in three positions of cervical rotation. Others have advocated for a more general strengthening and full body endurance program for rehabilitation of neck pain disorders.

Use of a problem-solving impairment approach tends to follow components of all three possible recommendations depending on the findings of the clinical examination and reexamination of patients as they proceed through the rehabilitation process. If weakness is noted in the deep neck flexors or parascapular muscles, specific exercises should be instructed to target the strength and endurance of these muscles. If tightness is noted in specific muscles of the upper quarter, specific stretching should be integrated into the treatment approach. Self-mobilization techniques for the thoracic spine (see Box 5-1 in Chapter 5) can also be helpful to enhance the patient's home program for pain control and thoracic mobility. As specific impairments are addressed, a general exercise program is recommended that includes endurance training to enhance the patient's tolerance to functional activities and to assist in pain control through the beneficial analgesic effects associated with aerobic exercise.

The ultimate goal of the rehabilitation program is to restore mobility, inhibit pain, and return the patient to full functional activity. In the process, the physical therapist provides the patient with strategies to self treat and maintain the improvements made in the physical therapy sessions. Early in the rehabilitation process, a good deal of manual therapy procedures are provided and only mild low-level exercises are instructed. As the physical therapy program progresses, less manual therapy is needed and the exercise program duration and intensity are progressed under the direction of the physical therapist. Once the patient is independent in the exercise program and in self-management principles, further skilled physical therapy is no longer needed.

Specific exercises emphasize cervical stabilization and control, thoracic mobility, and scapular muscle strengthening (Box 6-4). The primary goals of the exercise program are to enhance neuromuscular control of the upper quarter, correct posture, and maintain mobility attained with the manual therapy techniques. In addition to the specific strengthening program, most patients benefit from the addition of a low-impact aerobic exercise program with an exercise that interests the patient and can fit into the patient's lifestyle, such as a walking program or use of an elliptical trainer.

## CERVICOGENIC HEADACHE

Cervicogenic headaches are believed to originate from musculoskeletal dysfunction of the cervical spine.[66] The incidence of cervicogenic headache is estimated to be 14% to 18% of all chronic headaches.[67] Box 6-5 provides the diagnostic criteria developed by Sjaastad and colleagues[68] for diagnosis of cervicogenic headache, with one of the primary criteria being headache pain elicited by pressure on the posterior neck, especially at one of the three upper cervical joints.

The clinical tests that have been shown to further assist in differentiating patients with cervicogenic headache from patients with migraine with an aura and controls include, in patients with cervicogenic headache, less cervical range of motion flexion/extension, a significantly higher incidence of upper three cervical joint dysfunctions (facet joint hypomobility and tenderness to palpation assessed by manual examination), and muscle length limitations (tightness of upper trapezius, levator scapula, scalenes, and suboccipital extensor muscles). Zito[66] found that manual examination could discriminate the cervicogenic headache group from other subjects (migraine with an aura and control subjects combined) with an 80% sensitivity. Zito[66] found that not all hypomobile joints were painful, but all painful joints were hypomobile in the patients with cervicogenic headaches. However, no differences were found among groups in this study for examination results of static posture, pressure pain threshold, mechanosensitivity of neural tissues, and measures of cervical kinesthetic sense. The patients in the cervicogenic headache group demonstrated poorer performance in the craniocervical flexion test, but this finding did not reach statistical significance.[66] Therefore, patients with cervicogenic headache present with a similar set

**BOX 6-4** Therapeutic Exercises for Cervical Spine Disorders

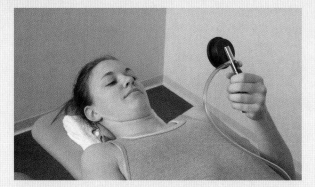

Supine craniocervical flexion (nodding)

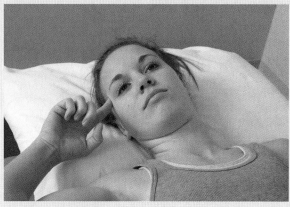

Supine cervical rotation with manual resistance

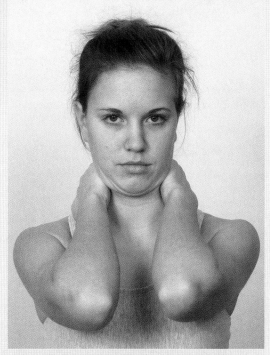

Standing craniocervical flexion with mid cervical manual stabilization

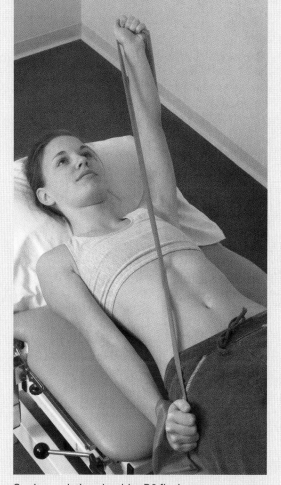

Supine resistive shoulder D2 flexion

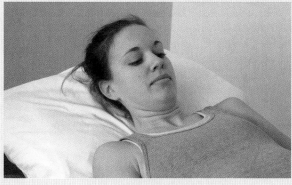

Supine craniocervical flexion with sustained lift

*Continued*

**BOX 6-4**    Therapeutic Exercises for Cervical Spine Disorders—cont'd

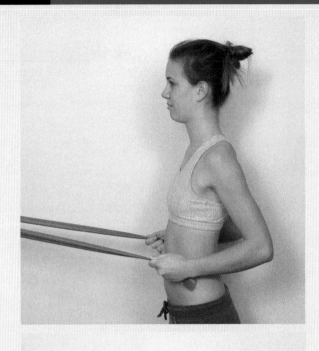

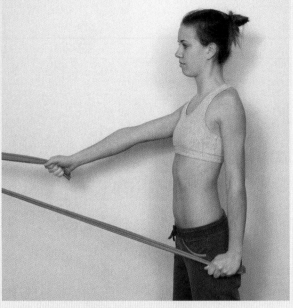

Standing resistive shoulder extension: reciprocal

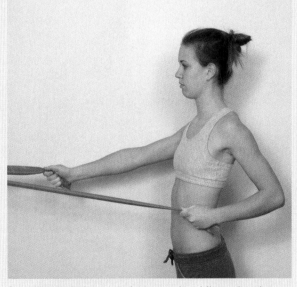

Standing resistive scapular retraction: bilateral and reciprocal

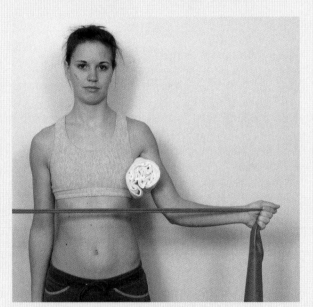

Standing resistive shoulder external rotation

| BOX 6-4 | Therapeutic Exercises for Cervical Spine Disorders—*cont'd* |
|---|---|

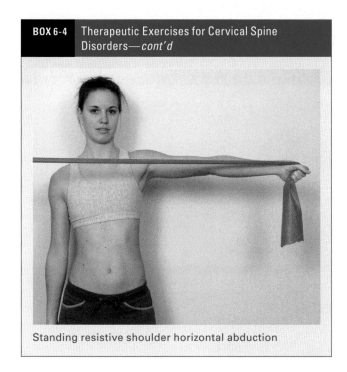

Standing resistive shoulder horizontal abduction

| BOX 6-5 | Diagnostic Criteria for Cervicogenic Headache |
|---|---|

**Major Criteria**
1. Symptoms and signs of neck involvement (one or more of points 1 (a-c) must be present to diagnose)
   a. Precipitation of head pain, similar to the usually occurring one, by:
      i. Neck movement or sustained awkward head positioning and/or
      ii. External pressure over the upper cervical or occipital region on the symptomatic side
   b. Restriction of range of motion in the neck
   c. Ipsilateral neck, shoulder, or arm pain
2. Confirmatory evidence by diagnostic anesthetic blocks (i.e., reduce headache with block of major or minor occipital nerves, C2 nerve root, or the third occipital nerve) necessary for research, but not clinical purposes to confirm diagnosis
3. Unilateral head pain without sideshift (i.e., primary headache is on one side of the head most of the time)
4. Head pain characteristics
   a. Moderate-severe, nonthrobbing and non-lancinating pain, usually starting in the neck
   b. Episodes of varying duration
   c. Fluctuating continuous pain

**Other Characteristics of Importance**
5. a. Only marginal effects or lack of effect of medication (indomethacin, ergotamine, and sumatriptan)
   b. Female sex
   c. Not infrequent history of head or indirect neck trauma, usually of more than medium severity

**Other Features of Lesser Importance**
6. Various attack-related phenomena, only occasionally present, and/or moderately expressed when present
   a. Nausea
   b. Phonophobia and photophobia
   c. Dizziness
   d. Ipsilateral blurred vision
   e. Difficulties swallowing
   f. Ipsilateral edema, mostly in the periocular area

Adapted from Sjaastad O, Fredriksen TA, Pfaffenrath V: *Headache* 38:442-445, 1998.

of impairments as do patients with cervical spine instability or hypomobility, but their primary complaint is headache.

Jull[55] completed a randomized controlled trial comparing physical therapy interventions for treatment of 200 patients who met the diagnostic criteria for cervicogenic headache developed by Sjaastad and collegues[68] who were randomly placed in one of the four physical therapy treatment groups of manual therapy, exercise therapy, combined manual therapy and exercise, and a control group. Beneficial effects were found for headache frequency and intensity and neck pain and disability for both manual therapy and exercise used alone and in combination at both 7 weeks and 12 months follow-up.[55] Of the participants receiving combined manual therapy and exercise, 10% more obtained good and excellent results, lending support for the combined use of specific therapeutic exercise and manual therapy to treat patients with cervicogenic headaches.[55]

The manual therapy procedures employed by the physical therapists participating in Jull's study[55] included both thrust and nonthrust manipulation techniques to the cervical spine. The therapeutic exercise regimen incorporated use of a pressure biofeedback unit to train the deep neck flexors, the longus capitus and colli, which are believed to be important in supporting the function of the cervical region.[55] Additionally, the exercise regimen included training the muscles of the scapula, particularly the lower trapezius and serratus anterior muscles, to hold scapular adduction and retraction postural positions.[55]

Postural instruction and training of the deep neck rotator muscles were also included in the exercise regimen.[55] Muscle-lengthening exercises were also incorporated based on the needs of the patient. Patients received 8 to 12 treatment sessions with a physical therapist over a 6-week period. The physical therapists were allowed to vary their treatments based on the initial examination and subsequent re-examinations of the patients in the treatment groups.[55] Jull's study illustrates the effectiveness of an impairment-based manual physical therapy approach that combines manual therapy and exercise for treatment of patients with cervicogenic headache.

## SELECTED SPECIAL TESTS FOR CERVICAL SPINE EXAMINATION

### Sharp-Purser Test  [DVD]

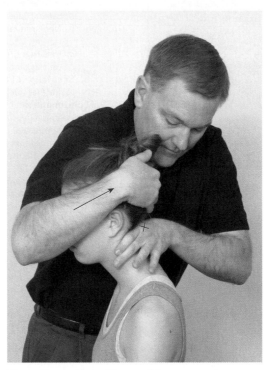

Sharp-Purser test with use of forearm and shoulder to glide head

| | |
|---|---|
| **PURPOSE** | This test is used to detect atlantoaxial instability. |
| **PATIENT POSITION** | The patient is seated and asked to relax the head in a semiflexed position. |
| **THERAPIST POSITION** | The therapist stands at the side of the patient. |
| **HAND PLACEMENT** | **Cranial hand:** The upper arm is placed across the front of the patient's forehead and the occiput is cupped with the hand. |
| | **Caudal hand:** The web space between the index finger and thumb is placed horizontally across the spinous process of C2. |
| **PROCEDURE** | The patient's forehead is pressed posteriorly with the cranial arm in a plane parallel with the superior aspect of C2 as the caudal hand provides a stabilizing force at C2. A sliding motion of the head posteriorly in relation to the axis is indicative of atlantoaxial instability. The manual maneuver reduces the atlantoaxial (AA) subluxation that occurs with a semi-flexed posture in patients with AA instability. Perception of excessive posterior glide of the cranium on the stabilized C2 or relief of pain with the manual gliding motion are considered positive findings. |
| **NOTES** | A positive Sharp-Purser test has been correlated with AA instability in patients with rheumatoid arthritis (RA) at a specificity of 96% and predictive value of 85%.[69] In this study, the results of the Sharp-Purser test were compared with flexion radiograph results and were considered positive for instability if the results measured greater than 4 mm at the interval between the anterior arch of the atlas and the axis. Positive Sharp-Purser test results indicate AA instability, which is a contraindication to cervical manipulation techniques that place strain through the craniovertebral region. Atlantoaxial instability is common in RA from weakening of the transverse portion of the cruciate ligament that stabilizes the dens to the anterior arch of the atlas. |

## Spurling's Test[70]

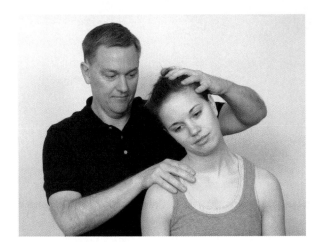

Spurling's test A

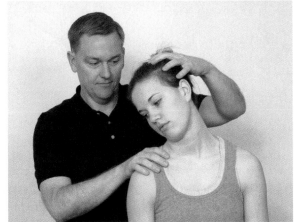

Spurling's test B

| | |
|---|---|
| **PURPOSE** | Results of this pain provocation test are considered positive for cervical nerve root irritation if the patient reports reproduction or intensification of peripheral symptoms with application of the test maneuver. |
| **PATIENT POSITION** | The patient is seated in a straight-backed chair. Having the patient face a mirror is also helpful to monitor pain facial expressions during the test. |
| **THERAPIST POSITION** | The therapist stands behind the patient. |
| **PROCEDURE** | The therapist passively side bends the head toward the symptomatic side and applies overpressure ($\approx$7 kg) to the patient's head in the direction of the side bending to perform Spurling's test A. |
| **NOTES** | If the patient reports neck or arm symptom reproduction related to the condition at any point during performance of the test, results are considered positive and no further application of force is needed. The procedure for Spurling's test B combines cervical extension and rotation with ipsilateral lateral flexion. Application of overpressure for Spurling's test B is the same as in Spurling's test A.[60] Wainner et al[60] reported Kappa of 0.60 (0.32, 0.87) for Spurling's test A and Kappa of 0.62 (0.25, 0.99) for Spurling's test B.<br><br>Spurling's test B was used on 255 patients who were referred for electrodiagnosis of the upper extremity nerve disorders.[71] Test results were scored positive if symptoms were reported beyond the elbow, and results were correlated with the results of the electrodiagnositic tests. The Spurling's test had a sensitivity of 30% and a specificity of 93%, which means that it is not a very useful screening tool but that it is clinically useful to help confirm cervical radiculopathy.[71]<br><br>Spurling's test A is one of the four findings for the clinical prediction rule for cervical radiculopathy.[60] |

## Shoulder Abduction Test

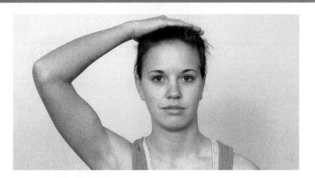

| | |
|---|---|
| **PURPOSE** | If this position alleviates the patient's radicular arm pain, nerve root irritation is suggested as the cause of the arm pain. |
| **PATIENT POSITION** | The patient is positioned sitting. |
| **PROCEDURE** | The patient is seated and asked to place the hand of the symptomatic extremity on the head. Positive test results occur with reduction or elimination of symptoms.[60] The therapist should ask open-ended questions with this test, such as, "Does this change your symptoms in any way?" |
| **NOTES** | Wainner et al[60] reported a Kappa value of 0.20 (0.00, 0.59). |

## Neck Distraction Test   (DVD)

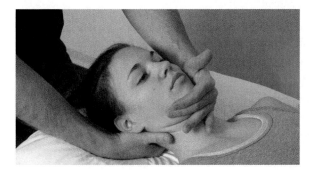
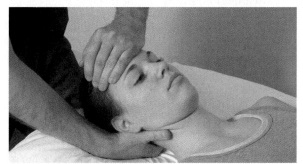

Neck distraction test with hand on forehead

| | |
|---|---|
| **PURPOSE** | Test results are positive if the patient reports a reduction of symptoms with application of cervical distraction force. The test is used to assist in diagnosis of cervical radiculopathy. |
| **PATIENT POSITION** | The patient is supine with the head resting on a small pillow and the crown of the head even with the top edge of the table. |
| **THERAPIST POSITION** | The therapist sits or stands at the head of the treatment table. |
| **HAND PLACEMENT** | **Dominant hand:** The fingers are together with the thumb spread across the occiput to cradle the posterior aspect of the patient's cranium. |
| | **Nondominant hand:** The therapist cups the patient's chin with the fingers or cups the anterior aspect of the patient's forehead. |
| **PROCEDURE** | The therapist flexes the patient's neck to a position of comfort by lifting the head off the pillow (20-25 degrees from horizontal) and gradually applies a distraction force up to 14 kg.[60] |
| **NOTES** | If this test alleviates symptoms, manual or mechanical cervical traction should be incorporated into the plan of care. The therapist should ask open-ended questions with this test such as, "Does this change your symptoms in any way?" Wainner et al[60] reported a Kappa value of 0.88 (0.64, 1.0). This test is one of the four findings for the clinical prediction rule to diagnose cervical radiculopathy.[60] |

## Neck Traction Test

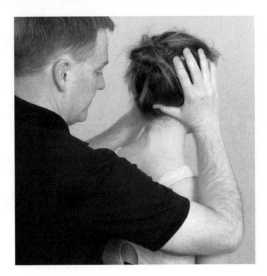

| | |
|---|---|
| **PURPOSE** | Test results are positive if the patient reports a reduction of upper-extremity radicular symptoms with application of cervical distraction force. The test is used to detect signs of cervical radiculopathy. |
| **PATIENT POSITION** | The patient sits or stands (preferably facing a mirror). |
| **THERAPIST POSITION** | The therapist sits or stands directly behind the patient. |
| **HAND PLACEMENT** | The thumbs and thenar eminences of both hands are molded across the inferior aspect of the patient's occiput and the mastoid processes, with the forearms placed across the superior aspect of the patient's shoulders. |
| **PROCEDURE** | The therapist gradually applies a distraction force by lifting the patient's head superiorly to create cervical traction. Test results are positive if the patient's symptoms are alleviated during the traction. |
| **NOTES** | If this test alleviates symptoms, manual or mechanical cervical traction should be incorporated into the plan of care. The therapist should ask open-ended questions with this test such as, "Does this change your symptoms in any way?" Bertilson, Grunnesjo, and Strender[72] reported Kappa scores of 0.49 if the therapist did not have knowledge of the patient's history and Kappa scores of 0.45 if the therapist had knowledge of the patient's history when this test was performed on 100 patients with neck or shoulder problems with or without radiating pain. |

## Vertebral Artery Test: Cervical Rotation Supine    DVD

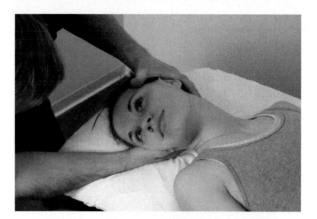

| | |
|---|---|
| **PURPOSE** | The purpose of this test is to screen for vertebral artery insufficiency and collateral circulation to the brain. |
| **PATIENT POSITION** | The patient is supine with the head on a pillow and the top of the head even with the top edge of the table. |
| **THERAPIST POSITION** | The therapist stands at the head of the patient. |
| **HAND PLACEMENT** | **Left hand:** The hand supports the left side of the patient's head with the fingers spread. |
| | **Right hand:** The hand supports the right side of the patient's head with the fingers spread. |
| **PROCEDURE** | The therapist must instruct the patient to look at the therapist's forehead throughout the procedure, and the therapist must move with the patient to maintain a clear view of the patient's eyes throughout the procedure to assess for nystagmus. The therapist must also continually seek verbal feedback from the patient throughout the test. A delayed response or a report of dizziness, lightheadedness, or nausea is considered positive. As the therapist supports the patient's head, the cervical spine is slowly rotated to the right to the end of available range. The therapist pauses in this position for 3 to 5 seconds to assess the patient's response. If the test results are still negative, the therapist gently adds lateral flexion to the right and extension and holds this position for 5 to 10 seconds. If the test results are negative, the therapist repeats to the opposite side. |
| **NOTES** | If the patient has a positive response, the therapist repositions the head to a neutral or slightly flexed position immediately and continues to monitor the patient. The therapist supports the patient's head on one or two pillows and passively positions the patient's legs in a 90/90 position either on a stool or on the therapist's shoulders. The therapist continues to monitor the patient until the positive response completely subsides. |
| | Cote et al[75] showed that this test has a sensitivity of approximately 0, which indicates a high likelihood of false-negative results from this commonly performed screening examination procedure. See Chapter 3 for more information regarding premanipulation screening. |

## Vertebral Artery Test: Standing (Body on Head Rotation Test)

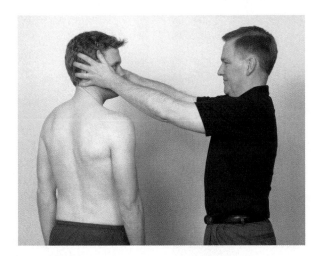

| | |
|---|---|
| **PURPOSE** | This test screens for vertebral artery insufficiency and collateral circulation to the brain while avoiding vestibular activation by avoiding inner ear movements. |
| **PATIENT POSITION** | The patient stands directly facing the therapist. |
| **THERAPIST POSITION** | The therapist stands in front of the patient and holds each side of the patient's head. |
| **PROCEDURE** | As the therapist holds the patient's head, the patient is asked to rotate the body fully toward one side and hold that position for 10 seconds as the therapist monitors the patient's response. The procedure is repeated toward the opposite direction. |
| **NOTES** | If this test provokes patient dizziness, the patient should be referred for a medical consultation to further assess the vertebral artery and collateral circulation to the brain. If dizziness is noted with the supine test but does not occur with this test, the patient may be a candidate for vestibular rehabilitation. |

## Upper Limb Neurodynamic Test 1[73,74]    🔘DVD

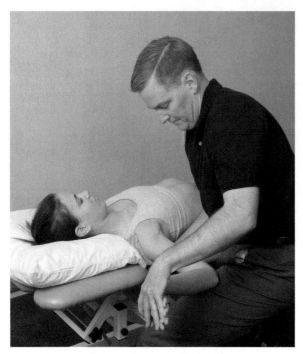

Upper limb neurodynamic test 1, start position

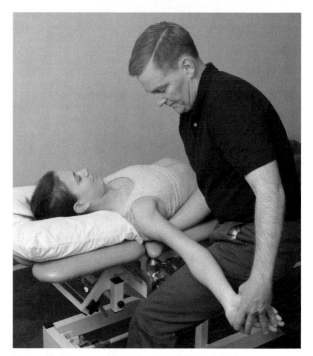

Upper limb neurodynamic test 1, end position

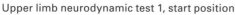

| | |
|---|---|
| **PURPOSE** | The purpose of this test is to apply tension though the brachial plexus and nerve root sleeves of the cervical spine to determine whether the cause of upper extremity symptoms originates from irritation of the cervical nerve roots and surrounding connective tissues. In theory, ULNT 1 is designed to focus tension on the median nerve and its corresponding nerve roots. |
| **PATIENT POSITION** | The patient lies supine with the arm to be tested in the start position of 90 degrees shoulder abduction, 10 degrees horizontal extension, and 90 degrees elbow flexion. |
| **THERAPIST POSITION** | The therapist stands with a diagonal stance on the side to be tested with the most lateral leg forward and the thigh positioned up against the inferior aspect of the upper arm and the patient's shoulder positioned at 90 degrees abduction. |
| **HAND PLACEMENT** | **Left hand:** The left hand reaches up and under the posterior aspect of the patient's scapula to place the hand across the posterior and superior aspect of the scapula to depress the shoulder girdle. |
| | **Right hand:** The therapist's other hand is placed across the palmar surface of the patient's left hand and fingers. |
| **PROCEDURE** | The therapist passively depresses the patient's scapula with the shoulder in 90 degrees abduction and 10 degrees horizontal extension and holds this position as the left hand sequentially: (1), supinates the patient's forearm; (2), laterally rotates the shoulder; (3), extends the wrist and fingers; and (4), extends the elbow. The patient is asked to report upper-extremity symptoms throughout the maneuver. Typically, symptoms occur during the final phase of the test with elbow extension. The therapist can document the test results as positive and note the degree of elbow extension where the symptoms occur. Both sides should be tested, and a difference between sides of greater than 10 degrees is considered a positive test result. |

## Upper Limb Neurodynamic Test 1—cont'd

**NOTES** If the test is nonprovocative, cervical lateral flexion to the contralateral side can be added before repeating the test to further sensitize the neural structures to attempt to elicit positive test results. If contralateral neck lateral flexion is needed to elicit a positive test, this is an indication of low level of irritability with the neural structures, and more vigorous neural mobilizing techniques can be used for treatment. Ipsilateral lateral neck flexion could also be added as a follow-up to a positive test to confirm the findings. If a greater degree of elbow extension is required to elicit positive test results when the neck is placed in ipsilateral lateral flexion, this confirms the positive test findings are from a neural dynamic disorder likely originating from the cervical spine rather than tight upper-extremity muscles. Further tension to the neural system can be added by having a second therapist add a passive straight leg raise on the ipsilateral side before retesting, which applies further tension to dural and neural structures to determine whether loss of central dural extensibility has occurred. Also, end range of motion sensations of tension, tautness, and tingling may be considered normal, especially if they are at the end of the test range and are present bilaterally. Wainner et al[60] reported a Kappa value of 0.76 (0.51, 1.0). This test is one of the four findings for the clinical prediction rule for cervical radiculopathy.[60]

## Upper Limb Neurodynamic Test 2a[73,74]    DVD

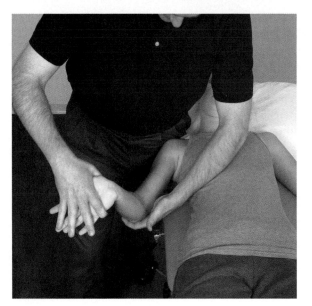

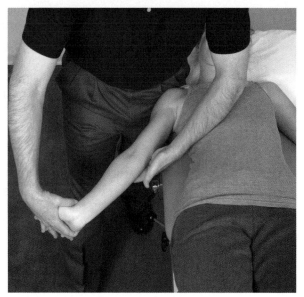

Upper limb neurodynamic test 2a, start position

Upper limb neurodynamic test 2a, end position

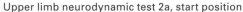

| | |
|---|---|
| **PURPOSE** | The test is used to apply tension though the brachial plexus and nerve root sleeves of the cervical spine to determine whether the cause of upper extremity symptoms originates from irritation of the cervical nerve roots and surrounding connective tissues. In theory, ULNT 2a is designed to focus tension on the median nerve and its corresponding nerve roots. |
| **PATIENT POSITION** | The patient lies supine with the arm to be tested positioned in a start position of 10 degrees shoulder abduction and 90 degrees elbow flexion. |
| **THERAPIST POSITION** | The therapist stands with a diagonal stance on the side to be tested with the left hip placed firmly across the superior aspect of the patient's shoulder girdle. |
| **HAND PLACEMENT** | **Left hand:** The left hand supports the patient's upper arm and elbow. |
| | **Right hand:** The therapist's right hand is placed across the palmar surface of the patient's right hand and fingers. |
| **PROCEDURE** | The therapist passively depresses the patient's scapula with the hip with the shoulder in 10 degrees abduction and 10 degrees horizontal extension and holds this position as the right hand sequentially: (1), supinates the patient's forearm; (2), laterally rotates the shoulder; (3), extends the wrist and fingers; and (4), extends the elbow. The patient is asked to report upper extremity symptoms throughout the maneuver. Typically, symptoms occur during the final phase of the test with elbow extension. The therapist can document the test results as positive and note the degree of elbow extension where the symptoms occur. Both sides should be tested, and a difference between sides of greater than 10 degrees is considered a positive test result. |
| **NOTES** | If the test is nonprovocative, cervical lateral flexion to the contralateral side can be added before repeating the test to further sensitize the neural structures to attempt to elicit positive test results. If contralateral neck lateral flexion is needed to elicit positive results, this is an indication of low level of irritability with the neural structures, and more vigorous mobilizing techniques can be used for treatment. Ipsilateral lateral neck flexion could also be added as a follow-up to a positive test to confirm the findings. If a greater degree of |

## Upper Limb Neurodynamic Test 2a—cont'd

elbow extension is needed to elicit positive test results when the neck is placed in ipsilateral lateral flexion, this confirms that the cause of the positive test findings is from a neural dynamic disorder likely originating from the cervical spine rather than tight upper-extremity muscles. Further sensitization can be added by having a second therapist add a passive straight leg raise on the ipsilateral side before retesting, which applies further tension to dural and neural structures to determine whether a loss of central dural extensibility has occurred. Also, end range of motion sensations of tension, tautness, and tingling may be considered normal, especially if they are at the end of the test range and are present bilaterally.

## Upper Limb Neurodynamic Test 2b[73,74]

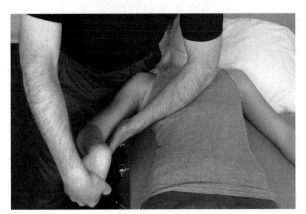
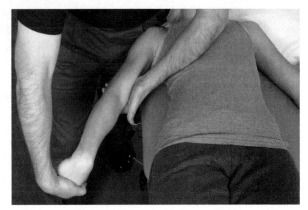

Upper limb neurodynamic test 2b, start position

Upper limb neurodynamic test 2b, end position

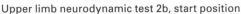

| | |
|---|---|
| **PURPOSE** | This test is used to apply tension though the brachial plexus and nerve root sleeves of the cervical spine to determine whether the cause of upper-extremity symptoms originates from irritation of the cervical nerve roots and surrounding connective tissues. In theory, ULNT 2b is designed to focus tension on the radial nerve and its corresponding roots. |
| **PATIENT POSITION** | The patient lies supine with the arm to be tested positioned in a start position of 10 degrees shoulder abduction and 90 degrees elbow flexion. |
| **THERAPIST POSITION** | The therapist stands with a diagonal stance on the side to be tested with the left hip placed firmly across the superior aspect of the patient's shoulder girdle. |
| **HAND PLACEMENT** | **Left hand:** The left hand supports the patient's upper arm and elbow. |
| | **Right hand:** The therapist's right hand is placed across the dorsal surface of the patient's right hand and fingers. |
| **PROCEDURE** | The therapist passively depresses the patient's scapula and holds this position with the front of the left hip and sequentially introduces: (1), shoulder medial rotation; (2), full elbow extension; and (3), wrist and finger flexion. The patient is asked to report any upper extremity symptoms throughout the maneuver. Typically, symptoms occur during the final phase of the test with wrist flexion. The therapist can document the test results as positive and note the degree of wrist flexion where the symptoms occurred. Both sides should be tested, and a difference between sides of greater than 10 degrees is considered a positive test result. |
| **NOTES** | If the test is nonprovocative, cervical lateral flexion to the contralateral side can be added before repeating the test to further sensitize the neural structures to attempt to elicit positive test results. If contralateral neck lateral flexion is needed to elicit positive test results, this is an indication of low level of irritability of the neural structures, and more vigorous neural mobilizing techniques may be needed for treatment. Ipsilateral lateral neck flexion could also be added as a follow-up to positive test results to confirm the findings. If a greater degree of wrist flexion is needed to elicit positive test results when the neck is placed in ipsilateral lateral flexion, this helps to confirm that the cause of the positive test findings is a neural tension disorder likely originating from the cervical spine rather than tight forearm muscles. Further sensitization can be added by having a second therapist add a passive straight leg raise on the ipsilateral side before retesting, which applies further tension to dural and neural structures to determine whether a loss of central dural extensibility has occurred. Wainner et al[60] reported a Kappa value of 0.83 (0.65, 1.0). |

## Upper Limb Neurodynamic Test 3[73,74]          (DVD)

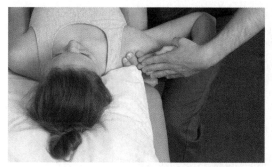
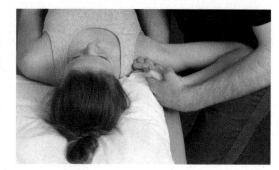

Upper limb neurodynamic test 3, start position          Upper limb neurodynamic test 3, end position

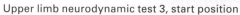

| | |
|---|---|
| **PURPOSE** | This test is used to apply tension through the brachial plexus and nerve root sleeves of the cervical spine to determine whether the cause of upper-extremity symptoms originates from irritation of the cervical nerve roots and surrounding connective tissues. In theory, ULNT 3 is designed to focus tension on the ulna nerve and its corresponding nerve roots. |
| **PATIENT POSITION** | The patient lies supine with the arm to be tested positioned in a start position of 10 degrees shoulder abduction and full elbow extension. |
| **THERAPIST POSITION** | The therapist stands with a diagonal stance on the side to be tested. |
| **HAND PLACEMENT** | **Left hand:** The therapist's left hand is placed across the palmar surface of the patient's right hand and fingers. |
| | **Right hand:** The right hand reaches up and under the posterior aspect of the patient's right scapula to place a hand across the posterior and superior aspect of the shoulder girdle to depress the scapula. |
| **PROCEDURE** | The therapist passively depresses the patient's scapula and holds this position as the left hand of the therapist sequentially introduces: (1), shoulder lateral rotation; (2), full elbow flexion; (3), forearm pronation; (4), wrist and finger extension; and (5), shoulder abduction (applied with the thigh of the therapist's front right leg). The patient is asked to report any upper extremity symptoms throughout the maneuver. Typically, symptoms occur during the final phase of the test with shoulder abduction. The therapist can document the test results as positive and note the degree of shoulder abduction where the symptoms occur. Both sides should be tested, and a difference between sides of greater than 10 degrees is considered to a positive test result. |
| **NOTES** | If the test is nonprovocative, cervical lateral flexion to the contralateral side can be added before repeating the test to further sensitize the neural structures to attempt to elicit positive test results. If contralateral neck lateral flexion is needed to elicit positive test results, this is an indication of low level of irritability with the neural structures, and more vigorous neural mobilizing techniques may be needed for treatment. Ipsilateral lateral neck flexion could also be added as a follow-up to positive test results to confirm the findings. If a greater degree of elbow flexion is needed to elicit positive test results when the neck is placed in ipsilateral lateral flexion, this helps to confirm that the cause of the positive test findings is a neurodynamic disorder likely originating from the cervical spine rather than tight upper-extremity muscles. Further sensitization can be added by having a second therapist add a passive straight leg raise on the ipsilateral side before retesting, which applies further tension to dural and neural structures to determine whether a loss of central dural extensibility has occurred. |

## Upper Trapezius Muscle Length Test and Hold/Relax Stretch

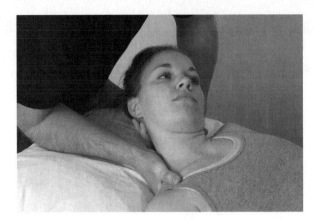

| | |
|---|---|
| **PURPOSE** | The purpose is to assess the length and stretch the upper trapezius muscle. |
| **PATIENT POSITION** | The patient is supine with the head resting on a pillow. |
| **HAND PLACEMENT** | **Left hand:** The left hand cradles the patient's occiput. |
| | **Right hand:** The web space and radial aspect of the metacarpal phalange joint are placed firmly across the superior aspect of the first rib and the superior aspect of the scapula. |
| **PROCEDURE** | The therapist depresses and holds the right shoulder girdle as the neck is moved into slight forward bending, full contralateral (left) lateral flexion, and ipsilateral (right) rotation. For the stretch, once positioned in the end-range position, the patient is asked to elevate the right shoulder as the therapist holds the shoulder into a depressed position to create an isometric contraction of the upper trapezius. After a 10-second isometric hold, the patient is instructed to relax and the tissue slack is taken up and held 10 seconds with further shoulder depression or further cervical left side bending, forward bending, or right rotation. This sequence is repeated for three to four repetitions and can be followed with instruction in a home stretching program, with the stretch position sustained for 30 to 60 seconds two to three times per day. |

## Levator Scapula Muscle Length Test and Hold/Relax Stretch (DVD)

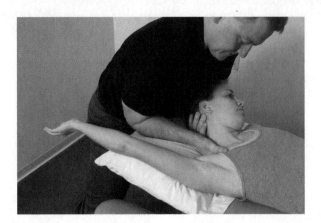

| | |
|---|---|
| **PURPOSE** | The purpose is to assess the length and stretch the levator scapula muscle. |
| **PATIENT POSITION** | The patient is supine with the head resting on a pillow with the ipsilateral (right) arm fully flexed. |
| **HAND PLACEMENT** | **Left hand:** The left hand cradles the patient's occiput. |
| | **Right hand:** The web space and radial aspect of the metacarpal phalange joint are placed firmly across the superior aspect of the first rib and superior medial angle of the scapula. |
| **PROCEDURE** | The therapist depresses and holds the right shoulder girdle as the neck is moved into slight forward bending, full contralateral (left) lateral flexion, and contralateral (left) rotation. For the stretch, once positioned in the end-range position, the patient is asked to elevate the right shoulder as the therapist holds the scapula into a depressed position to create an isometric contraction of the levator scapula. After a 10-second isometric hold, the patient is instructed to relax and the tissue slack is taken up and held 10 seconds with further shoulder depression or further cervical left side bending, forward bending, or left rotation. This sequence is repeated for three to four repetitions and can be followed with instruction in a home stretching program, with the stretch position sustained for 30 to 60 seconds two to three times per day. |

## PASSIVE INTERVERTEBRAL MOTION TESTING

### Craniovertebral Forward- and Backward-Bending Passive Physiological Intervertebral Motion (PPIVM) Test

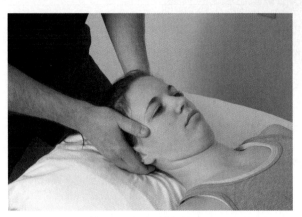

Craniovertebral forward-bending PPIVM test

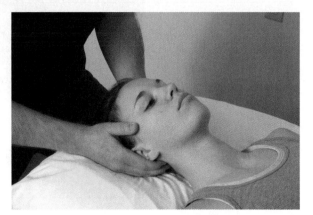

Craniovertebral backward-bending PPIVM test

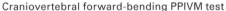

| | |
|---|---|
| **PURPOSE** | The purpose of this test is to evaluate the passive forward and backward bending of the cranium (C0) in relation to C1 and C2. |
| **PATIENT POSITION** | The patient is supine with the head on a pillow and the top of the head even with the edge of the table. |
| **THERAPIST POSITION** | The therapist stands at the head of the patient. |
| **HAND PLACEMENT** | Both hands gently grasp the posterior and lateral aspect of the cranium. |
| **PROCEDURE** | Both hands are used to gently isolate craniovertebral backward and forward bending while avoiding full cervical spine movement. Overpressure is applied to assess the end feel and the level of reactivity. |
| **NOTES** | The normal amount of craniovertebral forward and backward bending is approximately 10 to 30 degrees of each (see Table 6-2). Passive movement restrictions are commonly found with patients with cervicogenic headache, forward head posture, and mid cervical instability. The chin tends to deviate toward the side of the craniovertebral restriction with backward bending and away from the side of the restriction with forward bending. |

## Craniovertebral Side-Bending PPIVM Test (DVD)

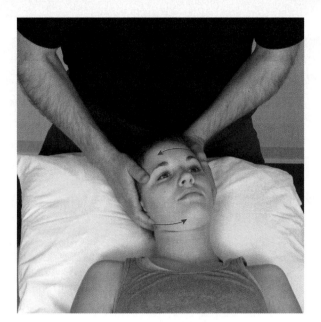

| | |
|---|---|
| **PURPOSE** | The test evaluates the passive side bending of the cranium (C0) in relation to C1 and C2. |
| **PATIENT POSITION** | The patient is supine with the head on a pillow and the top of the head even with the edge of the table. |
| **THERAPIST POSITION** | The therapist stands at the head of the patient. |
| **HAND PLACEMENT** | Both hands gently grasp the head. |
| **PROCEDURE** | Both hands are used to gently side bend the patient's head to the right while avoiding neck movement. The amount of passive side bending available to the right is noted. Overpressure is applied to assess the end feel and the level of reactivity. The procedure is repeated with side bending the head to the left. The amount of motion is noted and compared with the other side. Another variation of this technique is to attempt to palpate movement of transverse process of C1 toward the direction of the side-bending motion as passive side bending is induced. |
| **NOTES** | The axis of the movement should be through the patient's nose. The normal amount of craniovertebral side bending is approximately 5 to 15 degrees. Passive movement restrictions are commonly found with patients with cervicogenic headache, forward head posture, and mid cervical instability. |
| | This technique can be modified to assess the integrity of the alar ligament, which connects the occiput to C2, by palpating the lateral aspect of the C2 spinous process with the pad of the third digit as the therapist induces passive craniovertebral side bending. If the alar ligament is intact, the C2 spinous process moves the instant the cranium is passively side bent. |
| | Olson et al[40] assessed interrater reliability of craniovertebral side bending in five different positions and found poor interrater (Kappa values, −0.03 to 0.18) and intrarater (Kappa values, −0.02 to 0.14) reliability in all positions. The "Paris physiological position" with neck flexed approximately 20 degrees proved to be the most reliable position to test craniovertebral side bending.[40] Piva et al[76] reported Kappa values of 0.35 (0.15, 0.49) for assessment of mobility asymmetry and 0.35 (0.15, 0.55) for pain provocation intertester reliability tested on 30 patients. |

## Craniovertebral Rotation Passive Intervertebral Motion Test in Full Cervical Forward Bending

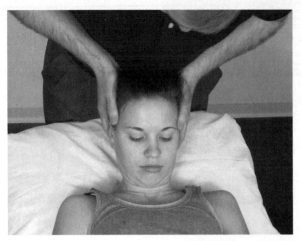

Start position for craniovertebral rotation PIVM test in full cervical forward bending

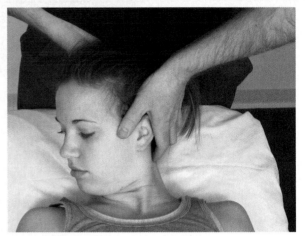

End position for craniovertebral rotation PIVM test in full cervical forward bending

| | |
|---|---|
| **PURPOSE** | The purpose is to evaluate the passive craniovertebral rotation primarily of the C1-C2 segment with the lower cervical spine locked with ligamentous tension. |
| **PATIENT POSITION** | The patient is supine with the head on a pillow and the top of the head even with the edge of the table. |
| **THERAPIST POSITION** | The therapist stand at the head of the patient. |
| **HAND PLACEMENT** | Both hands gently grasp the side of the patient's head. |
| **PROCEDURE** | The therapist holds the patient's head and neck in a fully flexed position with the posterior aspect of the cranium supported with the therapist's abdomen. While holding the head and neck in the fully flexed position, the therapist gently rotates the head to end range in one direction and then repeats in the other direction. Left versus right is compared. |
| **NOTES** | Asymmetry of movement or pain provocation is noted. Limitations in movement with this test are believed to be the result of stiffness of the C1-C2 spinal segment. |
| | Piva et al[76] reported Kappa values of 0.21 (0.08, 0.34) for assessment of mobility asymmetry and 0.36 (0.24, 0.49) for pain provocation intertester reliability tested on 30 patients. |

## Craniovertebral Rotation Passive Intervertebral Motion Test in Full Cervical Lateral Flexion

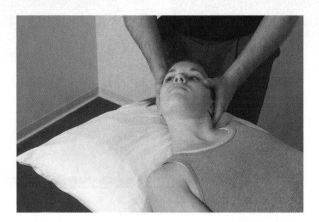

| | |
|---|---|
| **PURPOSE** | This test evaluates the passive craniovertebral rotation primarily of the C1-C2 segment with the lower cervical spine locked with ligamentous and joint capsular tension. |
| **PATIENT POSITION** | The patient is supine with the head on a pillow and the top of the head even with the edge of the table. |
| **THERAPIST POSITION** | The therapist stands at the head of the patient. |
| **HAND PLACEMENT** | Both hands gently grasp the side of the patient's head. |
| **PROCEDURE** | The therapist brings the patient's head and neck to a fully laterally flexed position and then gently rotates the head to the opposite direction of the lateral flexion to the end range in one direction and then repeats in the other direction. Left versus right is compared. |
| **NOTES** | Asymmetry of movement or pain provocation is noted. Limitations in movement with this test are believed to be the result of stiffness of the C1-C2 spinal segment. |
| | Piva et al[76] reported Kappa values of 0.30 (0.17, 0.43) for assessment of mobility asymmetry and 0.61 (0.5, 0.72) for pain provocation intertester reliability tested on 30 patients. |

## Cervical Downglide Passive Intervertebral Motion Test    🅓🅥🅓

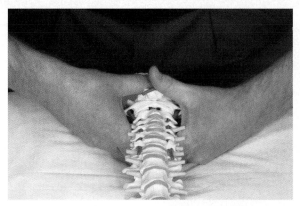

Hand placement for mid cervical downglide PIVM

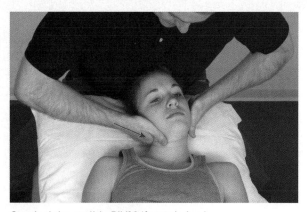

Cervical downglide PIVM (frontal view)

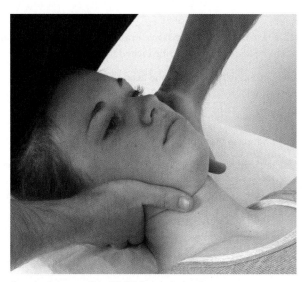

Cervical downglide PIVM (lateral view)

| | |
|---|---|
| **PURPOSE** | This test is used to evaluate the passive downglide of cervical segments C2-C3 through C7-T1. |
| **PATIENT POSITION** | The patient is supine with the head on a pillow and the top of the head even with the top edge of the table. |
| **THERAPIST POSITION** | The therapist stands at the head of the patient. |
| **HAND PLACEMENT** | **Left hand:** The radial border of the metacarpophalangeal joint of the index finger is used to contact the articular pillar of the specified segment, and the fourth and fifth fingers are used to support the patient's head. |
| | **Right hand:** The radial border of the metacarpophalangeal joint of the index finger is used to contact the articular pillar of the specified segment, and the fourth and fifth fingers are used to support the patient's head. |

## Cervical Downglide Passive Intervertebral Motion Test—cont'd

**PROCEDURE**

Both hands are used to gently grasp the patient's head and neck. The neck is brought into slight flexion (approximately 20 degrees), and the top of the patient's head rests on the therapist's abdomen. The radial border of the metacarpophalangeal joint of the index fingers on both hands is used to contact the articular pillars of C2. The fourth and fifth fingers of both hands are used to support the base of the patient's skull. Right side bending is induced by applying a force (through the contact point of the right hand) that is directed to the left and slightly caudally as the top of the patient's head continues to rest on the stationary therapist's abdomen. The amount of passive downglide available at the segment is noted. Also, any swelling or tenderness is noted. Left side bending is induced by applying a force (through the contact point of the left hand) that is directed to the right and slightly caudally as the top of the patient's head continues to rest on the stationary therapist's abdomen. The amount of passive downglide available is noted, as is any swelling or tenderness. The procedure is repeated with assessment of the mobility of the remaining cervical segments. The amount of passive downglide available at each segment and in each direction is noted and compared.

**NOTES**

This technique can be performed by starting at C2 and proceeding caudally. When the right C2 articular pillar is contacted, the segment being tested is described as a downglide PIVM test of the right C2-C3 facet joint. Counting down from C2 allows for easy location of the cervical vertebrae. When the patient's head is supported, the therapist does not apply excessive downward pressure through the abdomen. The top of the patient's head should not move, but rather, the side bending is induced from the passive downgliding motion imparted from the therapist's hand. Also, the therapist should be sure that the top of the patient's head is even with the edge of the table and not off the edge of the table. If this procedure induces a pain response at a particular spinal segment, the therapist should slightly readjust the hand placement cephalic or caudal or use the softer volar surface of the hand to induce the force. If the technique continues to cause pain, the cause is likely a reactive facet joint capsule at the level being tested. Smedmark, Wallin, and Arvidsson[77] reported a Kappa value of 0.43 and a 70% agreement for lateral flexion PIVM between two physical therapists when testing 61 patients with neck pain See Table 6-9 for interexaminer reliability for cervical spine PIVM testing.

## Cervical Downglide Passive Intervertebral Motion Test—cont'd

| TABLE 6-9 | Passive Intervertebral Motion Test Interexaminer Reliability for Patients with Neck Pain | | | | | |
|---|---|---|---|---|---|---|
| | | | INTEREXAMINER RELIABILITY VALUES | | | |
| | | | LIMITED MOVEMENTS | | PAIN | |
| **TEST AND MEASURE** | **TEST PROCEDURE AND DETERMINATION OF POSITIVE FINDINGS** | **POPULATION** | **RIGHT** | **LEFT** | **RIGHT** | **LEFT** |
| C0-C1[83] | Patient supine. Passive flexion is performed. Motion classified as limited or not limited, and patient pain response assessed on 11-point numeric pain rating (NPR) scale. | 32 Patients with neck pain. | $\kappa = 0.29$* | | ICC = 0.73 | |
| C1-C2[83] | Patient supine. Rotation is performed and classified as limited or not limited, and patient pain response assessed on 11-point NPR scale. | | $\kappa = 0.20$ | $\kappa = 0.37$ | ICC = 0.56 | ICC = 0.35 |
| C2-C3 | Patient supine. Fixation of lower segment with side bending to right and left. | | $\kappa = 0.34$ | $\kappa = 0.63$ | ICC = 0.50 | ICC = 0.78 |
| C3-C4 | Motion classified as limited or not limited, and patient pain response assessed on 11-point NPR scale. | | $\kappa = 0.20$ | $\kappa = 0.26$ | ICC = 0.62 | ICC = 0.75 |
| C4-C5 | | | $\kappa = 0.16$ | $\kappa = 0.09$ | ICC = 0.62 | ICC = 0.55 |
| C5-C6 | | | $\kappa = 0.17$ | $\kappa = 0.09$ | ICC = 0.66 | ICC = 0.65 |
| C6-C7 | | | $\kappa = 0.34$ | $\kappa = 0.03$ | ICC = 0.59 | ICC = 0.22 |
| C7-T1 | | | $\kappa = 0.08$ | $\kappa = 0.14$ | ICC = 0.45 | ICC = 0.34 |
| T1-T2[83] | | | $\kappa = 0.33$ | $\kappa = 0.46$ | ICC = 0.80 | ICC = 0.54 |

From Cleland J: *Orthopedic clinical examination: an evidence-based approach for physical therapists*, Carlstadt, NJ, 2005, Icon Learning Systems.
*Kappa and ICC values were calculated only for flexion of C0-C1. Data from Pool J, Hoving J, de Vet H, et al: *J Manipulative Physiol Ther* 27:84-90, 2003.
*ICC*, Interclass correlation coefficient.

## Cervical Upglide Passive Intervertebral Motion Test ⓓⱽᴰ

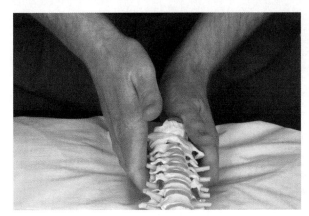 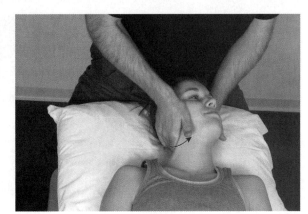

Finger placement for cervical upglide PIVM test

| | |
|---|---|
| **PURPOSE** | The purpose is to evaluate the passive upglide of cervical segments C2-C3 through T1-T2. |
| **PATIENT POSITION** | The patient is supine with the head on a small-sized to medium-sized soft pillow. |
| **THERAPIST POSITION** | The therapist stands at the head of the patient. |
| **HAND PLACEMENT** | **Right hand:** In testing of left rotation, the index finger is hooked around the posterior and lateral aspect of the articular pillar of the superior member of the segment; in testing of right rotation, the right hand is used to support the patient's head. |
| | **Left hand:** In testing of left rotation, the left hand is used to support the head; in testing right rotation, the index finger is hooked around the posterior and lateral aspect of the articular pillar of the segment. |
| **PROCEDURE** | The index finger of the right hand is used to palpate the right articular pillar of C2. The volar pad of the index finger is hooked posteriorly around the articular pillar and into the lamina. Left rotation is induced by pulling the articular pillar anteriorly cranially 45 degrees and across to the left side. The left hand is used to gently support the head to induce slight right side bending and backward bending and to return the head to midline after the rotation. The amount of passive rotation available at the segment is noted. The procedure is repeated with assessment of the left rotation at the remaining cervical segments. The amount of passive rotation available at each segment is noted and compared. The procedure is repeated with the index finger of the left hand passively rotating each segment to the right. The amount of passive rotation available at each segment and in each direction is noted and compared. |
| **NOTES** | This technique can be performed by starting at C2 and proceeding caudally, which allows for easy location of the cervical vertebrae (by counting down from C2). The therapist should ensure that the top of the patient's head is even with the edge of the table and not off the edge of the table. |

## Cervical Lateral Glide Passive Intervertebral Motion Test

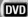

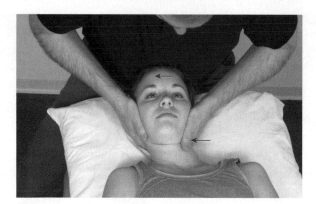

|  |  |
|---|---|
| **PURPOSE** | This test evaluates the passive lateral glide (joint play) of cervical segments C2-C3 through C7-T1. |
| **PATIENT POSITION** | The patient is supine with the head on a pillow and the top of the head even with the top edge of the table. |
| **THERAPIST POSITION** | The therapist stands at the head of the patient. |
| **HAND PLACEMENT** | **Left hand:** The radial border of the metacarpophalangeal joint of the index finger is used to contact the articular pillar of the specified segment, and the fourth and fifth fingers are used to support the patient's head. |
|  | **Right hand:** The radial border of the metacarpophalangeal joint of the index finger is used to contact the articular pillar of the specified segment, and the fourth and fifth fingers are used to support the patient's head. |
| **PROCEDURE** | Both hands are used to gently grasp the patient's head and neck. The neck is brought into slight flexion (approximately 20 degrees), but the top of the patient's head does not rest on the therapist's abdomen. The radial border of the metacarpophalangeal joint of the index fingers on both hands is used to contact the articular pillars of C2. The fourth and fifth fingers on both hands are used to support the base of the patient's skull. Right lateral glide is induced by applying a force (through the contact point of the left hand and with passive head movement) that is directed to the right. The amount of passive lateral glide available at the segment is noted. Also, tenderness or pain provocation is noted. Left lateral glide is induced by applying a force (through the contact point of the right hand) that is directed to the left. The cranial cervical spine segments and the head are allowed to move in the same lateral direction. The amount of passive lateral glide available is noted, as is any tenderness or pain provocation, and compared with the right side. The procedure is repeated with assessment of the mobility of the remaining cervical segments. The amount of passive lateral glide available at each segment and in each direction is noted and compared. |
| **NOTES** | This technique can be performed by starting at C2 and proceeding caudally, which allows for easy location of the cervical vertebrae (by counting down from C2). If this procedure induces a pain response at a particular spinal segment, the therapist should readjust the hand placement slightly cephalic or caudal or use the softer volar surface of the hand to induce the force. If the technique continues to cause pain, the cause is likely an irritable capsule tissue at the spinal segment being tested. The lateral glide is a general assessment of segmental joint play that tests the mobility of the uncovertebral joints, the facet joints, and neural tissues of the segment. If a restriction is found with the lateral glide PIVM test, graded end-range oscillations (grade III or IV manipulations) can be used with this same maneuver to free segmental restrictions. |

## Cervical Lateral Glide Passive Intervertebral Motion Test—cont'd

Fernandez-de-las-Penas, Downey, and Miangolarra-Page[78] compared cervical lateral glide test results with a radiographic assessment of segmental lateral flexion and found a strong correlation between the lateral glide PIVM test with the radiographic assessment in the 25 patients with neck pain assessed in the study.

## Lateral Glide Combined with Upper Limb Neurodynamic 1 Mobilization

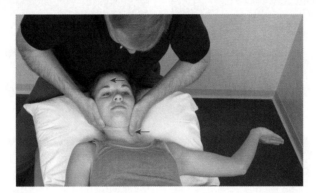

A lateral glide mobilization of the C5-C6 away from the symptomatic upper extremity can be used combined with ULNT 1 AROM to treat cervical radiculopathy. Typically, a sustained lateral glide stretch is used at the mid cervical spine as the patient moves the elbow in and out of end range elbow extension for 10 to 15 repetitions.

### Thoracic Passive Intervertebral Motion Testing and Manipulation

For completion of the cervical spine examination, palpation and PIVM testing must also be completed of the thoracic spine and rib cage. In addition, most patients with cervical spine disorders benefit from manual therapy techniques directed toward correction of thoracic spine dysfunctions. Chapter 5 provides a detailed description of examination and treatment procedures for the thoracic spine.

# CERVICAL SPINE MANIPULATION TECHNIQUES

## Cervical Spine Downglide Manipulation    DVD

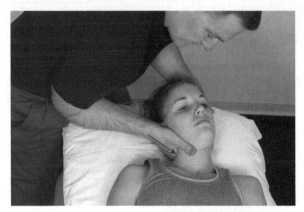

Cervical spine downglide manipulation (cradle hold)

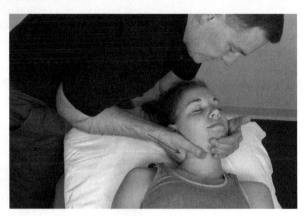

Cervical spine downglide manipulation (chin hold)

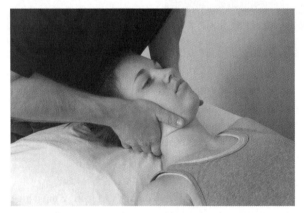

Cervical spine downglide manipulation (lateral view)

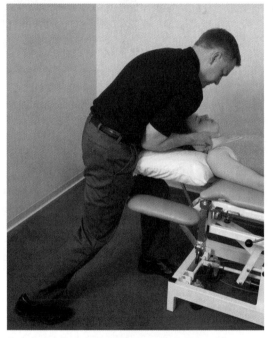

Cervical spine downglide manipulation with demonstration of therapist diagonal stance and forearm positioning

| | |
|---|---|
| **PURPOSE** | This technique is used to manipulate a specific cervical segment (C2-C3 though C7-T1) into side bending. |
| **PATIENT POSITION** | The patient is supine with the head on a pillow and the top of the head even with the top edge of the table. |
| **THERAPIST POSITION** | The therapist stands at the head of the patient. |
| **HAND PLACEMENT** | **Nonmanipulating hand:** This hand supports the patient's head and neck, with fingers draped across the occiput for the cradle hold or the hand wrapped across the chin and forearm across the posterior lateral aspect of the cranium for the chin hold. |

## Cervical Spine Downglide Manipulation—cont'd

**Manipulating hand:** The radial border of the metacarpophalangeal joint of the index finger is used to contact the articular pillar of the specified segment.

PROCEDURE

The radial border of the metacarpophalangeal joint of the index finger on the right hand is used to contact the right articular pillar of the specified cervical segment. The left hand supports the patient's head. Side bending of the patient's head slightly to the right is induced by taking up the joint motion in a downglide direction. The therapist then shifts the stance to the right and places the elbow at the hip with the forearm aligned with the direction of the force. The patient's neck is moved into rotation to the left down to the targeted spinal level. Further slack can be taken up by side gliding the neck away from the direction of side bending (to the left) and adding cervical distraction. The therapist manipulates into right side bending by applying a force through the contact point of the right hand that is directed to the left and slightly caudally toward the patient's axilla. On completion of the manipulation, right side bending is retested.

The therapist manipulates into left side bending by side bending the head slightly to the left and applying a force through the contact point of the left hand that is directed to the right and slightly caudally. On completion of the manipulation, left side bending is retested.

NOTES

Indication for use of this technique is decreased side bending (downglide) of a specific cervical segment (C2-C3 through C7-T1). Also, the top of the patient's head should be even with the edge of the table and not off the edge of the table. If the point of contact is uncomfortable for the patient, the therapist can attempt to adjust the position of the point of contact slightly superiorly or inferiorly or can attempt to use the volar aspect of the index finger metacarpal phalangeal joint to provide a softer point of contact. Once a firm barrier is attained, graded oscillations or a thrust may be used to manipulate the targeted spinal segment.

## Cervical Spine Upglide Manipulation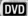

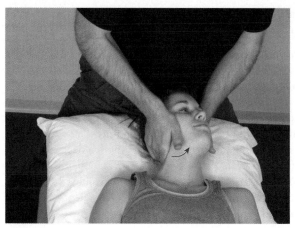

Mid cervical spine rotation/upglide manipulation (cradle hold)

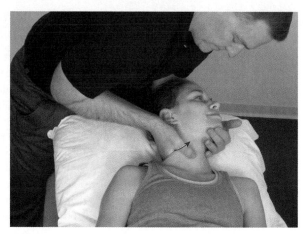

Mid cervical spine rotation/upglide manipulation (chin hold)

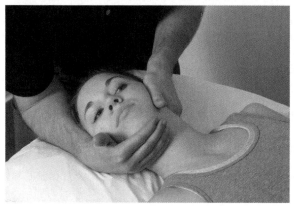

Mid cervical spine rotation/upglide manipulation with use of secondary levers

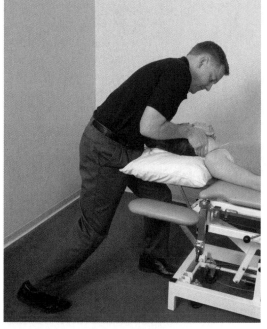

Mid cervical spine rotation/upglide manipulation with demonstration of therapist body and forearm position

| | |
|---|---|
| **PURPOSE** | The technique is used to manipulate a specific cervical segment (C2-C3 though C7-T1) into rotation. |
| **PATIENT POSITION** | The patient is supine with the head on a pillow. |
| **THERAPIST POSITION** | The therapist stands at the head of the patient in a diagonal athletic stance. |
| **HAND PLACEMENT** | **Left hand:** With manipulation into left rotation, the left hand supports the patient's head with fingers draped across the occiput for the cradle hold or the hand wrapped across the |

## Cervical Spine Upglide Manipulation—cont'd

chin and forearm across the posterior lateral aspect of the cranium for the chin hold; with manipulation into right rotation, the volar pad of the index finger is hooked around the posterior and lateral aspect of the articular pillar of the segment.

**Right hand:** With manipulation into right rotation, the right hand supports the patient's head with fingers draped across the occiput for the cradle hold or the hand wrapped across the chin and forearm across the posterior lateral aspect of the cranium for the chin hold; with manipulation into left rotation, the volar pad of the index finger is hooked around the posterior and lateral aspect of the articular pillar of the segment.

PROCEDURE The index finger of the right hand palpates the right articular pillar of the specified segment. The index finger hooks posteriorly around the articular pillar and into the lamina. The therapist manipulates into left rotation by lifting the articular pillar anteriorly cranially 45 degrees and across to the left side. The left hand supports the head and provides a counterforce to establish secondary levers of side bending to the right, side glide to the left, extension above the targeted level, and distraction. Once a firm barrier is established, the therapist oscillates or thrusts the targeted facet joint in the left rotation/upglide direction (i.e., primary lever). On completion of the manipulation, left rotation is retested.

The therapist manipulates into right rotation by repeating the procedure with the left hand to contact the left side of the specified segment. On completion of the manipulation, right rotation is retested.

The chin hold of the head creates a broader point of contact for the patient's head and may assist in control of the multiple planes of motion used to create the firm joint barrier, which may assist with patient relaxation during the manipulation.

NOTES Indication for use of this technique is decreased rotation (upglide) of a specific cervical segment (C2-C3 through C7-T1). The patient's head should be kept on the pillow during this technique. Also, the top of the patient's head should be even with the edge of the table and not off the edge of the table. The technique can be performed with very small oscillations at the end range (grade IV) or larger oscillations at end (III) or mid (II) range or with an end-range, small-amplitude, high-velocity thrust. Measurement with an inclinometer of supine cervical active rotation can be used as an effective premanipulation and postmanipulation range-of-motion test. Use of multiple planes of motion (levers) allows the therapist to create an effective firm manipulative joint barrier without extreme degrees of cervical rotation to take up the tissue slack. This technique builds safety into the technique by avoiding potential strain on the vertebral artery and other cervical soft tissue structures.

## Prone Cervical Unilateral (Upglide) Posterior-to-Anterior Passive Accessory Intervertebral Motion Test and Mobilization

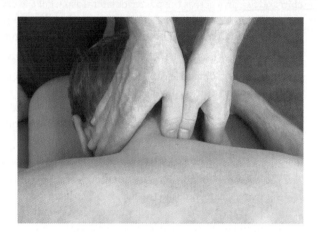

| | |
|---|---|
| **PURPOSE** | The test assesses the passive accessory motion in a posterior to anterior direction for segments C2-C3 through C7-T1 and manipulates a specific cervical or upper thoracic segment (C2-C3 through T3-T4) in a posterior to anterior direction. |
| **PATIENT POSITION** | The patient is prone with a pillow under the chest and the forehead resting on a towel and the cervical spine in a neutral position. |
| **THERAPIST POSITION** | The therapist stands in a diagonal athletic stance at the head of the patient. |
| **HAND PLACEMENT** | The therapist places both thumbs together with fingers in a mid/relaxed position across the posterior lateral aspect of the patient's neck. The tips of both thumbs are placed on the posterior aspect of the targeted articular pillar. |
| **PROCEDURE** | The therapist gently applies pressure in an anterior-posterior direction in the plane of the facet joint to assess mobility, resistance, end feel, and pain provocation. Gentle oscillations can be used to either inhibit pain (grade I and II) or restore motion (grades III and IV). Slight variations in depth and direction of force can be used to optimize the therapeutic effects of this technique. |
| **NOTES** | The forces used in this procedure are very gentle, and the patient should be monitored verbally throughout the procedure to ensure comfort. |

## Prone Cervical Unilateral (Upglide) Posterior-to-Anterior PAIVM Test and Mobilization: Alternative "Dummy Thumb" Method

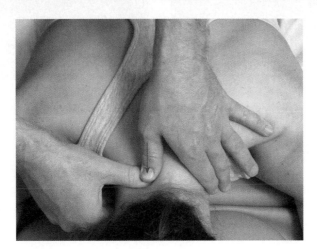

This procedure can be modified by having the therapist stand at the side of the patient with a diagonal stance with the more lateral leg forward and a dummy thumb hand placement. The more lateral hand is used as the dummy thumb that is placed at the posterior aspect of the articular pillar and the distal pad of the more medial thumb is placed across the top of the dummy thumb (on the thumb nail) to provide the manipulative force.

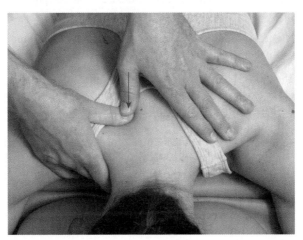

Prone upper thoracic unilateral (upglide) posterior-to-anterior PAIVM and mobilization with dummy thumb method

NOTES    This alternative method works well for lower cervical and upper thoracic spinal segments to maintain the force along the plane of the facet joint surfaces, which is 45 degrees in the mid cervical spine and 30 degrees in the upper thoracic spine.

## Suboccipital Release/Inhibitive Distraction

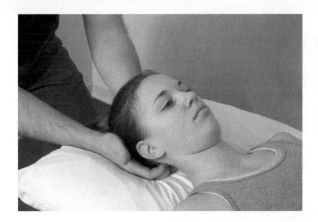

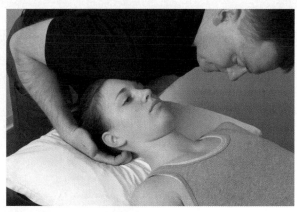

Suboccipital release/inhibitive distraction with shoulder counterpressure

| | |
|---|---|
| **PURPOSE** | The purpose is to relax the suboccipital muscles and distract the cranium from C1 to restore craniovertebral mobility. |
| **PATIENT POSITION** | The patient is supine with the head on a pillow. |
| **THERAPIST POSITION** | The therapist sits at the head of the treatment table. |
| **HAND PLACEMENT** | **Left hand:** This hand contacts the base of the occiput (just caudal to the nuchal line) with the tips of digits 2 to 5. |
| | **Right hand:** This hand contacts the base of the occiput (just caudal to the nuchal line) with the tips of digits 2 to 5. |
| **PROCEDURE** | The tips of digits 2 to 5 of both hands gently lift the patient's head anteriorly. The dorsum of the hands rest on the pillow. With the tips of the fingers only, the therapist gently pulls the head cranially as the patient's suboccipital muscles relax. The therapist continues with this position and takes up tissue slack with distraction as it becomes available. Distraction may continue for up to 5 minutes. Once relaxation of the suboccipital muscles is achieved, the therapist can position the anterior aspect of the shoulder across the patient's forehead to create a firm vice on the head and apply greater suboccipital distraction. |
| **NOTES** | Indications for use of this technique is decreased craniovertebral motion or muscle holding of the suboccipital muscles. During the performance of this technique, the forces should be applied to the base of the skull and not to C1. Patient relaxation is the key to the effectiveness of this technique. |

## Craniovertebral Distraction with C2 Stabilization

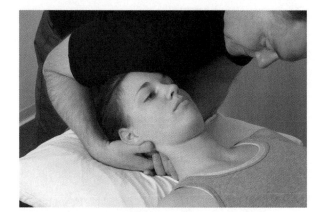

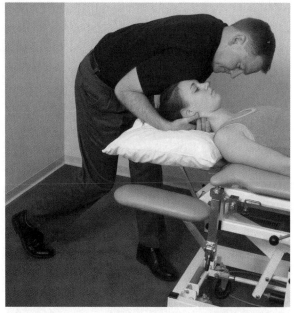

Craniovertebral distraction with C2 stabilization with demonstration of therapist stance and body position

| | |
|---|---|
| **PURPOSE** | The purpose is to distract the cranium and C1 from C2 to restore craniovertebral mobility. |
| **PATIENT POSITION** | The patient is supine with the head on a pillow. |
| **THERAPIST POSITION** | The therapist stands at the head of the patient. |
| **HAND PLACEMENT** | **Left hand:** The therapist uses the thumb and index finger to stabilize C2 (through the articular pillar and lamina). |
| | **Right hand:** The therapist uses the thumb and index finger to grasp the patient's occiput and the anterior shoulder to create a vice on the patient's forehead. |
| **PROCEDURE** | The thumb and index finger of the left hand are used to stabilize C2. The thumb and index finger of the right hand are used to grasp the patient's occiput. The right anterior shoulder is used to create a vice on the patient's forehead. The right hand distracts the cranium. This technique can be performed with a sustained stretch or slow grade III oscillations. |

## Occipitoatlantal Distraction Manipulation (DVD)

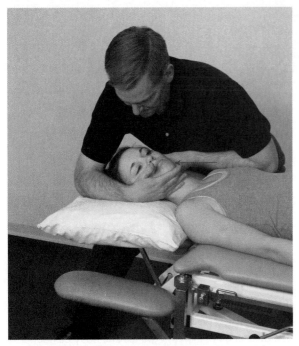 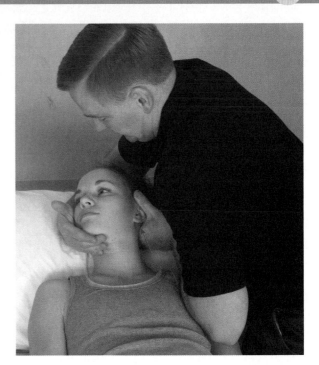

Occipitoatlantal distraction manipulation with demonstration of therapist body positioning

| | |
|---|---|
| **PURPOSE** | The technique is used to distract/stretch the occipitoatlantal (OA) joint. |
| **PATIENT POSITION** | The patient is supine with the head on a pillow and positioned with the head slightly side bent toward and rotated away from the side to be manipulated. |
| **THERAPIST POSITION** | The therapist stands at the side of the patient's head with the legs in a lunge position. |
| **HAND PLACEMENT** | **Left hand:** The hand contacts the occiput with the volar surface of the MC-P joint and forearm in a sagittal plane. |
| | **Right hand:** The hand and forearm support the patient's head and chin. |
| **PROCEDURE** | The therapist take up the slack with a distractive force with the left hand. Next, to create a more effective barrier, the therapist side glides the patient's head and neck toward the side of rotation to further lock the mid cervical spine. As the position of the head is held firm, the weight is shifted quickly onto the cranial foot with a lunging motion to create a thrust. Most of the force is applied with the left hand into the patient's occiput. |

## Cervical Spine Rotation Isometric Manipulation in Supine

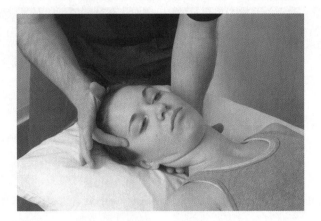

| | |
|---|---|
| **PURPOSE** | This technique is used to restore (mobilize) the downglide component of cervical rotation. |
| **PATIENT POSITION** | The patient is supine with the head on a medium-sized pillow. |
| **THERAPIST POSITION** | The therapist stands or sits at the head of the treatment table. |
| **HAND PLACEMENT** | **Right hand:** This hand guides the head movements and applies resistance at the patient's temple on the side of the rotation motion that is limited. |
| | **Left hand:** The thumb and index or third finger stabilize the posterolateral aspect (articular pillars) of the caudal member of the segment. |
| **PROCEDURE** | The thumb and index finger of the left hand palpate and stabilize the posterolateral aspect (articular pillars) of C3. The right hand guides the patient's head into right rotation with slight ipsilateral side bending to the point of resistance or pain. This procedure is repeated throughout the cervical segments, stabilizing the caudal member of the segment, until the position of the limited or painful motion is located. Once the painful or restricted segment is located, the thumb and index finger of the left hand are used to stabilize the caudal member of the segment. The patient's head is guided into the right rotated position to the point of pain or resistance and backed off slightly. A light resistance with the pad of the index finger of the right hand is applied at the patient's temple toward left rotation, and the patient is asked to hold against that resistance for 10 seconds. The head is guided slightly farther into the right rotation, and the isometric resistance is repeated. This motion is repeated for a total of four to five repetitions. On completion of the technique, the painful segment is reexamined. |
| **NOTES** | Indication for use of this technique is a positive Spurling's B test result for neck pain or mid cervical pain reported on the same side of neck rotation tested in supine or standing. Follow-up of this technique with manual cervical distraction or manual resistive cervical rotation in the supine position is often useful. |

## Cervical Spine Isometric Manipulation in Sitting      DVD

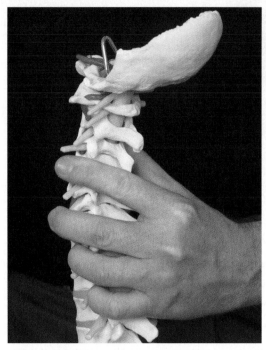

Inferior hand placement for cervical spine isometric manipulation in sitting

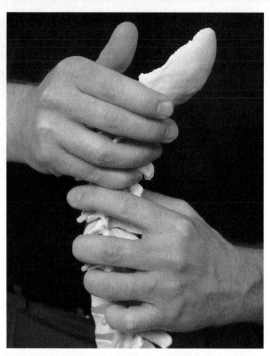

Bilateral hand placement for cervical spine isometric manipulation in sitting

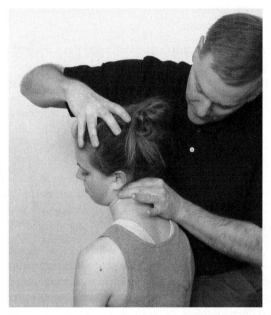

Cervical spine downglide PIVM in sitting

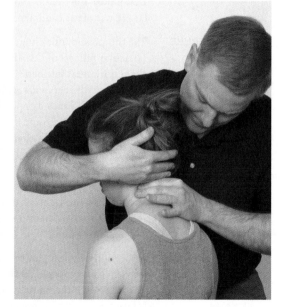

| | |
|---|---|
| **PURPOSE** | The purpose is to restore the downglide component of pain-free cervical side bending and rotation. |
| **PATIENT POSITION** | The patient is in a sitting position. |
| **THERAPIST POSITION** | The therapist stands to the side of the patient on the opposite side of the joint to be manipulated. |
| **HAND PLACEMENT** | **Right hand:** This hand guides the head movements and applies resistance (with the fifth finger contacting the cranial member of the segment's articular pillar). |

## Cervical Spine Isometric Manipulation in Sitting—cont'd

**Left hand:** The thumb and index finger are used to stabilize the posterolateral aspect (articular pillars) of the caudal member of the segment.

PROCEDURE

The therapist stands on the patient's right side and uses the thumb and index finger of the left hand to palpate and stabilize the posterolateral aspect (articular pillars) of C3. The right hand guides the patient's head into the left posterior quadrant (side bending combined with ipsilateral rotation and backward bending). This procedure is repeated throughout the cervical segments, stabilizing the caudal member of the segment, until the position of the painful entrapment (motion limited by pain/guarding) is located. Once the painful or restricted segment is located, the thumb and index finger of the left hand stabilize the caudal member of the segment. The patient's head is guided into the left posterior quadrant to the point of pain and backed off slightly. The cranial member of the segment is contacted with the volar aspect of the right fifth finger (the remaining fingers and palm contact the posterolateral aspect of the patient's head). With the contact points of the right hand, the therapist gently pulls the patient's head out of the left posterior quadrant (into forward bending, side bending, and rotation) while the patient isometrically resists. The position is held for 10 seconds. The head is guided slightly farther into the left posterior quadrant, and the isometric resistance is repeated. The motion is repeated for a total of four to five repetitions. On completion of the technique, the painful segment is reexamined.

If the painful entrapment is located on the patient's right side, the procedure is repeated with the therapist standing on the patient's left side and reversing the roles of the hands.

NOTES

Indication for use of this technique is a Spurling's B test result that is positive for neck pain. One should note the placement of the caudal hand of this technique: the thumb and index fingers of the caudal hand should be stabilizing the posterolateral aspect of the caudal vertebral member of the segment.

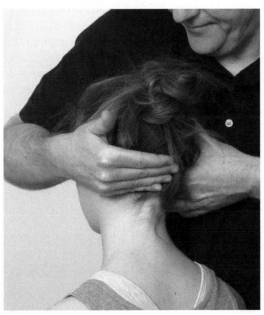

Cervical manual distraction in sitting

Follow-up of the cervical spine isometric manipulation sitting technique with manual cervical distraction or manual resistive cervical rotation either in the supine or sitting position is often useful. The sitting cervical distraction technique should be combined with deep breathing. The head should be held firmly, with the hands positioned at the patient's mastoid processes, as the patient lets the air out.

## Craniovertebral Rotation Isometric Manipulation in Supine

**DVD**

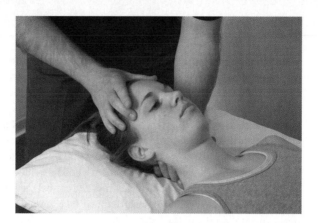

| | |
|---|---|
| **PURPOSE** | The purpose is to restore craniovertebral rotation. |
| **PATIENT POSITION** | The patient is supine with the head on a medium-sized pillow. |
| **THERAPIST POSITION** | The therapist stands or sits at the head of the treatment table. |
| **HAND PLACEMENT** | **Left hand:** The thumb and index or third finger stabilize the posterolateral aspect (articular pillars) of the axis (C2 vertebra). |
| | **Right hand:** This hand is spread across the patient's forehead to guide cervical rotation. |
| **PROCEDURE** | The thumb and index finger of the left hand palpate and stabilize the posterolateral aspect (articular pillars) of C2. The right hand guides the patient's head into right rotation with slight ipsilateral side bending to the point of resistance or pain, and the patient is asked to hold that position. A light resistance with the pad of the index finger of the right hand is applied at the patient's temple toward left rotation, and the patient is asked to hold against that resistance for 10 seconds. The head is guided farther into the right rotation, and the isometric resistance is repeated. The motion is repeated for a total of four to five repetitions. On completion of the technique, craniovertebral rotation is reexamined. |
| **NOTES** | Follow-up of this technique with manual craniovertebral distraction or manual resistive cervical rotation in the supine position is often useful. |

## Craniovertebral Side-Bending (Lateral Flexion) Isometric Manipulation in Supine

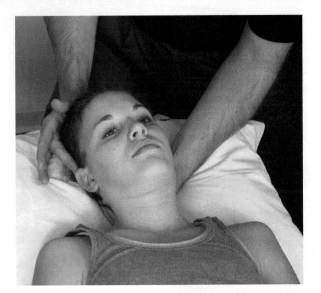

| | |
|---|---|
| **PURPOSE** | The purpose is restoration of craniovertebral side bending. |
| **PATIENT POSITION** | The patient is supine with the head on a medium-sized pillow. |
| **THERAPIST POSITION** | The therapist stands or sits at the head of the treatment table. |
| **HAND PLACEMENT** | **Left hand:** The thumb and index or third finger stabilize the posterolateral aspect (articular pillars) of the axis (C2 vertebra). |
| | **Right hand:** The hand is spread across the top of the patient's head to guide craniovertebral side bending. |
| **PROCEDURE** | The thumb and index finger of the left hand palpate and stabilize the posterolateral aspect (articular pillars) of C2. The right hand guides the patient's head into right craniovertebral side bending (lateral flexion) to the point of resistance or pain, and the patient is asked to hold that position. A light resistance with the pad of the index finger of the right hand is applied just above the patient's right ear, and the patient is asked to hold against the resistance for 10 seconds. The head is guided farther into the right lateral flexion, and the isometric resistance is repeated. The motion is repeated for a total of four to five repetitions. On completion of the technique, craniovertebral side bending (lateral flexion) is re-examined. |
| **NOTES** | Follow-up of this technique with manual craniovertebral distraction and the active craniocervical flexion exercise is often useful. |

## First Rib Depression Manipulation

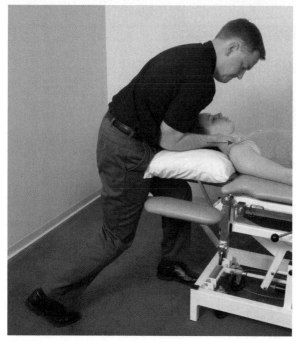
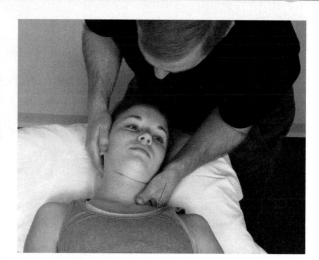

First rib depression manipulation with demonstration of therapist body and forearm position

| | |
|---|---|
| **PURPOSE** | The purpose is to manipulate (depress) a hypermobile first rib to restore first rib mobility. |
| **PATIENT POSITION** | The patient is supine with the head on a pillow. |
| **THERAPIST POSITION** | The therapist stands with a diagonal stance at the head of the patient toward the side to be manipulated. |
| **HAND PLACEMENT** | **Left hand:** The radial or volar aspect of the index finger metacarpophalangeal joint manipulates the left first rib. |
| | **Right hand:** The radial or volar aspect of the index finger metacarpophalangeal joint manipulates the right first rib. |
| **PROCEDURE** | The radial or volar aspect of the index finger metacarpophalangeal joint of the right hand palpates the right first rib. The first rib is located in the space lateral to the C7 transverse process, posterior to the clavicle and anterior to the scapula. The therapist side bends and rotates the head and neck slightly towards the right and takes up the slack and oscillates the first rib. The manipulation is coordinated with the patient's breathing, with progressive oscillation into slightly more depression with each oscillation. The procedure is repeated through three breathing cycles. On completion of the manipulation, the mobility of the right first rib is retested. |
| | The therapist manipulates the left first rib by repeating the procedure with the radial or volar aspect of the index finger metacarpophalangeal joint of the left hand to contact the left first rib. On completion of the manipulation, the mobility of the first rib is retested. |
| **NOTES** | Indication for use of this technique is elevation and decreased mobility of the first rib. During the performance of this technique, the manipulating hand is reinforced with bracing the elbow with the ipsilateral hip. The direction of the manipulating force should be toward the patient's umbilicus. An elevated and hypomobile first rib is commonly associated with signs and symptoms characteristic of thoracic outlet syndrome. |

## First Rib Posterior Glide Manipulation in Supine

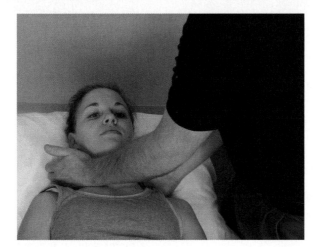

| | |
|---|---|
| **PURPOSE** | The purpose is manipulation of a stiff first rib and restoration of first rib and T1-T2 rotation mobility. |
| **PATIENT POSITION** | The patient is supine with the head on a pillow. |
| **THERAPIST POSITION** | The therapist stands on the opposite side to be manipulated. |
| **HAND PLACEMENT** | **Left hand:** The ulnar aspect of the left hand on the anterior aspect of the right first rib just superior and posterior to the clavicle manipulates the right first rib. |
| | **Right hand:** The pad of the long finger is placed at the left lateral aspect of the T2 spinous process to block T2 rotation. |
| **PROCEDURE** | The ulnar aspect of the fifth metacarpal of the left hand provides an anterior-to-posterior force into the first rib as the right hand blocks T2. The therapist takes up the slack and oscillates the first rib. The manipulation is coordinated with the patient's breathing, with progressive oscillation into slightly more posterior glide with each oscillation. The procedure is repeated through approximately three breathing cycles. On completion of the manipulation, the mobility of the right first rib is retested. |
| **NOTES** | Indication for use of this technique is decreased mobility of the first rib and limited rotation of the T1-T2 spinal segment. Ipsilateral pain and limited motion at the cervicothoracic junction during cervical rotation AROM testing is an indication of this technique. Supine cervical rotation AROM can be used as a pretest and posttest for this manipulation. |

# CASE STUDIES AND GROUP PROBLEM SOLVING

The following patient case reports can be used by the student to develop problem-solving skills by considering the information provided in the patient history and tests and measures and developing appropriate evaluations, goals, and plans of care.

## MS. HEAD ACHE

### History
A 32-year-old female secretary has a diagnosis of cervicogenic headache with pain focused in the right ocular area and the right upper cervical spine.

### Tests and Measures
- Structural examination: Moderate forward head posture (FHP) with protracted scapulas
- Cervical AROM: 75% Left side bending and left rotation, 50% right side bending and right rotation with provocation of pain, 60% forward bending with deviation to the right
- Cervical passive range of motion (PROM): Overpressure to right rotation increases pain and has a capsular end feel
- Shoulder AROM and strength: Normal
- Muscle length: Moderately tight right levator scapula and minimally tight bilateral pectoralis major and minor muscles
- Strength: 3+/5 Bilateral lower trapezius, middle trapezius, and serratus anterior
- Spurling's B test: Positive to the right for provocation of neck pain
- Distraction test: Decreased pain in the head and neck
- Neurological screen: Negative
- Palpation: Tender and guarded in area of right C2-C3 facet joint and right suboccipital muscles
- Passive intervertebral motion tests: Hypomobility right C23 upglide and downglide and craniovertebral right sidebending

### Evaluation
Diagnosis
Problem list
Goals

### Treatment Plan/Intervention

## MS. WHIP LASH

### History
A 16-year-old female high school student has a diagnosis of neck pain with pain focused in the left mid cervical region after a motor vehicle accident caused a whiplash injury 4 weeks before the initial visit. The patient has been using a Philadelphia collar since the injury.

### Tests and Measures
- Structural examination: Moderate FHP with protracted scapulas
- Cervical AROM in standing: 50% in all planes of motion with provocation of pain at the end of range of motions with poor control noted
- Cervical AROM in supine: 80% in all planes with less pain reported
- Cervical PROM: Overpressure to left and right rotation increased pain with a muscle holding end feel
- Shoulder AROM and strength: Normal
- Muscle length: Moderately tight right levator scapula and minimally tight bilateral pectoralis major and minor
- Strength: 3+/5 Bilateral lower trapezius, middle trapezius, and serratus anterior; 2/5 longus capitis, longus colli, and cervical multifidus; poor control with craniocervical test and unable to hold contraction for 10 seconds beyond 22 mm Hg
- Spurling's B test: Positive bilaterally for provocation of neck pain
- Distraction test: Decreased pain in the head and neck
- Neurological screen: Negative
- Palpation: Tender and guarded and inflammation throughout the mid cervical facet joints and surrounding muscle/soft tissues
- Ligament stability tests: Alar and Sharp-Purser tests are both negative
- Passive intervertebral motion tests: Hypomobility T2-T3 and T3-T4 left and right rotation

### Evaluation
Diagnosis
Problem list
Goals

### Treatment Plan/Intervention

## MR. NECK A. ARMPAIN

### History

A 55-year-old male police officer has a diagnosis of neck and arm pain with the pain focused in the right lateral upper arm, right shoulder, right scapula, and right cervical/thoracic junction.

### Tests and Measures

- Structural examination: Moderate FHP with protracted scapulas; holds the right arm close to the body and supports it with the opposite arm
- Cervical AROM in standing: 50% in all planes of motion with provocation of pain at the end of range of motions with poor control noted; upper thoracic mobility is 25% of expected range of motion
- Cervical AROM in supine: 45 degrees right rotation, 55 degrees left rotation
- Cervical PROM: Overpressure to left and right rotation increased pain with a capsular end feel
- Right shoulder screen:
  - AROM: 120 flexion and 110 abduction with pain arm pain at end range
  - PROM: 120 flexion and 110 abduction with pain arm pain at end range
  - Tissue tension signs: Strength was normal and pain free with resistance
  - Accessory motion tests: Normal for right shoulder
  - Nerve tension tests: Positive ULNT 1 at −60 elbow extension
- Muscle length: Moderately tight right levator scapula and minimally tight bilateral pectoralis major and minor
- Strength: 3+/5 Bilateral lower trapezius, middle trapezius, and serratus anterior; 3/5 longus capitis, longus colli, and cervical multifidus
- Spurling's A: Positive right for provocation right arm pain
- Distraction test: Decreased arm pain
- Neurological screen: Diminished biceps reflex, but normal sensation
- Palpation: Tender and guarded and inflammation at the right C5-C6 and C6-C7 facet joints and surrounding muscle/soft tissues
- Passive intervertebral motion tests: Hypomobility T3-T4 and T4-T5 left and right rotation

### Evaluation

Diagnosis
Problem list
Goals

### Treatment Plan/Intervention

## REFERENCES

1. Shekelle PG, Markovich M, Louis R: An epidemiologic study of episodes of back pain care, *Spine* 20:1668-1673, 1995.
2. Wright A, Mayer TG, Gatchel RJ: Outcomes of disabling cervical spine disorders in compensation injuries: a prospective comparison to tertiary rehabilitation response for chronic lumbar spinal disorders, *Spine* 24(2):178-183, 1999.
3. Bovin G, Schrader H, Sand T: Neck pain in the general population, *Spine* 19:1307-1309, 1994.
4. Cote P, Cassidy JD, Carroll L: The Saskatchewan Health and Back Pain Survey: the prevalence of neck pain and related disability in Saskatchewan adults, *Spine* 23:1689-1698, 1998.
5. Lethbridge-Cejku M, Schiller JS, Bernadel L: Summary health statistics for US adults: National Health Interview Survey, 2002, *Vital Health Stat* 10:1-151, 2004.
6. Nygren A, Berglund A, von Koch M: Neck and shoulder pain, an increasing problem: strategies for using insurance material to follow trends, *Scand J Rehabil Med Suppl* 32:107-112, 1995.
7. Jette A, Delitto A: Physical therapy treatment choices for musculoskeletal impairments, *Phys Ther* 77(2):145-154, 1997.
8. Youdas JW, Garret TR, Suman VJ, et al: Normal range of motion of the cervical spine: an initial goniometric study, *Phys Ther* 72(11):770-780, 1992.
9. Mercer SR, Jull GA: Morphology of the cervical intervertebral disc: implications for McKenzie's model of the disc derangement syndrome, *Man Ther* 2:76-81, 1996.
10. Williams PL, Dyson M, Bannister LH, editors: *Gray's anatomy*, ed 37, New York, 1989, Churchill Livingstone.
11. Penning L: Normal movement in the cervical spine, *Am J Roentgenol* 130:317-326, 1978.
12. Dvorak J, Panjabi MM, Novotny JE, et al: In vivo flexion/extension of the normal cervical spine, *J Orthop Res* 9:828-834, 1991.
13. Mimura M, Hideshige M, Tsuneo W, et al: Three-dimensional motion analysis of the cervical spine with special reference to the axial rotation, *Spine* 14(11):1135-1139, 1989.
14. Werne S: Studies in spontaneous atlas dislocation, *Acta Orthop Scand* (Suppl):23, 1957.
15. Dumas J, Sainte Rose M, Dreyfus P, et al: Rotation of the cervical spinal column: a computed tomography in vivo study, *Surg Radiol Anat* 15:333-339, 1993.
16. Lysell: Motion in the cervical spine: an experimental study on autopsy specimens, *Acta Orthop Scand* Suppl (123): 1969.
17. Penning L, Wilmink JT: Rotation of the cervical spine: a CT study in normal subjects, *Spine* 12(8):732-738, 1987.
18. Jarrett JL, Olson KA, Bohannon RW: Reliability in examining cranioverterbral sidebending, University of St. Augustine for Health Sciences, Master's thesis, 2004.
19. Neumann DA: *Kinesiology of the musculoskeletal system: foundations for physical rehabilitation*, St Louis, 2002, Mosby.
20. Stiell I, et al: The Canadian C-spine rule for radiography in alert and stable trauma patients, *JAMA* 286(15):1841-1848, 2001.
21. Childs JD, Fritz JM, Piva SR, et al: Proposal of a classification system for patients with neck pain, *JOSPT* 34(11):686-700, 2004.
22. Fritz JM, Brennan GP: Preliminary examination of the validity of a proposed classification system for patients receiving physical therapy interventions for neck pain, *Phys Ther* 87(5):513-524, 2007.
23. Barnsley L, Lord S, Bogduk N: Clinical review: whiplash injury, *Pain* 58:283-307, 1994.

24. Sterling M: A proposed new classification system for whiplash associated disorders: implications for assessment and management, *Man Ther* 9:60-70, 2004.
25. Sterling M, Jull G, Kenardy J: Physical and psychological factors maintain long-term predictive capacity post-whiplash injury, *Pain* 122:102-108, 2006.
26. McKinnry LA: Early mobilization and outcome in acute sprains of the neck, *BMJ* 299:1006-1008, 1989.
27. Rosenfeld M, Bunnarsson R, Borenstein P: Early intervention in whiplash-associated disorders: a comparison of two treatment protocols, *Spine* 25:1782-1787, 2000.
28. Jull G, Kristjansson E, Dall'Alba P: Impairment in cervical flexors: a comparison of whiplash and insidious onset neck pain patients, *Man Ther* 9:89-94, 2004.
29. O'Leary S, Jull G, Kim M, et al: Specificity in retraining craniocervical flexor muscle performance, *JOSPT* 37(1):3-9, 2007.
30. Cleland JA, Childs JD, Fritz JM, et al: Development of a clinical prediction rule for guiding treatment of a subgroup of patients with neck pain: use of thoracic spine manipulation, exercise, and patient education, *Phys Ther* 87(1):9-23, 2007.
31. Panjabi MM: The stabilizing system of spine: part II: neutral zone and instability hypothesis, *J Spinal Disord* 5:390-397, 1992.
32. Panjabi MM: The stabilizing system of the spine: part I: function, dysfunction, adaptation, and enhancement, *J Spinal Disord* 5:383-389, 1992.
33. Panjabi MM, Lydon C, Vasavada A, et al: On the understanding of clinical instability, *Spine* 23:2642-2650, 1994.
34. Oxland TR, Panjabi MM: The onset and progression of spinal injury: a demonstration of neutral zone sensitivity, *J Biomechanics* 25:1165-1172, 1992.
35. Hohl M: Normal motions in the upper portion of the cervical spine, *J Bone Joint Surg* 46-A(8):1777-1779, 1978.
36. Panjabi MM, Krag MH, Chung TQ: Effects of disc injury on mechanical behavior of the human spine, *Spine* 9:707-713, 1984.
37. White AA III, Johnson RM, Panjabi MM, et al: Biomechanical analysis of clinical instability in the cervical spine, *Clin Orthop Related Res* 109:85-96, 1975.
38. Frymoyer JW, Selby DK: Segmental instability: rationale for treatment, *Spine* 10:280-286, 1985.
39. Ogon M, Bender BR, Hooper DM, et al: A dynamic approach to spinal instability, part I: sensitization of intersegmental motion profiles to motion direction and load condition by instability, *Spine* 22:2841-2858, 1997.
40. Paris SV, Loubert PV: *Foundations of clinical orthopaedics*, St Augustine, Florida, 1986, Institute Press.
41. Fritz JM, Erhard RE, Hagen BF: Segmental instability of the lumbar spine, *Phys Ther* 78:889-896, 1998.
42. Shippel AH, Robinson GK: Radiological and magnetic resonance imaging of cervical spine instability: a case report, *J Manipulative Physiol Ther* 10:317-322, 1987.
43. Twomey LT: A rationale for the treatment of back pain and joint pain by manual therapy, *Phys Ther* 72:885-892, 1992.
44. Olson KA, Joder D: Cervical spine clinical instability: a resident's case report, *J Orthop Sports Phys Ther* 31(4):194-206, 2001.
45. Gonnella C, Paris SV, Kutner M: Reliability in evaluating passive intervertebral motion, *Phys Ther* 62:436-444, 1982.

46. Richardson CA, Jull GA: Muscle control-pain control: what exercises would you prescribe? *Man Ther* 1:2-10, 1995.

47. Tippets RH, Apfelbaum RI: Anterior fusion with the caspar instrumentation system, *Neurosurgery* 22:1008-1013, 1988.

48. Cook C, Brismee JM, Fleming R, et al: Indentifiers suggestive of clinical cervical spine instability: a Delphi study of physical therapists, *Phys Ther* 85(9):895-906, 2005.

49. Jull G, Bogduk N, Marsland A: The accuracy of manual diagnosis for cervical zygapophysial joint pain syndromes, *Med J Aust* 148:233-236, 1988.

50. Pope MH, Frymoyer JW, Krag MH: Diagnosing instability, *Clin Orthop Related Res* 279:60-67, 1992.

51. Herkowitz HN, Rothman RH: Subacute instability of the cervical spine, *Spine* 9:348-357, 1984.

52. Paris SV: Cervical symptoms of forward head posture, *Topics Geriatr Rehabil* 5(4):11-19, 1990.

53. Falla D: Unraveling the complexity of muscle impairment in chronic neck pain, *Man Ther* 9:125-133, 2004.

54. Ylinen J. Takala EP, Nydanen M, et al: Active neck muscle training in treatment of chronic neck pain in women: a randomized controlled trial, *JAMA* 289(19):2509-2516, 2003.

55. Jull G, Trott P, Potter H, et al: A randomized controlled trial of physiotherapy management for cervicogenic headache, *Spine* 27:1835-1843, 2002.

56. Torrens M: Adult: cervical spondylosis: part I: pathogenesis, diagnosis, and management options, *Current Orthop* 8:255-263, 1994.

57. Cleland JA, Whitman JM, Fritz JM, et al: Manual physical therapy, cervical traction, and strengthening exercises in patients with cervical radiculopathy: a case series, *JOSPT* 35(12):803-811, 2005.

58. Radhakrishnan K, Litchy WJ, O'Fallan M, et al: Epidemiology of cervical radiculopathy: a population-based study from Rochester, Minnesota, 1976-1990, *Brain* 117:325-335, 1994.

59. Shelerud RA, Paynter KS: Rarer causes of radiculopathy: spinal tumors, infections, and other unusual causes, *Phys Med Rehabil Clin North Am* 13:645-696, 2002.

60. Wainner RS, Fritz JM, Irrgang JJ, et al: Reliabilty and diagnostic accuracy of the clinical examination and patient self-report measures for cervical radiculopathy, *Spine* 28(1):52-62, 2003.

61. Waldrop MA: Diagnosis and treatment of cervical radiculopathy using a clinical prediction rule and a multimodal intervention approach: a case series, *JOSPT* 36(3):152-159, 2006.

62. Hoving JL, Koes BW, de Vet HCW, et al: Manual therapy, physical therapy, or continued care by a general practitioner for patients with neck pain: a randomized controlled trial, *Ann Intern Med* 136:713-722, 2002.

63. Korthals-de Bos IBC, Hoving JL, van Tulder MW, et al: Cost effectiveness of physiotherapy, manual therapy, and general practitioner care for neck pain: economic evaluation alongside a randomized controlled trial, *BMJ* 326:1-6, 2003.

64. Gross AR, Hoving JL, Haines TA, et al: A Cochrane review of manipulation and mobilization for mechanical neck disorders, *Spine* 29(14):1541-1548, 2004.

65. Tseng YL, Wang WTF, Chen WY, et al: Predictors for the immediate responders to cervical manipulation in patients with neck pain, *Man Ther* 11:306-315, 2006.

66. Zito G, Jull G, Story I: Clinical tests of musculoskeletal dysfunction in the diagnosis of cervicogenic headache, *Man Ther* 11:118-129, 2006.

67. Pfaffenrath V, Kaube H: Diagnostics of cervicogenic headache, *Funct Neurol* 5:159-64, 1990.

68. Sjaastad O, Fredriksen TA, Pfaffenrath V: Cervicogenic headache: diagnostic criteria, *Headache* 38:442-445 1998.

69. Uitvlugt G, Indenbaum S: Clinical assessment of atlantoaxial instability using the sharp-purser test, *Arthritis Rheum* 31(7):918-922, 1988.

70. Spurling RG, Scoville WB: Lateral rupture of the cervical intervertebral discs: a common cause of shoulder and arm pain, *Surg Gynecol Obstet* 78:350-358, 1944.

71. Tong HC, Haig AJ, Yamakawa K: The Spurling test and cervical radiculopathy, *Spine* 27(2):156-159, 2002.

72. Bertilson B, Grunnesjo M, Strender L: Reliability of clinical tests in the assessment of patients with neck/shoulder problems: impact of history, *Spine* 28:2222-2231, 2003.

73. Butler D, Gifford L: The concepts of adverse mechanical tension in the nervous system: part 1: testing for 'dural tension,' *Physiotherapy* 75(11):622-628, 1989.

74. Elvey RL: Treatment of arm pain associated with abnormal brachial plexus tension, *Aust J Physiother* 32:224-229, 1986.

75. Cote P, Kreitz BG, Cassidy JD, et al: The validity of the extension-rotation test as a clinical screening procedure before neck manipulation: a secondary analysis, *J Manipulative Physiol Ther* 19:159-164, 1996.

76. Piva SR, Erhard RE, Childs JD, et al: Inter-rater reliability of passive intervertebral and active movements of the cervical spine, *Man Ther* 11(4):321-330, 2006.

77. Smedmark V, Wallin M, Arvidsson I: Inter-examiner reliability in assessing passive intervertebral motion of the cervical spine, *Man Ther* 5:97-101, 2000.

78. Fernandez-de-las-Penas C, Downey C, Miangolarra-Page JC: Validity of the lateral gliding test as tool for the diagnosis of intervertebral joint dysfunction in the lower cervical spine, *J Manipulative Physiol Ther* 28(8):610-616, 2005.

79. Panjabi M, Dvorak J, Duranceau J, et al: Three-dimensional movements of the upper cervical spine, *Spine* 13(7):726-730, 1988.

80. Kottke FJ, Mundale MO: Range of mobility of the cervical spine, *Arch Phys Med Rehabil* 379-382, 1959.

81. White A, Panjabi MM: Kinematics of the spine. In White A, Panjabi MM, editors: *Clinical biomechanics of the spine*, Philadelphia, 1978, Lippincott.

82. Spitzer W, Skovron M, Salmi L, et al: Scientific monograph of Quebec Task Force on whiplash associated disorders: redefining "whiplash" and its management, *Spine* 20:1-73, 1995.

83. Pool J, Hoving J, de Vet H, et al: The interexaminer reproducibility of physical examination of the cervical spine, *J Manipulative Physiol Ther* 27:84-90, 2003.

## CHAPTER 7

# Temporomandibular Disorders

## CHAPTER OVERVIEW

This chapter includes descriptions of the kinematics and functional anatomy of the temporomandibular joint (TMJ) and related structures and the examination, diagnostic classification, and treatment of temporomandibular disorders (TMD).

## OBJECTIVES

- Describe the functional anatomy and kinematics of the TMJ
- Identify the classification of TMD and describe the components of each disorder
- Perform a comprehensive examination of the TMJ and related structures
- Perform treatment procedures for TMD, including soft tissue mobilization, joint mobilization/manipulation, and exercise instruction
- Describe the functional interrelationships between the TMJ and the cervical spine and identify why examination and treatment of the cervical spine are important to include with the management of TMDs

## SIGNIFICANCE OF THE PROBLEM

More than 17 million people in the United States are estimated to have temporomandibular disorders (TMDs).[1] The lifetime incidence rate of TMD is reported to be 34%, with a 2% annual incidence rate.[2] Dworkin and LeResche[2] estimate that 178 lost activity days per 1000 persons per year can be attributed to TMD. Although temporomandibular joint (TMJ) problems can occur in individuals of any age, they are most common in individuals 13 to 35 years of age and are four times more prevalent in women than in men.[3] Temporomandibular disorder is a musculoskeletal condition that results in craniofacial pain, functional limitations, and disability.[4] Symptoms associated with TMD can include TMJ pain, decreased jaw motion, joint clicking, headaches, neck pain, facial pain, and pain with chewing.[5] Temporomandibular disorders may be the result of osteoarthritic degeneration, articular disc subluxation, or muscle guarding of the muscles of mastication.[5]

Treatment options for TMD include surgery, injections, medications, intraoral appliances, biofeedback, and physical therapy. Outcomes reported with the use of surgery and intraoral appliances in treatment of TMD have been disappointing. A retrospective cohort study revealed that at a 6-month follow-up examination only 50% of patients who underwent TMJ arthroplasty viewed the outcome as favorable.[6] Intraoral appli-

ances, which are used in theory to create a natural resting position of the mandible to inhibit excessive tension in the muscles of mastication and relieve pain, have been shown to be less effective than a manual physical therapy approach in the management of TMJ articular disc anterior displacement without reduction syndrome.[7] The group that used manual therapy combined with active exercise showed significant reductions in pain and increases in range of motion (ROM), and the group with the soft repositioning splint did not show significant changes in either dependent measure.[7]

This chapter focuses on the physical therapy diagnosis and management of TMJ conditions. High-quality randomized controlled studies are not available to guide treatment decision making for TMD. However, published case series studies support the use of an impairment-based manual physical therapy approach for treatment of TMD and form the basis for the approach presented in this chapter.[8-10]

## TEMPOROMANDIBULAR KINEMATICS: FUNCTIONAL ANATOMY AND MECHANICS

The temporomandibular joint is a synovial articulation between the mandible and the temporal bone of the cranium with an articular disc interposed between the two bony structures. The articular disc divides the joint into an upper and lower compartment. The TMJ is classified as a hinge joint with a moveable socket because of the hinge-like motion of the lower compartment and the gliding movement of the upper compartment.[11] The articular disc is biconcave, with the thin intermediate portion composed of an avascular and aneural fibrous structure that is well suited for the stresses of the joint surfaces.[12] The anterior and posterior portions of the disc are two to three times thicker than the intermediate portion and have vascular and nerve supplies.[13] The biconcave shape of the disc offers congruency of the articular surfaces and contributes greatly to the stability of the TMJ.

The posterior aspect of the TMJ is referred to as the bilaminar region and is composed of the posterior ligament, which has two heads: the inferior stratum, which attaches the disc to the neck of the mandibular condyle; and the superior stratum, which attaches the disc to the posterior aspect of the temporal bone. The retrodiscal pad is interspersed between the two heads of the posterior ligament and includes highly vascularized and innervated loose connective tissue that attaches to the posterior wall of the capsule.[11] The superior head of the lateral pterygoid muscle attaches to the anterior medial portion of the disc, and additional fibrous capsular tissues attach to the anterior portion of the disc.[11] The lateral and medial collateral ligaments connect the disc to the lateral and medial poles of the condyle to form a bucket-handle configuration, which allows the disc to slide anterior/posterior on the condyle.[12] The fibrous joint capsule envelops the entire joint and is reinforced laterally by the temporomandibular ligament. With hypermobility of the TMJ, the posterior ligament and collateral ligaments tend to lose their ability to stabilize the disc on the mandibular condyle and the lateral pterygoid tends to pull the disc anterior and medially as the disc dysfunction progresses to cause a disc dislocation.[12]

The innervation of the TMJ is from the auriculotemporal and masseteric branches of the mandibular nerve, and the blood supply is from the superficial temporal and maxillary arteries.[11]

The osteokinematics of the mandible include depression (opening), elevation (closing), protrusion, retrusion, and lateral excursion. Mandibular depression is measured as the space between the maxillary and mandibular incisors; normal range of motion can vary from 35 mm to 50 mm, depending on the size and shape of the mouth and teeth.[11,13] Lateral excursion and protrusion motions are approximately 10 mm. A 4 : 1 ratio of depression to lateral excursion is considered ideal and is an important consideration in restoration of motion to a stiff TMJ.[12]

Arthrokinematically, mandibular depression begins with the first 25 mm of opening that occurs primarily as a rotational motion (roll-gliding) of the condyle in the inferior joint space (Figure 7-1). Once the collateral ligaments tauten, the opening continues as primarily a translatory gliding motion in the upper joint space until 35 mm is reached and the posterior and collateral ligaments are taut. Opening greater than 35 mm results from further translation with overrotation and further stretching applied to the posterior and collateral ligaments.[12] The lateral pterygoid, inferior head, provides a protracting force on the condyles and discs; the geniohyoid and digastic muscles produce a depressing and retracting force on the chin; and the mylohyoid muscle pulls downward on the body of the mandible to combine to produce the rotatory and translatory movements of the jaw that occur with mandibular depression[12] (Figure 7-2).

Elevation of the mandible to close the mouth is initiated by the posterior fibers of the temporalis muscle contracting to retract the condyle of the mandible and clear the articular eminence of the temporalis bone. The temporalis, masseter, and

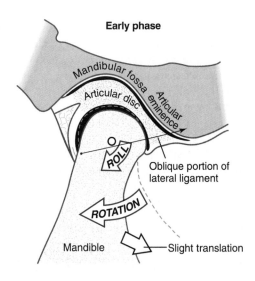
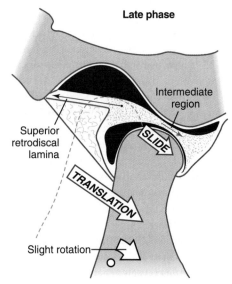

**FIGURE 7-1** Arthrokinematics of opening mouth: early phase and late phase. From Neumann DA: *Kinesiology of the musculoskeletal system. foundations for physical rehabilitation*, St Louis, 2002, Mosby.

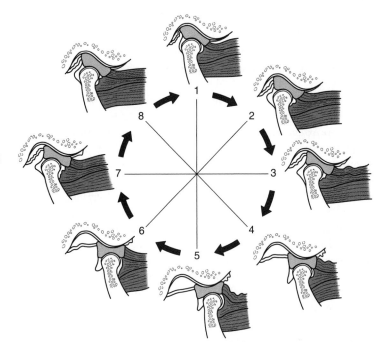

**FIGURE 7-2** Normal functional movement of condyle and disc during full range of opening and closing. From Magee DJ: *Orthopedic physical assessment*, ed 5, Philadelphia, 2008, Saunders.

medial pterygoid contract on both sides to elevate the mandible, and the lateral pterygoid stabilizes the disc/condyle complex against the articular eminence during closing.[11,12]

Protusion of the mandible is created with symmetrical anterior translation of both condyle/disc complexes on the articular eminence, and the motion occurs at the superior joint space. Protrusion is created by contraction of the inferior head of the lateral pterygoid and holding action of the masseter and medial pterygoid muscles.[12] The lateral pterygoid pulls the condyle and disc forward and down along the articular eminence while the elevator and depressor muscles maintain the mandibular position.[12] Retrusion is the return to rest position from the protrusion position and is created by the contraction of the middle and posterior fibers of both temporalis muscles while the depressors and elevators maintain a slight opening of the mouth.[12]

Lateral excursion occurs when the condyle and disc of the contralateral side are pulled forward, downward, and medially along the articular eminence. The condyle on the ipsilateral side performs minimal rotation around a vertical axis and a slight lateral shift.[12] These motions take place primarily in the upper joint space. Lateral excursion is created by contraction of the lateral pterygoid muscles on the contralateral side of the direction of the motion combined with the ipsilateral side temporalis muscle contracting to hold the rest position of the condyle to prevent the mandible from deviating anteriorly.[12]

## Cervical Spine Influence on the Temporomandibular Joint

The cervical spine can influence TMJ function in a variety of ways, and postural interrelationships have been noted through a series of studies. McClean et al[14] found that occlusional contacts change as the body position is altered on a tilt table. The

mandible was consistently in a more retruded position with the subjects in supine, and the occlusional contact became more anterior as the subjects assumed a more upright position.[14]

Funakoshi et al[15] measured jaw muscle activity changes associated with head position and found that with cervical forward bending, increased electromyographic (EMG) activity was noted in the bilateral digastric muscles. With cervical backward bending, increased EMG activity was noted in the bilateral temporalis muscles. With cervical rotation and side bending, increased EMG activity was noted in the ipsilateral temporalis, masseter, and digastric muscles. This increased EMG activity was believed to occur in an attempt to maintain the rest position of the mandible in various head and neck postural positions.[15]

Darling et al[16] showed that head and neck postural positioning could be improved with 4 weeks of physical therapy and that an increase in the vertical postural position of the mandible occurred as the head and neck postural positioning improved. The vertical postural position is the rest position of the mandible in which the teeth are not occluded, the lips are in light contact, and only minimal amount of muscular activity occurs to maintain and balance the postural position. In other words, as the patient's head and neck posture improved, the mandible assumed a more relaxed neutral position.

Goldstein et al[17] found that the vertical distance of mandibular closure from the rest position of the mandible decreased significantly as a maximum forward head posture was assumed in comparison with the same subjects in their best "normal" posture. As a result, they also saw a change in trajectory of mandibular occlusion with forward head posture positioning and a change in initial tooth contact.[17] These postural influences on mandibular function have been postulated as causing a "pseudomalocclusion" that could contribute to increased strain on the joint capsule and myofascial structures associated with TMJ function.[18]

Not only can head and neck posture affect TMJ function, but also mandibular rest position change can affect head and neck posture. Daly[19] had 30 subjects sit with an 8-mm spacer between the teeth for 1 hour and found that all subjects had an altered craniovertebral angle after 1 hour, with 27 subjects having a more extended position of the head on the neck and three subjects assuming a more flexed position. One hour after removal of the spacer appliance, all subjects showed at least partial recovery toward the original head position.[19] These study results reinforce the interdependence of cervical, cranial, and mandibular positioning and function and may assist in explaining why patients occasionally have worse symptoms in the head and neck after initiation of an intraoral appliance therapy.

The cervical spine can also be a source of referred pain to the head and face and must be thoroughly screened as part of the comprehensive examination of a patient with symptoms of head and facial pain. The most likely anatomical sources of referred pain to the head and face include impairments of the suboccipital muscles and the upper cervical and C2-C3 facet joints and entrapment neuropathies of the greater and lesser occipital nerves. The strain associated with suboccipital muscle guarding may impinge on the greater occipital nerve and may result in referred pain into the craniofacial region, most typically into the distribution of the trigeminal nerve.[20] In a study by Aprill, Axinn, and Bogduk,[21] 21 of 34 participants who underwent a nerve block to C1-C2 had complete resolution of headache symptoms. These findings suggest a high prevalence rate of headache and facial pain symptoms referred from the upper cervical spine.

Therefore, palpation and provocation tests for the both the TMJ and upper cervical spine must be completed to differentiate the source of the symptoms. A thorough examination of the cervical and thoracic spine is a necessary component of examination of patients with primary symptoms of headaches and facial pain to differentiate the source of the symptoms and biomechanical factors that could potentially contribute to perpetuation of a temporomandibular disorder.

## TEMPOROMANDIBULAR DISORDERS

The classification system presented in this chapter is useful to guide clinical decision making in management of TMD. Table 7-1 provides a summary of the common signs and symptoms associated with each disorder. Patients may have a combination of temporomandibular disorders, which makes management of this condition challenging.

### Capsulitis/Synovitis

Capsulitis/synovitis is an inflammatory condition of the articular capsule and soft tissues that surround the TMJ, especially the highly vascularized and innervated extracapsular articular tissues. The patient has pain with palpation and loading the TMJ. Pain may also be noted with accessory motion testing.

| TABLE 7-1 | Signs and Symptoms of Temporomandibular Disorders |
|---|---|
| **TMD CLASSIFICATION** | **SIGNS AND SYMPTOMS** |
| Capsulitis/synovitis | Tender to palpation at TMJ lateral condyle or posterior compartment<br>Pain with biting on opposite side<br>Pain with retrusive overpressure<br>Pain with accessory motion testing |
| Capsular fibrosis | Limited AROM mandibular dynamics<br>Limited mobility with TMJ accessory motion tests<br>No joint sounds<br>Deviation of mandible with opening toward limited side<br>History of trauma or surgery |
| Masticatory muscle disorders | No joint sounds<br>Pain with palpation muscles of mastication<br>Inconsistent alterations in mandibular control<br>Parafunctional oral behaviors<br>Pain with biting on same side of facial pain |
| Hypermobility | Excessive AROM with opening >40 mm<br>Joint sound at end range of opening<br>Hypermobility with accessory motion testing |
| Anterior disc displacement with reduction | Reciprocal joint sound with opening and closing<br>S curve with opening<br>Full AROM (unless combined with acute capsulitis) |
| Anterior disc displacement without reduction | History of joint sounds<br>Limited opening <25 mm if acute<br>Deviation of mandible with opening toward limited side |
| Osteoarthritis | TMJ crepitus as noted with stethoscope<br>Pain with TMJ palpation<br>Radiographic evidence of osteoarthritis |

Chewing and biting down with the molars on the contralateral side of the involved TMJ tend to be painful. If capsulitis continues chronically over time, capsular fibrosis could form. Capsulitis can be combined with any of the other common TMJ disorders or can present in isolation.

The cause of capsulitis/synovitis has been explained as microtrauma or macrotrauma.[12] Microtrauma includes low-level repeated stresses and strains on the TMJ and surrounding tissues that may occur with parafunctional habits, such as clenching and grinding the teeth, chewing gum, or chewing on a pencil. Macrotrauma occurs with greater force, such as a blow to the jaw or surgery to the TMJ.

Antiinflammatory treatment, such as iontophoresis, gentle range of motion activities, and ice, can often be helpful. In a study by Majwer and Swider,[22] 27 of 32 cases of posttraumatic TMD benefited with decreased pain from the application of dexamethasone (n = 8) or xylocane (n = 24) through iontophoresis. Reduction of the parafunctional activities through behavior modification may assist as well. Creation of a good environment for proper TMJ function, such as postural correction exercises and treatment of cervical and upper thoracic impairments, can also facilitate the rehabilitation process.

Furto et al[8] had successful outcomes that included reduction of pain and disability in a case series of 15 patients with TMD as the primary symptoms. At a 2-week follow-up examination, the group had received a mean of 4.3 physical therapy treatment sessions. Specific interventions included manual physical therapy techniques, such as intraoral soft tissue mobilization and nonthrust joint mobilization/manipulation to the cervical spine, TMJ, and thoracic spine. Five of the patients also received iontophoresis with dexamethasone to the symptomatic TMJ. Eighty percent of the patients received instruction in TMJ proprioception and postural exercises. The mean TMD disability index (Box 7-1) scores were 32.1% at baseline and 18.3% at the 2-week follow-up examination, an improvement of 13.9% (confidence interval [CI], 8.2%, 19.5%; $P < .05$). Eleven patients (73%) reported they were "somewhat better" to "a very great deal better" on the global rating of change questionnaire, and Patient Specific Functional Scale (PSFS) scores improved 3.1 points (CI, 2.3, 3.9; $P < .05$).[8] The treatment approach used in this case series is representative of an impairment-based approach in which manual physical therapy and exercise interventions were used to address the specific impairments noted at the cervical spine and craniomandibular region. Iontophoresis was used as an adjunct to reduce the pain and inflammation at the TMJ capsular tissues.

Furto et al[8] used a TMJ exercise program developed by Rocabado[23] to facilitate dynamic neuromuscular control through the use of repetitive lateral deviation motions with a 0.5-inch piece of surgical tubing placed between the incisors to assist with mobility, proprioception, and pain inhibition. Box 7-2 provides an illustration of TMJ proprioception exercises. The first (ROM) phase involves active range of motion lateral excursion while the surgical tubing is rolled between the incisors, with movement away from the side of TMJ pain or hypermobility; the second (bite) phase involves a submaximal biting down contraction in the lateral excursion position with the bite let off before a return to midline; and the third phase involves biting down on the tube with the lateral excursion motion and with return to midline. In theory, the biting with motion recruits the muscles of mastication to apply a compressive force to the disc to improve the condylar-disc-eminence congruency and TMJ function.[23] Phases 4 to 6 of this program involve a similar progression with mandibular protrusion active motions. Patients are instructed to perform six repetitions every 2 hours. Although limited evidence exists to support the theoretical effect of this treatment approach, the patients in the case series had improvements in function, pain, and disability.[8]

## Capsular Fibrosis

Capsular fibrosis is characterized by a mandibular opening of less than 25 mm because of adhesions that limit extensibility of the TMJ capsule. The mandible deviates toward the side of the restricted TMJ with opening, lateral excursion to the opposite side of the stiff joint is limited, and protrusion deviates toward the affected side. Accessory motion testing of the TMJ shows hypomobility. The causes of capsular fibrosis may include a chronic inflammatory condition, trauma, immobilization, or a subluxed articular disc without reduction relationship that places the mandibular head in a posterior and superior position.[12]

When the capsular fibrosis is coupled with capsulitis or a masticatory muscle disorder, these conditions need to be addressed as part of the treatment. Cervical spine and postural disorders should also be appropriately addressed if present with TMD. Joint mobilization/manipulation, active and passive mandibular range of motion exercises, and sustained TMJ stretching techniques are indicated to restore TMJ mobility. Sustained TMJ stretching can be accomplished with a stack of tongue depressors placed between the molars on the ipsilateral side of the stiff TMJ (Box 7-3; see p. 316). The patient is instructed to maintain the stretch for 15 to 20 minutes, three times per day. This technique can be combined with a heat modality, such as moist heat or therapeutic ultrasound. TMJ range of motion and proprioception exercises for opening and lateral excursion should be performed at least five to six times per day.

## Masticatory Muscle Disorders

Masticatory muscle disorders are most commonly associated with painful guarded muscles of mastication and may progress to include tendonitis, commonly of the temporalis tendon. Palpation of the involved muscles and chewing/biting on the ipsilateral side of the pain provoke the symptoms. Neuromuscular control deficits may also be noted with altered trajectory of opening and closing with inconsistent S and Z movement patterns in the absence of joint sounds. TMJ palpation, compression, and accessory motion tests are nonprovocative if the masticatory muscle disorder is present in isolation. Masticatory muscle disorders can occur in isolation or can be combined with other TMJ disorders. The most common cause is parafunctional behaviors that cause irritation and inflammation of the muscles of mastication; most commonly, the closing/clenching muscles are involved, especially the masseter, temporalis, and lateral pterygoid muscles. Oral habits such as gum chewing, chewing on ice, repetitive nonfunctional jaw movements, and frequent leaning of the chin on the palm have been associated with the presence of TMJ disorders in females of high school age.[24]

Treatment may include use of heat modalities, such as moist heat, therapeutic ultrasound, or warm water rinses. Instruction in proper tongue/teeth/lip positioning and isometric opening exercises may assist in inhibition of the guarded closing/clenching muscles. The controlled mandibular opening exercise can facilitate muscle relaxation and strengthen the proper tongue function and placement (Box 7-4; see p. 317). Intraoral and extraoral soft tissue mobilization (STM) techniques are also indicated. The patient can be instructed in self-STM techniques and educated to inhibit parafunctional activities. Muscle reeducation and TMJ proprioception exercises can assist to improve masticatory muscle control and function.

## BOX 7-1   Temporomandibular Disorder Disability Index

Please check the statement that best pertains to you (not necessarily exactly) in each of the following categories.

**1. Communication (talking).**
—I can talk as much as I want without pain, fatigue, or discomfort.
—I can talk as much as I want, but it causes some pain, fatigue, or discomfort.
—I can't talk as much as I want because of pain, fatigue, or discomfort.
—I can't talk much at all because of pain, fatigue, or discomfort.
—Pain prevents me from talking at all.

**2. Normal living activities (brushing teeth/flossing).**
—I am able to care for my gums and teeth in a normal fashion without restriction and without pain, fatigue, or discomfort.
—I am able to care for all my teeth and gums, but I must be slow and careful, otherwise pain/discomfort or jaw tiredness results.
—I do manage to care for my teeth and gums in a normal fashion, but it usually causes some pain/discomfort or jaw tiredness no matter how careful I am.
—I am unable to properly clean all my teeth and gums because of restricted opening or pain.
—I am unable to care for most of my teeth and gums because of restricted opening or pain.

**3. Normal living activities (eating, chewing).**
—I can eat and chew as much of anything I want without pain/discomfort or jaw tiredness.
—I can eat and chew most anything I want, but it sometimes causes pain/discomfort or jaw tiredness.
—I can't eat much of anything I want because it often causes pain/discomfort or jaw tiredness or because of restricted opening.
—I must eat only soft foods (consistency of scrambled eggs or less) because of pain/discomfort, jaw fatigue, or restricted opening.
—I must stay on a liquid diet because of pain or restricted opening.

**4. Social/recreational activities (singing, playing musical instruments, cheering, laughing, social activities, playing amateur sports/hobbies, etc).**
—I am enjoying a normal social life or recreational activities without restriction.
—I participate in a normal social life or recreational activities, but pain/discomfort is increased.
—The presence of pain or fear of likely aggravation only limits the more energetic components of my social life (sports, exercise, dancing, playing musical instruments, singing).
—I have restrictions socially as I can't even sing, shout, cheer, play, or laugh expressively because of increased pain/discomfort.
—I have practically no social life because of pain.

**5. Nonspecialized jaw activities (yawning, mouth opening, and opening my mouth wide).**
—I can yawn in a normal fashion, painlessly.
—I can yawn and open my mouth fully wide open, but sometimes there is discomfort.
—I can yawn and open my mouth wide in a normal fashion, but it almost always causes discomfort.
—Yawning and opening my mouth wide are somewhat restricted by pain.
—I cannot yawn or open my mouth more than two finger widths (2.8 to 3.2 cm) or, if I can, it always causes greater than moderate pain.

**6. Sexual function (including kissing, hugging, and any and all sexual activities to which you are accustomed).**
—I am able to engage in all my customary sexual activities and expressions without limitation or causing headache, face, or jaw pain.
—I am able to engage in all my customary sexual activities and expressions, but it sometimes causes some headache, face, or jaw pain or jaw fatigue.
—I am able to engage in all my customary sexual activities and expressions, but it usually causes enough headache, face, or jaw pain to markedly interfere with my enjoyment, willingness, and satisfaction.
—I must limit my customary sexual activities and expressions because of headache, face, or jaw pain or limited mouth opening.
—I abstain from almost all sexual activities and expression because of the head, face, or jaw pain it causes.

**7. Sleep (restful, nocturnal sleep pattern).**
—I sleep well in a normal fashion without any pain medication, relaxants, or sleeping pills.
—I sleep well with the use of pain pills, antiinflammatory medication, or medicinal sleeping aids.
—I fail to realize 6 hours of restful sleep even with the use of pills.
—I fail to realize 4 hours of restful sleep even with the use of pills.
—I fail to realize 2 hours of restful sleep even with the use of pills.

**8. Effects of any form of treatment, including, but not limited to, medications, in-office therapy, treatments, oral orthotics (e.g., splints, mouthpieces), ice/heat, etc.**
—I do not need to use treatment of any type to control or tolerate headache, face, or jaw pain and discomfort.
—I can completely control my pain with some form of treatment.
—I get partial, but significant, relief through some form of treatment.
—I don't get "a lot" of relief from any form of treatment.
—There is no form of treatment that helps enough to make me want to continue.

**9. Tinnitus, or ringing in the ear(s).**
—I do not experience ringing in my ear(s).
—I experience ringing in my ear(s) somewhat, but it does not interfere with my sleep or my ability to perform my daily activities.
—I experience ringing in my ear(s) and it interferes with my sleep or daily activities, but I can accomplish set goals and can get an acceptable amount of sleep.
—I experience ringing in my ear(s), and it causes a marked impairment in the performance of my daily activities or results in an unacceptable loss of sleep.
—I experience ringing in my ear(s), and it is incapacitating or forces me to use a masking device to get any sleep.

**10. Dizziness (lightheadedness, spinning, or balance disturbance).**
—I do not experience dizziness.
—I experience dizziness, but it does not interfere with my daily activities.
—I experience dizziness that interferes somewhat with my daily activities, but I can accomplish my set goals.
—I experience dizziness that causes a marked impairment in the performance of my daily activities.
—I experience dizziness that is incapacitating.

Adapted from Streigerwald DP, Maher JH: The Streigerwald/Maher TMD disability questionnaire, *Today Chiropract* 26:86-91, 1997.

**BOX 7-2** Temporomandibular Joint Proprioception Exercises with a Rubber Tube

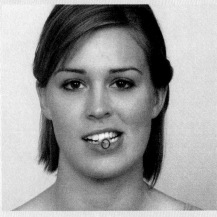

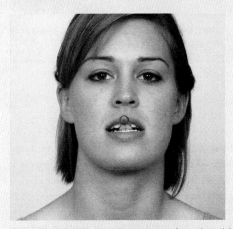

Bite phase (phase 2): At end of lateral deviation ROM, patient applies submaximal bite onto tube and holds bite for 5 seconds. Mandible is then returned to midline. This is repeated for five to six repetitions. Next progression (phase 3) is to maintain bite as mandible is returned to midline.

Start position for TMJ proprioception exercises with rubber tube.

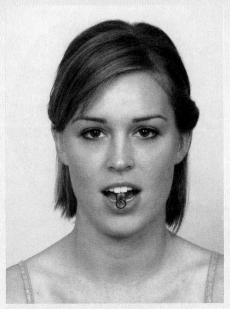

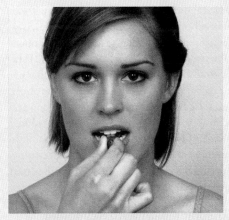

Phases 4 to 6: Protrusion range of motion, bite at end range, and bite as return to starting position can be progressed in similar fashion to lateral deviation progression.

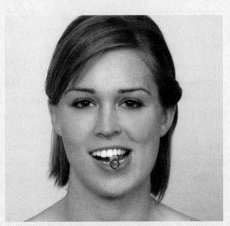

ROM phase (phase 1): Perform active lateral deviation away from painful TMJ within pain-free range of motion and without joint sounds.

Final progression is to gently pull tube and resist in either protrusion or laterally deviated position.

**BOX 7-3** Passive Mandibular Range of Motion and Sustained Mandibular Stretching

Finger position to offer active assistive and passive mandibular depression ROM.

Stack of wooden tongue blades can be used to apply sustained stretch to facilitate mandibular depression.

## Hypermobility

Hypermobility of the TMJ is characterized by a mandibular opening greater than 40 mm with an end range opening click and chin deviation away from the hypermobile joint that clicks. The joint sound in this case is the result of the mandibular condyle snapping across the distal edge of the articular crest. Hypermobility also is noted with accessory motion testing. Hypermobility of the TMJ may be asymptomatic unless combined with a capsulitis/synovitis condition and is postulated as being a precursor to articular disc displacement conditions.[12] Treatment is a TMJ stabilization treatment program with an emphasis on multidirectional mandibular isometric exercises, proprioception exercise, and education to avoid full wide opening (see Box 7-4). Five to 10 repetitions of each of the TMJ stabilization exercises should be performed at least 5 to 6 times per day. The isometric exercises are held 5 to 6 seconds each. Short, frequent doses of exercise can assist in muscle reeducation and pain inhibition. A strategy that is often helpful to avoid end range stresses on the TMJ is to instruct the patient to maintain the tip of the tongue up on the roof of the mouth with yawning. Cervical spine impairments should also be addressed as part of the rehabilitation program of all TMDs.

## Articular Disc Displacement with Reduction

Articular disc displacement with reduction is considered a progression of the dysfunction of a hypermobile TMJ. As the joint becomes more lax, the posterior ligament and collateral ligaments elongate and are unable to maintain the articular disc in its ideal position in relation to the mandibular condyle throughout the range of mandibular motion. As the mouth closes, the disc tends to slide forward and medial, which produces a joint noise.[12] With mandibular depression, a joint sound occurs as the condyle translates far enough anterior to recapture the disc–condyle relationship to create an opening click. The mandible tends to deviate to the ipsilateral side because of the in-itial restriction of condyle anterior translation by the anterior medial position of the disc. Once the disc is recaptured, a joint click is produced at the apex of the mandibular deviation and then the mandible moves back toward midline as the opening proceeds. The greater the degree of ligamentous laxity, the later in the range of the motion the joint sound occurs with mandibular depression (Figure 7-3).[12] The most reliable method to detect joint sounds is to use a stethoscope (Figure 7-4; see p. 319).

Treatment is similar to TMJ hypermobility with an attempt to stabilize the joint and improve the neuromuscular control. If capsulitis or masticatory muscle involvement is evident, these conditions also need to be addressed. Education on joint stress reduction (Box 7-5; see p. 319) combined with an exercise program is used to prevent the condition from progressing to an acute articular disc displacement without reduction.

The proprioception exercises described in Box 7-2 can be modified first to protrude the mandible to recapture the disc and then to perform the lateral excursion progression of ROM, ROM with the end range bite, and ROM with the sustained bite. Rocabado[25] theorizes that this exercise regimen can assist in remodeling the disc and reeducating the local TMJ muscles

**BOX 7-4** Temporomandibular Joint Stabilization Exercises

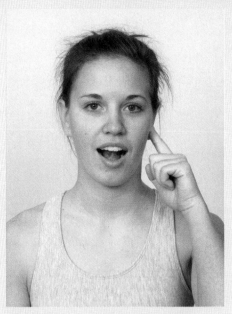

TMJ controlled opening with tongue up and palpation to isolate spinning of condyle and limit excessive translation. Mirror can be used to assist in retraining symmetrical opening. Keeping tongue up strengthens tongue and avoids excessive translation of TMJ.

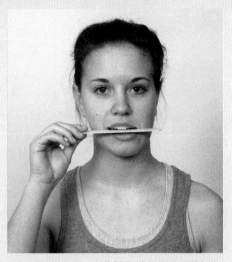

Lateral excursion AROM with tongue blade guidance.

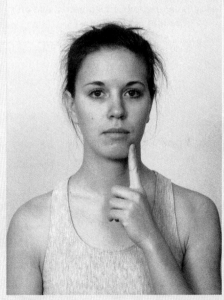

Mandibular lateral excursion isometric; use only force of weight of finger.

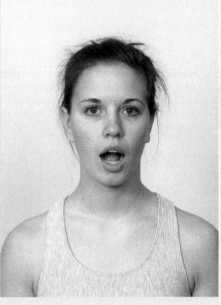

TMJ controlled opening with tongue up.

*Continued*

**BOX 7-4**    Temporomandibular Joint Stabilization Exercises—cont'd

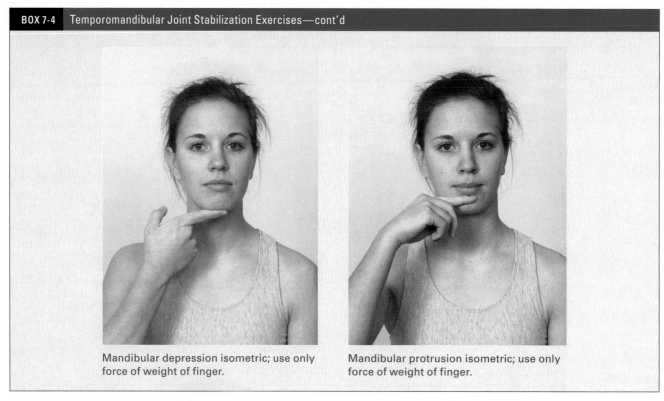

Mandibular depression isometric; use only force of weight of finger.

Mandibular protrusion isometric; use only force of weight of finger.

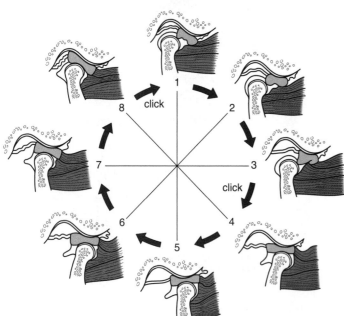

**FIGURE 7-3** Anterior disc dislocation with reduction. Note joint sound that occurs with opening as disc is reduced and joint sound with closing that occurs as disc dislocates. From Magee DJ: *Orthopedic physical assessment*, ed 5, Philadelphia, 2008, Saunders.

to attempt to correct and stabilize the disc displacement. If the disc displacement is a more chronic condition, TMJ capsular tightness may be evident as a result of the tendency of the mandibular condyle to rest in a more superior, retracted position with the disc displaced.[25] TMJ distraction mobilization techniques may be needed to assist in restoration of normal capsular mobility.

In a randomized clinical trial, Yoda et al[26] compared an exercise program with an education program for patients with anterior disc displacement with reduction. The results showed that the exercise program group had better outcomes for decreased pain and increased ROM ($P = .0001$).[26] Forty-two patients participated in the study; 61.9% of the exercise group had favorable outcomes (13/21 patients), and 0% of the control (education program) group had favorable results.[26] Success was measured on the severity of joint sounds or pain with maximal mouth opening. Of the 13 patients with a successful outcome, only three patients' TMJ articular discs (23.1%) were recaptured with reexamination with magnetic resonance imaging (MRI).[26]

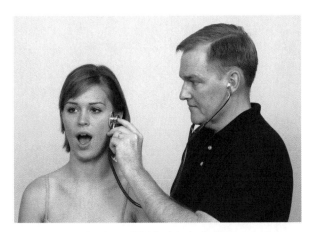

**FIGURE 7-4** Auscultation of TMJ with stethoscope during mandibular AROM testing can assist in identification of joint sounds.

| **BOX 7-5**   TMJ Education |
| --- |
| ■ Limit parafunctional activities: nail biting, gum chewing, clenching and grinding teeth |
| ■ Tongue position: at rest, the tip of the tongue should be at the ridge of the roof of the mouth with the front one third of the tongue on the roof of the mouth |
| ■ Teeth position: the teeth should be 2 to 3 mm apart at rest |
| ■ Lips should be lightly together with breathing through the nose |
| ■ Keep the tip of the tongue up on the roof of the mouth when yawning |
| ■ Avoid sleeping in the prone position |
| ■ Do not rest chin in hands |
| ■ Soft diet: avoid hard crunchy foods |
| ■ Cut food up into small pieces |
| ■ Warm water rinses |
| ■ Postural exercises 5 to 6 times per day |

Likewise, Nicolakis et al[10] reported on the outcomes of 30 patients with TMJ anterior disc displacement with reduction who underwent treatment with temporomandibular joint and soft tissue mobilization, range of motion and isometric exercises, and postural education for an average of nine visits with a physical therapist. Seventy-five percent of the patients had successful outcomes in this case series, with outcome measures that included pain level and mouth opening measurements at the 6-month follow-up examination; 13% had reduction in TMJ sounds.[10] This study supports the use of exercise combined with gentle manual therapy techniques for treatment of anterior disc displacement with reduction.

## Articular Disc Displacement without Reduction

Articular disc displacement without reduction is a progression of articular disc displacement with reduction. When the condition is acute, the opening is limited to less than 25 mm with an end range deviation toward the affected joint, limited contralateral lateral excursion, and with deviation of the mandible toward the affected side with protrusion. Because this pattern of limited mandibular AROM is the same as with capsular fibrosis, a history of joint sounds can help to distinguish the likelihood of a disc displacement without reduction. The disc displacement without reduction disorder typically has a history of an opening and closing joint sound, but the joint sounds disappear when the acute limitation in mandibular motion occurs. This condition occurs when the articular disc displaces anterior to the condyle and is unable to be reduced with movement of the mandible. The disc blocks further anterior translation with opening, contralateral lateral excursion, and protrusion (Figure 7-5). Accessory motions of the affected joint are also limited. When the condition is chronic, the posterior ligament and capsular tissues can be stretched to allow nearly full normal mandibular motion.

Cleland and Palmer[27] showed a good clinical outcome in a single case design study of a patient with bilateral articular disc displacement without reduction that was confirmed with MRI.

The treatment approach included TMJ mobilization techniques, cervical spine mobilization/manipulation techniques, postural and neck exercises, and patient education regarding parafunctional habits, soft diet, relaxation techniques, activity modification, and tongue resting position. The patient had a return of normal mouth opening and a reduction in pain and disability measures as a result of the physical therapy approach.[27]

Patients with anterior disc displacement without reduction can make functional and symptomatic improvements with the use of joint mobilization and therapeutic exercise. Over time, the shape of the articular disc tends to change and the likelihood of reducing and maintaining a normal disc condyle relationship is minimal. Some speculation exists that over time the posterior ligament can become more fibrous and function similar to a disc. However, without a properly positioned and functioning disc, the TMJ may be more susceptible to development of osteoarthritic changes. On occasion, the anterior disc displacement begins to reduce again and the joint sounds return as the range of motion and function of the mandible improves. In this situation, the rehabilitation program should progress as outlined for an anterior disc displacement with reduction.

## Temporomandibular Joint Osteoarthritis

Osteoarthritis (OA) of the TMJ is common and may be an added source of pain and limited mandibular motion. Joint crepitus is present with OA of the TMJ and is best noted with use of a stethoscope (see Figure 7-4). Radiographs or arthoscopic visualization are needed to confirm the diagnosis. Israel et al[28] tested 84 subjects with symptoms of TMJ pain with auscultation for crepitus with a stethoscope and compared the findings with arthroscopic visualization results to find a sensitivity of 0.70, a specificity of 0.43, a positive likelihood ratio (+LR) of 1.23, and a negative likelihood ratio (−LR) of 0.70 for detection of OA with positive findings of TMJ crepitus.

Nicolakis et al[9] had successful outcomes in a series of 20 patients with OA of the TMJ with improved measures of pain at

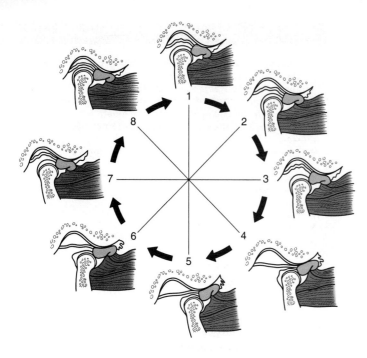

**FIGURE 7-5** Anterior disc dislocation without reduction. Disc remains dislocated anterior and medial to the condyle, which limits the distance the condyle can translate forward. From Magee DJ: *Orthopedic physical assessment*, ed 5, Philadelphia, 2008, Saunders.

rest, incisional opening, and function. The interventions included joint mobilization of the TMJ, soft tissue techniques, active and passive TMJ exercises, and postural exercises.[9] Data collected on these patients at a 12-month follow-up examination continued to suggest favorable results for the use of exercise and manual physical therapy in the management of TMD.[10]

## Postsurgical Temporomandibular Joint

A variety of surgical procedures are performed to treat TMDs. A detailed surgical report and the surgeon's postsurgical precautions should be obtained. A common example of TMJ surgery is an arthroscopy procedure in which a small scope is used to remove joint adhesions. After TMJ surgery, the patient often has findings similar to the capsulitis/synovitis classification; therefore, interventions to reduce inflammation and restore joint function are indicated. In addition, underlying impairments may be present, such as articular disc, muscle, and postural/cervical spine disorders that need to be addressed as part of the overall treatment plan. Education as outlined in Box 7-5 can assist with management of postsurgical conditions. TMJ range of motion exercises also are a vital part of the treatment approach. Joint mobilization techniques and sustained stretching with tongue depressors are indicated if joint mobility restrictions are present and the surgeon has cleared the patient for passive stretching techniques.

In addition to the normal physical therapy examination questions as outlined in Chapter 2, the TMJ examination should include completion of the TMJ disability questionnaire (see Box 7-1) and additional TMD history questions (Box 7-6) for identification of whether the facial and jaw pain originates from the TMJ and for determination of whether the patient has parafunctional oral habits that could be perpetuating the TMD. The TMJ disability questionnaire[29] is scored 1 through 5 for each of the 10 categories, and these numbers are added and multiplied by 2 to report the percentage score for the questionnaire. If categories are not marked, the score is divided by the total possible score to determine the percentage. The TMJ disability questionnaire is interpreted in a similar fashion to the neck disability index and Oswestery LBP questionnaires as described in Chapter 2, but the psychometric properties of the TMJ disability questionnaire have not been established. The TMJ examination should also include a thorough cervical spine and upper thoracic examination as described in Chapters 2, 5, and 6.

| BOX 7-6 | History/Interview Questions for a TMJ Examination |
| --- | --- |

**I. SUBJECTIVE EXAMINATION**

**A. PAIN**

1. Jaw pain with opening, closing, chewing, or yawning?

2. Ear symptoms of pain, fullness, or ringing?

3. Headaches?                                                                 If yes, where _____

**B. FUNCTION**

1. Difficulty opening?

2. History of locking?

3. Joint sounds, such as popping, clicking, or grinding?

4. Recent changes in occlusion (the way teeth seem to come together)?

5. Difficulty swallowing?

6. Parafunctional habits, such as clenching, grinding, nail biting, smoking, pen chewing, or other?

7. Sleeping posture?

Supine_____ Prone_____                Side: Right_____ Left_____

Assessment of teeth and occlusion should also be completed; obvious malocclusions, such as premature contact or worn patterns characteristic of bruxism, should be noted and brought to the attention of the patient's dentist.

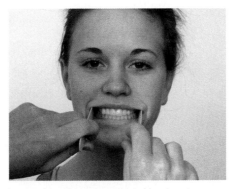

Occlusion and teeth assessment. Use two tongue depressors to move lips and cheeks out of the way to allow inspection of occlusion. Note signs of premature contacts, crossbite, or teeth wear patterns characteristic of bruxism.

The following is a detailed description of TMJ examination procedures, including active range of motion (AROM), palpation, provocation tests, and accessory motion tests, which when completed and considered in clusters of positive findings should allow the therapist to properly diagnose/classify the TMD and create a problem list that can be addressed with physical therapy interventions.

# TEMPOROMANDIBULAR JOINT ACTIVE RANGE OF MOTION AND MAPPING MOTION

Each mandibular active range of motion is tested at least three times. With the first trial of AROM, the therapist observes for the quality and range of motion. With the subsequent trials, the therapist palpates the TMJ to attempt to identify joint sounds and notes at what point in the range of motion the joint sound occurs. The therapist should note whether the joint sound occurs during opening or closing and whether deviation from midline occurs with the joint sound. These deviations and joint sounds are mapped on the mandibular dynamics chart. With the final trial, a millimeter ruler is used to measure the range of motion.

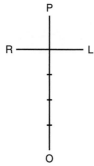

Mandibular dynamics mapping chart: line is drawn to document path of opening and closing and "x" is used to mark joints sounds within range of motion. Small slash mark is used to mark end of range of motion. Therapist should also note whether pain is provoked with each motion.

The amount of mandibular depression has been found to be affected by the head and neck position; therefore, the patient should be instructed to attain and hold the best natural comfortable postural position before and throughout the testing of mandibular AROM.[30] The postural position should be reproduced for subsequent reassessments of mandibular AROM to attain a valid measure of the effects of the therapy.

## Mandibular Protrusion

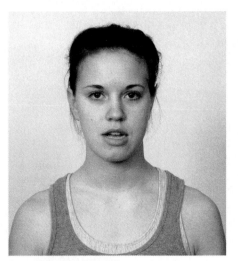

Mandibular protusion AROM.

| | |
|---|---|
| **PATIENT POSITION** | The patient sits or stands with good postural alignment. |
| **THERAPIST POSITION** | The therapist stands or sits in front of the patient. |
| **PROCEDURE** | Protrusion refers to the anterior movement of the mandible in the horizontal plane. The patient is instructed to actively protrude the mandible. The therapist observes for symmetrical protrusion. A deviation to either side during protrusion is noted. (Deviation usually occurs toward the side of TMJ restriction.) The amount of protrusion is noted with a millimeter ruler to measure the distance between the maxillary and mandibular central incisors. |
| **NOTES** | This motion is difficult to measure, but the mandibular incisors should move past the maxillary incisors by several millimeters. Walker, Bohannon, and Cameron[31] used a millimeter ruler to measure protrusion on 15 subjects with TMD and 15 subjects without TMD and reported an ICC for interexaminer reliability of 0.95 for subjects without TMD and 0.98 for subjects with TMD. The presence of a joint sound should also be noted. Interexaminer reliability for detection of joint sounds has been reported as a Kappa value of 0.47 on 79 patients referred to a craniomandibular disorder clinic.[32] |

## Mandibular Depression

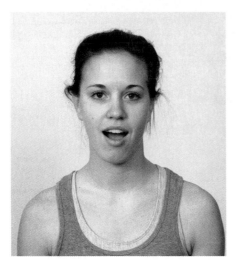

Mandibular depression AROM.

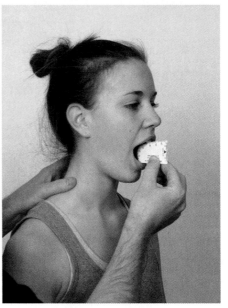

Interincisor measurement of mandibular depression with millimeter ruler.

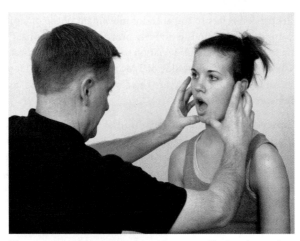

Therapist positioning for mapping mandibular dynamics.

| | |
|---|---|
| **PATIENT POSITION** | The patient sits or stands with good postural alignment. |
| **THERAPIST POSITION** | The therapist stands or sits in front of the patient. |
| **PROCEDURE** | Depression refers to opening the mouth in the sagittal plane. The patient is instructed to actively open the mouth as wide as possible. The therapist observes for symmetrical opening. A deviation to either side during opening is noted. (Deviation usually occurs to the side of TMJ restriction.) The amount of mandibular depression is noted with a millimeter ruler to measure the distance between the maxillary and mandibular central incisors. |
| **NOTES** | The distance between the incisors at maximal opening should be 35 to 50 mm, and the mandible should track in midline throughout the AROM. Walker, Bohannon, and Cameron[31] used a millimeter ruler to measure the opening on 15 subjects with TMD and 15 subjects without TMD and reported an interclass correlation coefficient (ICC) for inter- |

## Mandibular Depression—cont'd

examiner reliability of 0.98 for subjects without TMD and 0.99 for subjects with TMD. Of the six motions measured (opening, left excursion, right excursion, protrusion, overbite, and overjet) by two therapists in this study, mouth opening (mandibular depression) was the only TMJ ROM measurement to discriminate between subjects with and without TMJ disorders (mean, 36.2 ± 6.4 mm versus 43.5 ± 6.1 mm).[31] The presence of a joint sound should also be noted. Interexaminer reliability for detection of joint sounds has been reported as a Kappa value of 0.24 on 79 patients referred to a craniomandibular disorder clinic.[32] The presence of an audible palpable joint click has been correlated with MRI confirmation of an anterior disc displacement with reduction in 146 patients seen at a craniofacial pain clinic with a sensitivity of 0.51, a specificity of 0.83, a +LR of 3.0, and a −LR of 0.59. No clicking with opening has been correlated with an anterior disc displacement without reduction with a sensitivity of 0.77, a specificity of 0.24, a +LR of 1.01, and a −LR of 0.96.[33] Box 7-7 provides an illustration of use of a stethoscope to facilitate identification of a TMJ sound with mandibular AROM testing.

| BOX 7-7 | Auscultation of the Temporomandibular Joint with Stethoscope for Detection of Joint Sounds |

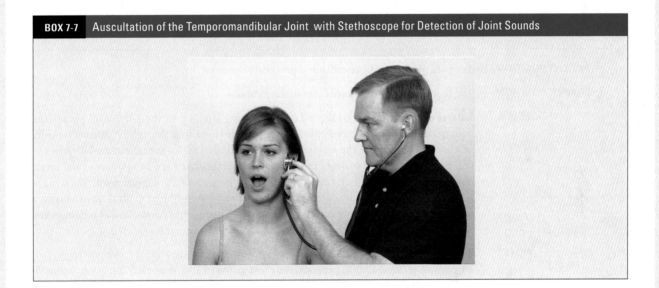

## Mandibular Lateral Excursion

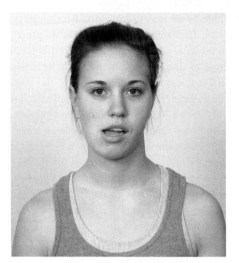

Mandibular lateral excursion AROM.

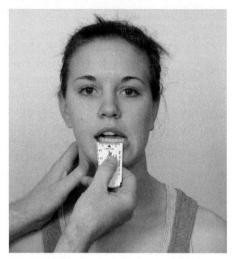

Mandibular lateral excursion measurement with millimeter ruler.

| | |
|---|---|
| **PATIENT POSITION** | The patient sits or stands with good postural alignment. |
| **THERAPIST POSITION** | The therapist stands or sits in front of the patient. |
| **PROCEDURE** | Lateral excursion refers to the mandible moving laterally in the horizontal plane. The patient is instructed to actively move the mandible laterally to the right. A millimeter ruler can be used to measure the amount of lateral excursion with use of the space between the two central maxillary incisors as a landmark for measurement in relation to the space between the two mandibular central incisors. A more accurate measurement can be made with marking a vertical line along the maxillary and mandibular central incisors with a marking pencil while in a neutral position and measuring the horizontal distance between the two marks at the end range of lateral excursion left and right. |
| **NOTES** | This motion is difficult to measure, but the mandibular canine should move past the maxillary canine by several millimeters. Lateral excursion of 10 mm in each direction is considered a normal range of motion. Most importantly, the motion should be equal in each direction. Walker, Bohannon, and Cameron[31] used a millimeter ruler to measure lateral excursion on 15 subjects with TMD and 15 subjects without TMD and reported an ICC for interexaminer reliability of 0.95 for subjects without TMD and 0.94 for subjects with TMD for left lateral excursion and reported an ICC for interexaminer reliability of 0.90 for subjects without TMD and 0.96 for subjects with TMD for right lateral excursion. The presence of a joint sound should also be noted. Interexaminer reliability for detection of joint sounds has been reported as a Kappa value of 0.50 on 79 patients referred to a craniomandibular disorder clinic.[32] |

# PALPATION

## Muscles of Mastication External Palpation

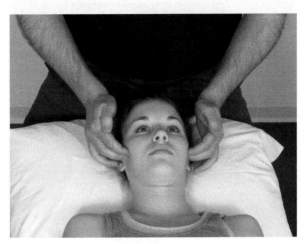

Palpation of the muscles of mastication.

| | |
|---|---|
| **PATIENT POSITION** | The patient is supine with the head on a pillow. |
| **THERAPIST POSITION** | The therapist stands at the head of the patient. |
| **PROCEDURE** | The therapist uses the pads of the second and third digits to palpate the temporalis, the masseter, the suprahyoid muscles, and the infrahyoid muscles. Swelling, tenderness, or excessive tension in the muscles is noted. |
| **NOTES** | Cacchiotti et al[34] examined 41 subjects who sought treatment for TMD and 40 normal subjects and graded the results of palpation examination on a 0 to 3 scale, with 0 indicating no response and 3 indicating that the patient pulled the head away in anticipation of palpation and reported significant pain. The results for use of palpation of the muscles of mastication for identification of patients with TMD were sensitivity of 0.76, specificity of 0.90, +LR of 7.6, and −LR of 0.27. |

## Muscles of Mastication Intraoral Palpation

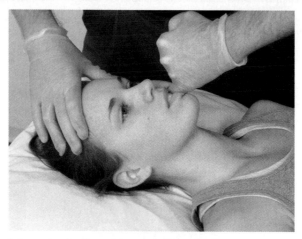

Intraoral palpation of muscles of mastication.

| | |
|---|---|
| **PATIENT POSITION** | The patient is supine with the head on a pillow. |
| **THERAPIST POSITION** | The therapist stands next to the patient. |
| **PROCEDURE** | The therapist wears a latex glove and uses the tip of the fifth digit to palpate the upper lateral corner of the patient's mouth between the teeth and cheek. Pain provocation and swelling, tenderness, or excessive tension in the muscles are noted. The therapist palpates and compares both sides. |
| **NOTE** | This technique is designed to palpate the lateral pterygoid muscle, but debate exists as to whether the fifth digit can actually reach far enough to palpate this muscle.[35] The tendon of the temporalis is also near this site of palpation, as is the masseter muscle. This palpation can be turned into a trigger point soft tissue mobilization treatment technique by simply sustaining the pressure for 30 to 90 seconds until tension and tenderness ease with the pressure. Dworkin et al[36] reported a Kappa value of 0.90 for intraoral palpation interexaminer reliability on 64 healthy volunteers. |

## Temporomandibular Joint Lateral Pole Palpation

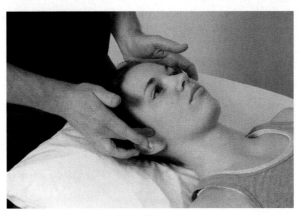

Palpation of the lateral condyle.

| | |
|---|---|
| **PATIENT POSITION** | The patient is supine with the head on a pillow. |
| **THERAPIST POSITION** | The therapist stands at the head of the table. |
| **PROCEDURE** | The pad of the third digit is used to palpate the lateral pole of the TMJ just anterior to the ear. Any swelling or tenderness is noted. The therapist palpates the opposite side, noting any swelling or tenderness. |
| **NOTE** | Tenderness of the lateral pole is an indication of inflammation of the TMJ capsule or lateral TMJ ligament. de Wiker[37] reported a Kappa value of 0.33 for interexaminer reliability for pain provocation with palpation of the lateral pole of the TMJ on 79 patients referred to a TMJ disorder and orofacial pain department. Manfredini et al[38] reported intraexaminer reliability of Kappa of 0.53 for pain provocation for palpation of lateral pole of the TMJ on 61 patients with TMJ pain and correlated pain with palpation with the presence of joint effusion as seen on MRI findings with a sensitivity of 0.83, a specificity of 0.69, a +LR of 2.68, and a −LR of 0.25. |

## Posterior Compartment Palpation

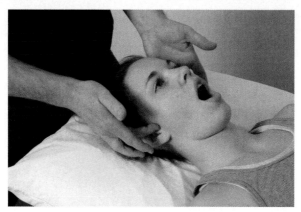

Palpation of posterior compartment of TMJ.

**PATIENT POSITION**  The patient is supine with the head on a pillow.

**THERAPIST POSITION**  The therapist stands at the head of the table.

**PROCEDURE**  The pad of the third digit palpates just posterior to the condyle of the mandible. The patient is instructed to actively open the mouth. The therapist palpates for tenderness or swelling of the posterior compartment during opening of the mouth. The procedure is repeated with assessment of the opposite side. Any differences between right and left sides are noted.

**NOTES**  Tenderness and swelling of the posterior compartment of the TMJ is an indication of inflammation/irritation of the posterior ligaments and joint capsule of the TMJ. Manfredini et al[38] reported intraexaminer reliability of Kappa of 0.48 for pain provocation with palpation of the posterior compartment of the TMJ on 61 patients with TMJ pain and correlated pain with palpation with presence of joint effusion as seen on MRI findings with a sensitivity of 0.85, a specificity of 0.62, a +LR of 2.24, and −LR of 0.24.

# PROVOCATION TESTS

## Forced Retrusion (Compression) Temporomandibular Joint Provocation Test

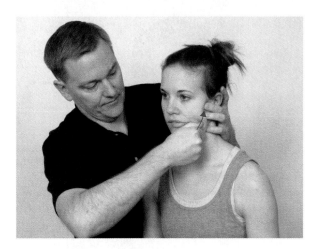

| | |
|---|---|
| **PATIENT POSITION** | The patient is in a sitting position. |
| **THERAPIST POSITION** | The therapist stands in front of the patient and on the opposite side of the TMJ to be tested. |
| **PROCEDURE** | The thumb and index finger are used to grasp the patient's chin. The opposite hand stabilizes the back of the patient's head. With the patient relaxed and the teeth slightly apart, the therapist applies a pressure directed posteriorly and slightly superiorly. Pain provocation is noted. |
| **NOTES** | Test results are considered positive if the test increases or reproduces the patient's symptoms. This test is not specific to either the right or left TMJ, but the force can be directed toward one joint at a time to attempt to isolate each joint. de Wiker[37] reported a Kappa value of 0.47 for interexaminer reliability of pain provocation with a TMJ compression test on 79 patients referred to a TMJ disorder and orofacial pain department. |

## Forced Biting Provocation Test

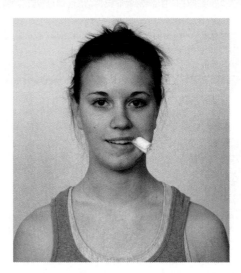

| | |
|---|---|
| **PATIENT POSITION** | The patient is in a sitting position. |
| **THERAPIST POSITION** | The therapist stands in front of the patient. |
| **PROCEDURE** | The therapist places gauze, a cotton ball, or a tongue depressor between the patient's back molars. The patient is instructed to bite down. Pain provocation is noted. Test results are considered positive if the test increases or reproduces the patient's symptoms. |
| **NOTES** | If pain is produced in the ipsilateral side, it is likely from muscle/tendon irritation; if the pain is reproduced on the contralateral TMJ, it is likely from TMJ capsulitis/synovitis. |

# ACCESSORY MOTION TESTS AND MOBILIZATIONS

## Temporomandibular Joint Distraction Accessory Motion Test and Mobilization (DVD)

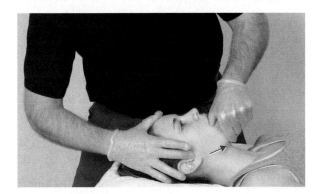
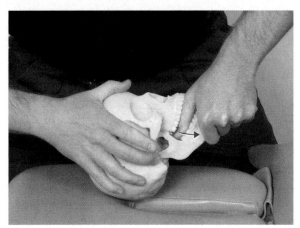

Distraction accessory motion test and mobilization of TMJ with hand placement on model.

| | |
|---|---|
| **PATIENT POSITION** | The patient is supine with the head on a pillow. |
| **THERAPIST POSITION** | The therapist stands next the patient on the side opposite the TMJ to be tested or mobilized. |
| **PROCEDURE** | The therapist stands on the patient's left side and inserts the left thumb into the patient's mouth. The thumb is placed on top of the patient's right mandibular molars, and digits 2 to 5 are gently folded around the lateral inferior aspect of the mandible (externally). The thumb is used to apply an inferior scooping force against the molars along the ramus of the mandible to distract the joint. The pad of the third digit of the right hand is used to palpate the right TMJ (externally). The amount of motion available at the joint is noted, and the procedure is repeated with assessment of the left side. The therapist stands on the patient's right side and uses the right thumb on the right mandibular molars. Pain provocation and the amount of motion available at the joint are noted and compared with the left side. |
| | This technique can be turned into a nonthrust manipulation with application of a sustained stretch to the joint or with oscillation of the joint. Thrust manipulation to the TMJ is rarely indicated. A successful outcome can be obtained with gentle nonthrust manipulation techniques. |
| **NOTES** | The therapist stands on the side opposite of the joint to be assessed. The therapist should wear a latex glove during this technique. Gentle forces are used to assess and manipulate the joint. The amount of accessory motion of a normally functioning TMJ is very small. Manfredini et al[38] correlated pain with joint distraction and joint effusion as seen on MRI findings on 61 patients with TMJ pain with a sensitivity of 0.80, a specificity of 0.39, a +LR of 1.31, and a −LR of 0.51; joint play intraexaminer reliability was reported as Kappa of 0.20. Lobbezoo-Scholte et al[32] reported a Kappa value of 0.46 for interexaminer reliability for testing of TMJ joint play on 79 randomly selected patients referred to a craniomandibular disorder department. |

## Temporomandibular Joint Lateral Glide Accessory Motion Test and Mobilization

DVD

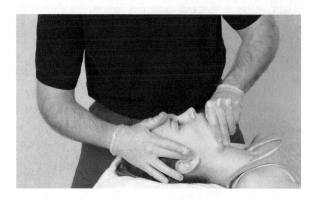

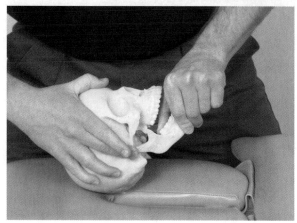

TMJ lateral glide accessory motion test and mobilization with hand placement on model.

| | |
|---|---|
| **PATIENT POSITION** | The patient is supine with the head on a pillow. |
| **THERAPIST POSITION** | The therapist stands next to the patient on the side opposite the TMJ. |
| **PROCEDURE** | The therapist stands on the patient's left side and inserts the left thumb into the patient's mouth. The pad of the thumb is used to contact the medial aspect of the patient's right mandibular molars. The thumb is used to apply a lateral force towards the patient's right side, and the pad of the third digit of the right hand is used to palpate the TMJ (externally). The amount of motion available at the joint is noted, and the procedure is repeated with assessment of the left side. The therapist stands on the patient's right side and uses the right thumb to contact the left mandibular molars. Pain provocation and the amount of motion available at the joint are noted and compared with the other side. This technique can be turned into a nonthrust manipulation with application of a sustained stretch to the joint or with oscillation of the joint. |
| **NOTES** | The therapist stands on the side opposite the joint to be assessed and wears a latex glove during this technique. Gentle forces are used to assess and manipulate the joint. The amount of accessory motion of a normally functioning TMJ is very small. Lateral glide is a joint play motion for the TMJ being tested. |

## Temporomandibular Joint Medial Glide Accessory Motion and Joint Mobilization

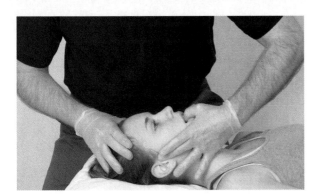

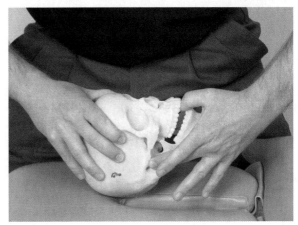

TMJ medial glide accessory motion and joint mobilization with hand placement on model.

| | |
|---|---|
| **PATIENT POSITION** | The patient is supine with the head on a pillow. |
| **THERAPIST POSITION** | The therapist stands next to the patient on the side opposite of the TMJ. |
| **PROCEDURE** | While standing on the patient's left side, the therapist places the left thumb between the patient's maxillary and mandibular incisors. The pads of the second and third digits are used to contact the lateral pole of the right TMJ. The third digit applies a medial force toward the patient's left side. The amount of motion available at the joint is noted, and the procedure is repeated with assessment of the left side. The therapist stands on the patient's right side and uses the pad of the third digit of the right hand to apply a medial force to the lateral pole of the left TMJ. Pain provocation and the amount of motion available at the joint are noted and compared with the other side. |
| | This technique can be turned into a nonthrust manipulation with application of a sustained stretch to the joint or with oscillation of the joint. |
| **NOTES** | The therapist stands on the side opposite of the joint to be assessed and wears a latex glove during this technique. Gentle forces are used to assess and manipulate the joint. The amount of accessory motion of a normally functioning TMJ is very small. Medial glide is a joint play motion for the TMJ being tested. |

# Case Studies and Problem Solving

The following patient case reports can be used by the student to develop problem-solving skills by considering the information provided in the patient history and tests and measures and developing appropriate evaluations, goals, and plans of care.

## Ms. TMJ Dysfunction

### History

A 23-year-old college student has tightness, discomfort, and clicking in the right TMJ with intermittent occipital headaches. Pain is provoked with stressful situations and with chewing meat and crunchy foods.

### Tests and Measures

- Structural examination: Moderate forward head posture (FHP) with protracted scapulas
- Cervical AROM in standing: 85% in all planes of motion and pain free except for backward bending, which is 50% and provokes occipital area pain
- Thoracic AROM: 75% to 85% in all planes of motion and pain free
- Mandibular dynamics: Opening to 35 mm with mid range deviation to the right and return to midline after a mid range of opening joint sound; joint sound also noted at mid range closing; lateral deviation is limited to the left with a joint sound; protrusion also has a mid range click
- Passive intervertebral motion (PIVM) testing: Limited craniovertebral forward bending, right side bending, and left rotation; mid cervical spine PIVM testing reveals hypermobility; upper thoracic is slightly restricted at T1-T2 left and right rotation and forward bending
- Shoulder screen: Full and pain-free bilateral shoulder AROM
- Muscle length: Mild tightness right levator scapula and minimally tight bilateral pectoralis major and minor
- Strength: Lower and middle trapezius are 4−/5; deep neck flexors are 3+/5
- Neurological screen: Negative
- Special tests:
  - Forced biting: Painful right TMJ with biting on left side
  - Retrusive overpressure: Provokes pain on right TMJ

- Palpation: Tender and guarded right muscles of mastication with internal (intraoral) and external palpation, tender at lateral pole right TMJ, and tender at C2-C3 facet joint right

### Evaluation

Diagnosis
Problem list
Goals

### Treatment Plan/Intervention

## Mr. Stiff TMJ

### History

A 50-year-old construction worker has difficulty opening his mouth after trauma to his jaw from being hit in the jaw during a bar fight 3 months before the initial evaluation. The patient has no history of TMJ sounds. Recent radiographic results were negative for signs of mandibular fracture.

### Tests and Measures

- Structural examination: Mild FHP with protracted scapulas
- Cervical AROM in standing: 85% in all planes of motion and pain free
- Thoracic AROM: 75% upper thoracic rotation motion and pain free
- Mandibular dynamics: 20 mm opening with deviation to the right, 5 mm left lateral excursion, 8 mm right lateral excursion, 4 mm protusion with deviation to the right; no joint sounds noted
- Accessory motion testing TMJ: Hypomobility with lateral and medial glide and joint distraction right TMJ
- PIVM testing: Slight hypomobility craniovertebral forward bending and right side bending; hypomobility T1-T2 left and right rotation

- Shoulder screen: Active shoulder range of motion is full and pain free with normal strength
- Muscle length: No limitations noted
- Strength: Lower and middle trapezius are 4−/5; deep neck flexors are 3+/5
- Neurological screen: Negative
- Special tests:
  - Forced biting: Negative
  - Retrusive overpressure: Negative

- Palpation: Tender and guarded right muscles of mastication internally (intraoral) and externally and tender at right lateral mandibular condyle

## Evaluation

Diagnosis
Problem list
Goals

## Treatment Plan/Intervention

# References

1. Dodson TB: Epidemiology of temporomandibular disorders. In Fonseca RJ, editor: *Oral and maxillofacial surgery: temporomandibular disorders*, vol 4, Philadelphia, 2000, Saunders.

2. Dworkin SF, LeResche L: Temporomandibular disorder pain: epidemiologic data, *Am Pain Soc Bull* April-May:12-13, 1993.

3. Helkimo M: Epidemiological surveys of dysfunction of the masticatory system. In Zarb G, Carlsson G, editors: *Temporomandibular joint dysfunction*, St Louis, 1979, Mosby.

4. Merskey H, Bogduk N: *Classification of chronic pain*, Seattle, 1994, IASP Press.

5. Kraus SL: *Clinics in physical therapy: temporomandibular joint disorders*, New York, 1994, Churchill Livingstone.

6. Godden DRP, Robertson JM: The value of patient feedback in the audit of TMJ arthroscopy, *Br Dent J* 188:125, 2000.

7. Carmeli E, Sheklow S, Bloomenfeld I: Comparative study of repositioning splint therapy and passive manual range of motion techniques for anterior displaced temporomandibular discs with unstable excursive reduction, *Physiotherapy* 87:26-36, 2001.

8. Furto ES, Cleland JA, Whitman JM, et al: Manual physical therapy interventions and exercise for patients with temporomandibular disorders, *J Craniomandib Dis* 24(4):283-291, 2006.

9. Nicolakis P, Burak EC, Kollmitzer J, et al: An investigation of the effectiveness of exercise and manual therapy in treating symptoms of TMJ osteoarthritis, *Cranio* 19:26-32, 2001.

10. Nicolakis P, Erdogmus B, Kopf A, et al: Effectiveness of exercise therapy in patients with internal derangement of the temporomandibular joint, *J Oral Rehabil* 29:362-368, 2002.

11. Williams PL, Warwick R: *Gray's anatomy*, ed 37, London, 1989, Churchill Livingstone.

12. Rocabado M, Inglarsh A: *Musculoskeletal approach to maxillofacial pain*, Philadelphia, 1991, Lippincott.

13. Neumann DA: *Kinesiology of the musculoskeletal system: foundations for physical rehabilitation*, St Louis, 2002, Mosby.

14. McClean LF, et al: Effects of changing body position on dental occlusion, *J Dent Res* 52(5):1041-1045, 1973.

15. Funakoshi M, et al: Relations between occlusal interference and jay muscle activities in response to changes in head position, *J Dent Res* 55(4):686-690, 1976.

16. Darling DW, et al: Relationship of head posture and the rest position of the mandible, *J Prosth Dent* 52(1):111-115, 1984.

17. Goldstein DF, Krauss S, Williams WB, et al: Influence of cervical posture on mandibular movement, *J Prosth Dent* 52(3):421-426, 1984.

18. Krauss SL: *TMJ disorders: management of the craniomandibular complex*, New York, 1988, Churchill Livingstone.

19. Daly P: Postural response of the head to bite opening in adult males, *Am J Orthodont* 82:157-160, 1982.

20. Packard RC: The relationship of neck injury and post-traumatic headache, *Curr Pain Headache Rep* 6:1-7, 2002.

21. Aprill C, Axinn M, Bogduk N: Occipital headaches stemming from the lateral atlanto-axial (C1-C2) joint, *Cephalalgia* 22:15-22, 2002.

22. Majwer K, Swider M: Results of treatment with iontophoresis of posttraumatic changes of temporomandibular joints with an apparatus of own design, *Protet Stomatol* 39:172-176, 1989.

23. Rocabado M: *Intermediate craniofacial: course manual*, International Fundamental Orthopedic Rocabado Center, Tucson, Arizona, 2003.

24. Gavish A, Halachmi M, Winocur E, et al: Oral habits and their association with signs and symptoms of temporomandibular disorders in adolescent girls, *J Oral Rehabil* 27:22-32, 2000.

25. Rocabado M: *Key note address*, St Louis, 2007, AAOMPT annual conference.

26. Yoda T, Sakamoto I, Imai H, et al: A randomized controlled trial of therapeutic exercise for clicking due to disk anterior displacement with reduction in the temporomandibular joint, *Cranio* 21:10-16, 2003.

27. Cleland J, Palmer: Effectiveness of manual physical therapy, therapeutic exercise, and patient education on bilateral disc displacement without reduction of the temporomandibular joint: a single-case design, *J Orthop Sports Phys Ther* 34:535-548, 2004.

28. Israel H, Diamond B, Saed-Nejad F, et al: Osteoarthritis and synovitis as major pathoses of the temporomandibular joint: comparison of the clinical diagnosis with arthroscopic morphology, *J Oral Maxillofac Surg* 56:1023-1028, 1998.

29. Steigerwald DP, Maher JH: The Steigerwald/Maher TMD disability questionnaire, *Today Chiropract* July-August:86-91, 1997.

30. Higbie EJ, Seidel-Cobb D, Taylor LF, et al: Effect of head position on vertical mandibular opening, *JOSPT* 29:127-130, 1999.

31. Walker N, Bohannon RW, Cameron D: Discriminant validity of temporomandibular joint range of motion measurements obtained with a ruler, *JOSPT* 30:484-492, 2000.

32. Lobbezoo-Scholte AM, de Wijer A, Steenks MH, et al: Interexaminer reliability of six orthopaedic tests in diagnostic subgroups of craniomandibular disorders, *J Oral Rehabil* 21:273-285, 1994.

33. Orsini MR, Kuboki T, Terada S, et al: Clinical predictability of temporomandibular joint disc displacement, *J Dent Res* 78:650-660, 1999.

34. Cacchiotti DA, Plesh O, Bianchi P, et al: Signs and symptoms in samples with and with out temporomandibular disorders, *J Craniomandib Disord* 5:167-172, 1991.

35. Johnstone J: The feasibility of palpating the lateral pterygoid muscle, *J Prosth Dent* 44(3):318-323, 1980.

36. Dworkin SF, LeResche L, DeRouen T, et al: Assessing clinical signs of temporomandibular disorders: reliability of clinical examiners, *J Prosthet Dent* 63:574-579, 1990.

37. de Wiker A, Lobbezoo-Scholte AM, Steenks MH, et al: Reliability of clinical findings in temporomandibular disorders, *J Orofac Pain* 9:181-191, 1995.

38. Manfredinin D, Tognini F, Zampa V, et al: Predictive value of clinical findings for temporomandibular joint effusion, *Oral Surg Oral Med Oral Pathol* 96:521-526, 2003.

# Index

Note: Page numbers followed by f indicate figures; t, tables; and b, boxed material.